AUTISM - PARADIGMS, RECENT RESEARCH AND CLINICAL APPLICATIONS

Edited by **Michael Fitzgerald** and **Jane Yip**

Autism - Paradigms, Recent Research and Clinical Applications
http://dx.doi.org/10.5772/63171
Edited by Michael Fitzgerald and Jane Yip

Contributors

Renee Cachia, Timo Lorenz, Nomi Reznik, Kathrin Heinitz, Pamela Bryden, Marwa Saleh, Aya Adel, Alina Simona Rusu, Aj Russo, Felwah Al-Zaid, Michael Fitzgerald, Huub Savelkoul, Anna Cieslinska, Jannicke Simmelink, Gosia Teodorowicz, Hans Verhoef, Hilde Tobi, Elena Predescu, Roxana Sipos, María Carmen Carrascosa-Romero, Carlos De Cabo De La Vega, Daina Crafa, M.Sc., M.Sc., Adriana Tapus, Pauline Chevalier, Jean-Claude Martin, Brice Isableu, Christophe Bazile, Elizabeth Hughes Fong, Helen Lee, Touraj Shafai

Published by InTech

Janeza Trdine 9, 51000 Rijeka, Croatia

Publishing Process Manager Iva Lipovic
Technical Editor SPi Global
Cover InTech Design team

First published April, 2017
Printed in Croatia
Legal deposit, Croatia: National and University Library in Zagreb

Additional hard copies can be obtained from orders@intechopen.com

Autism - Paradigms, Recent Research and Clinical Applications, Edited by Michael Fitzgerald and Jane Yip
p. cm.
Print ISBN 978-953-51-3079-6
Online ISBN 978-953-51-3080-2

For EU product safety concerns:
IN TECH d.o.o., Prolaz Marije Krucifikse Kozulić 3, 51000 Rijeka, Croatia,
info@intechopen.com or visit our website at intechopen.com.

Meet the editors

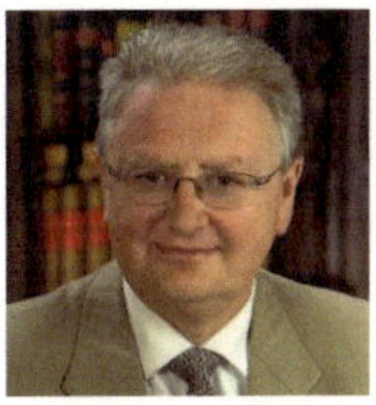

Professor Michael Fitzgerald was the first Professor of Child and Adolescent Psychiatry in Ireland, specialising in Autism Spectrum Disorders. He trained at the Chicago Medical School, the Maudsley Hospital, London, Kings College Hospital London and the National Hospital for Nervous Diseases, London. He has a Doctorate in Autism. He has a large number of peer-reviewed publications and thirty books written, co-written or co-edited, including Japanese and Polish translations of some books. Professor Simon Baron-Cohen of the University of Cambridge described one of his books on Autism as "the best book I have read on Autism". He also described him as an "exceptional scholar". He has diagnosed just under 4,000 persons with Autism Spectrum Disorder since 1973. He has lectured extensively throughout the world including The Royal Society/British Academy, The British Library in London and also in New York, Buenos Aires, Tbilisi, Melbourne and many European countries as well as China, Malaysia and Hawaii.

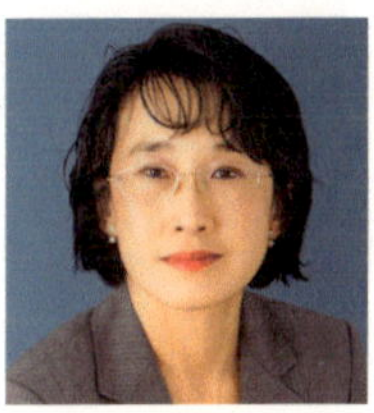

Jane Yip obtained her PhD from the University of Newcastle, Australia, specializing in neuropharmacology. She completed her post-doctoral training at Eli Lilly and Company, Indianapolis, USA. Her research is on the brain circuit that underlies neurological disorders including autism, schizophrenia, and depression. She has published in peer-review journals. Although trained in drug development, she emphasizes the application of the science of behavior to treat mental disorders, and uses natural environment modification as a treatment modality. She pioneered the use of portable brain imaging to guide behavior treatment in autism. She has a practice that offers brain mapping. The practice also treats patients with autism using applied behavior analysis (ABA). She is the director of a clinical center for the treatment of autism, Autism Parent Care. As a member of ABA international, multicultural alliance, and an NGO member of United Nations, she works on outreach projects in Asia to advance the Universal Declaration of Human Rights Bill aiming to promote better recognition of individuals with mental disabilities, including autism. Her overarching aim to is advance treatment intervention for autism.

Contents

Foreword

Autism Spectrum Disorders (ASD) are complex, brain-based disorders that affect a person's behavior. The Centers for Disease Control describes ASDs as: "developmental disabilities that cause substantial impairments in social interaction and communication and the presence of unusual behaviors and interests. People with ASDs have unusual ways of conducting themselves: they learn differently, may not pay attention and react unusually to different sensations. Thinking and learning abilities of people with ASDs can range from gifted or savant to severely challenged. ASD is noticeable since early childhood – usually before the age of 3 and lasts throughout a person's life."

Autism is four times more likely to affect boys than girls, and is prevalent across all racial, ethnic, and social groups, and affects all nations in the world. There is no known single cause for autism, although the best available science points to important genetics and in interaction with the environment (epigenetics).

ASD symptoms are difficult for families due to significant impairments in social interaction and communication skills, and by the presence of extremely challenging behaviors including aggression, property destruction and self-injury. In addition, socially inappropriate actions make these children stand out: repetitive motor behaviors (hand flapping, body rocking). They often insist on sameness and are ritualistic to the point of disruption to family routines. Many individuals with ASD have significant cognitive impairments making learning a challenge, although some have typical or even above average IQs. Among the ASD population, as many as 30-50% have seizures.

Dr. Leo Kanner first described autism in 1943. At first, autism was thought to be an early form of schizophrenia, which led to the belief that its onset could be caused by negative experience or bad parenting. We now know that this is not the case. ASD can be debilitating and is rising in prevalence. On March 27, 2014, the Centers for Disease Control and Prevention (CDC) reported that 1 in 68 children (1 in 42 boys and 1 in 189 girls) as having autism spectrum disorder (ASD) for the United States. This figure is an increased from the 2004 census of 1 in 166.

Even though the incidence of autism is rising, there is a lack of research writings concerning treatment. Most of the scientific research centers around biochemistry, neurology, and genetics. The important subject of treatment, the concerns of parents and caregivers who have children on the ASD spectrum, are often left to the private investigations of the families who often had to turn to ad hoc Google searches.

This book attempts to introduce some available approaches in the treatment domain. Beyond enduring the daily onslaught of the symptoms, parents are challenged to treat, live with, face other family members, and prepare a future for their special needs children within a social-cultural context. The quality of life for the individual affected is not separate from the quality of life for the family. Understanding these social context makes possible the process of treatment that is located both in clinics and in society. ASD is primarily a social disorder, and hence the diagnosis has to be approached more than nosologically, or merely as a medical condition to be treated. The neuro-diversity of people who are different from mainstream has to be integrated into society. Certain strengths and abilities of ASD individuals can be beneficial. It is up to society to be proactive in setting aside space for the neuro-diverse individual; a failure to do so will result in a social impasse as large numbers ASD individuals will likely face a fate in institutions or at homes idle.

The attempt to treat means to carefully analyze the cognitive processing of the ASD mind. Joint attention, sensory processing, and theory of mind are discussed. In considering the common struggles of ASD individuals with anxiety, some authors wrote about mindfulness training and physical activities as conjunctive therapy. The use of robotics and animal-assisted therapies are raised as a tool to foster communication.

Perhaps the most important by-product of this book is a closer interaction between a variety of approaches. Each discipline understands a certain aspect of ASD and its implication to treatment, but they often fail to address the full function of the person as a whole. A book that provides a smorgasbord of approaches on the treatment of autism is a much-needed supplement. For the parent and/or caregiver, it should aid in clarifying what could have looked like a confusing array of possibilities in treatment. For the professionals, this book should ideally function as an encouragement towards work as a team, as each discipline complements each other for the benefit of the patient. For this teamwork to occur, each specialist must comprehend the other's language. To this end, the authors in this book have made their respective language understandable; their effort is applauded.

Autism is not a disease with recovery as an endpoint. Unlike other disease states, the journey does not end at a certain point but continues. The more treatment one embarks on, the more one becomes gracious, optimistic, and informative.

Most of all, this book is an expression that there is hope in the development of ever better treatment.

Jane Yip, PhD
Autism Parent Care, USA
Purdue University, USA

Preface

Autism is one of the most important conditions for psychiatrists, psychologists, teachers, speech therapists and occupational therapists today. It is a common disorder at 1/68 according to the Centre for Diseases and Control. It is probably the most commonly missed diagnosis in psychology/psychiatry and in children in education, as well as adults attending occupational health settings. It is a clinical diagnosis as pointed out by the National Institute for Clinical Excellence. Unfortunately, a commonly used instrument called The Autism Diagnostic Instrument, (ADI/R), as reported by Feinstein, (2010) in his book, "Autism in History", that many of the critics at an International Meeting for Autism Research in London, "lambasted the tool, (ADI/R) for missing many cases of Autism", and that this instrument was an expensive and, "ineffective instrument". This problem has now become a serious public health problem. It is critical that children are diagnosed as early as possible, to have the best outcome.

Autism is probably one of the most complex phenomena that exists and this is so whether one considers it a disorder, (DSM V/ICD X), or a point of diversity on a neurodiversity spectrum. Both points of view are described in this book. Many persons with high functioning autism are part of this neurodiversity spectrum, when they have no need or contact with professionals in psychiatry/psychology, etc. When they become seriously anxious or depressed, they have a need for professional intervention. It's only then that their condition becomes a disorder.

The profile of autism is far wider and more complex than described in DSM V, as described in the chapter in this book called "The Clinical Gestalts of Autism: Over 40 years of Clinical Experience with Autism".

The chapters on interventions in this book range from pioneering and complex, for example robots in ASD therapy, to the simple physical activity with persons with ASD, with other chapters focusing on mindfulness and animal assisted activities with persons with autism.

Joint attention problems are central to understanding autism and this chapter will be very well worth reading, as is the chapter on proprioception and kinematic profiles.

Other correlations with autism have individual chapters including sex bias, month of birth and migration.

The neurobiology of autism is well covered in the chapters on epigenetics and intracellular pathways. Interventions are also dealt with by the chapters on socio-cultural perspectives, feeding issues and quality of life also have individual chapters.

The book is focused on recent advances in Autism Spectrum Disorders and will give the reader a unique up to date perspective on the topic of autism. The pace of new work on autism is now so fast that there is a need for a new book like this at relatively short intervals to keep professionals up to date and these professionals will include psychologists, psychiatrists, speech therapists, occupational therapists, teachers and all professionals including researchers working in the area of autism.

References

[1] American Psychiatric Association [2013]: Diagnostic and Statistical Manual of Mental Disorders, (Fifth Edition), Arlington, V.A: American Psychiatric Publishing.

[2] Feinstein A. [2010]: A history of Autism. Chichester: Wiley – Blackwell.

[3] World Health Organisation [1992]: The ICD 10 Classification of Mental and Behavioural Disorders: Clinical Descriptions and Diagnostic Guidelines. Geneva: World Health Organisation.

[4] Centres for Disease Control and Prevention [2017]: Autism Spectrum Disorder. CDC.Gov, downloaded, 22nd January 2017.

Professor Michael Fitzgerald
Department of Psychiatry
Trinity College, Dublin 2
Ireland

Section 1

Assessment and Neurodiversity

Chapter 1

A Different Point of View: The Neurodiversity Approach to Autism and Work

Timo Lorenz, Nomi Reznik and Kathrin Heinitz

Additional information is available at the end of the chapter

http://dx.doi.org/10.5772/65409

Abstract

With this chapter, we want to open up the debate whether neurodiversity might be the next step of diversity. The term neurodiversity was first established in the online autism community in the 1990s and has since spread both off- and online. It describes the idea that, throughout the human population, different brain developments and structures exist. Neuronal variances such as Autism are therefore not to be seen as disorders but as variations different from the neurotypical brain. Instead of being considered ill and cure-worthy, neurodiverse people should be included and integrated into society. In our current research, we follow the neurodiversity approach and focus on the subject of autism in the work context. We found that certain strengths and abilities are most prominent in autistic people (such as logical reasoning, visual perception) and that autistic people are able to find different effective solutions to overcome the barriers detaining them from entering the job market. Furthermore, while many autistic individuals are employed in regular competitive jobs, more focus on autism-specific job environments is needed. These findings lead us to the conclusion that autistic individuals have potential that is beneficial for society.

Keywords: autism, neurodiversity, employment

1. Introduction: color, gender, brain?

Neurodiversity is a much-discussed topic in today's Autism Spectrum Condition research (e.g., [1]). In this chapter, we will shed some light on the relationship of individuals with Autism with the Autism community, the workplace, and the scientific community.

The term neurodiversity originated from the autism online community in the late 1990s with sociologist Judy Singer commonly referred to as the creator of the word [2]. It is important to note that even now, about twenty years since its first use, there is still no proper scientific definition of neurodiversity. In this chapter, we define the neurodiversity concept simply as the fact that there are differences in brain structures among the population [2, 3] just as there are different skin colors and genders between people—a diverse neurology.

Of course, there is more to the topic than the fact that peoples' brains are physically different, that their amygdalae may or may not differ in size [4]. The neurodiversity movement (NDM) focuses on a positive, strengths-based approach. It has two major claims [3]: firstly, deviations from the standard neurotypical brain that result in differing behavioral patterns are natural variations, not disorders or illnesses. Therefore, autism is seen as a different nuance of human behavior with its very own set of strengths [5]. Many individuals with autism see their condition as a crucial part of their individual identity, not as a mere illness they happen to suffer from [6].

The NDM's second claim follows logically from this mindset: If neurological differences are not disorders or illnesses, but merely variations, neurodiverse people are to be treated equally to neurotypical individuals [3]. This, of course, is related to all kinds of human interaction, including the workplace. We therefore argue that neurodiversity should be the logical next step in diversity. There are many conditions that fall into the neurodiverse category—e.g., Tourette's syndrome or ADHD [2]. The debate on which conditions have to be included and which don't is still going on [2]. In this chapter, we, however, decided to focus solely on autism.

2. From the inside: the autism community and neurodiversity

As stated above, the NDM is no scientific invention, but stems from the 1990s autism online community [2]. Since then, the Internet as a whole and online communication specifically has changed, become more accessible and part of everyday life [7]. To paint a picture of the current situation, we will introduce some of the bigger networks, how they operate, and their opinion on the neurodiversity concept.

2.1. Autistic Self Advocacy Network (ASAN)

The probably most popular and best-known autism-related website is the Autistic Self Advocacy Network (ASAN) with its slogan "nothing about us without us". ASAN is a nonprofit organization "by and for autistic people" (autisticadvocacy.org) founded in 2006. They give advice on public policy advocacy, provide information about Autism to fight the public misconceptions on the condition, develop cultural activities for autistic people, and actively take part in advancing autism-related disability rights. They also work for a better employment situation for autistic people, as well as for a fairer, more equal approach to accepting autistic people in Academia. ASAN has a very inclusive point of view: Co-Founder and current president of ASAN, Ari Ne'eman, who himself is on the spectrum, serves on the National Council on Disability since 2010 and supports the neurodiversity concept.

2.1.1. Autism Asperger's Digest

Autism Asperger's Digest (AAD), a division of Future Horizons Inc., is a magazine about all autism-related topics. They reach out to autistic individuals, their parents, and their therapists to spread information and provide a network.

Various other online platforms, such as Art of Autism, also provide insights on Autism for neurodiverse people and everyone who takes an interest in the condition. Considering this broad base of neurodiversity-based autism resources, it is noteworthy that the autism online community does not wholeheartedly agree about the concept and its political implications. A rather controversial topic is the genetic cause of autism. Current research seems to agree that autism is, in fact, highly genetic [3]. Those who consider autism a variation rather than a disorder have voiced their concern about how this information is handled—fearing the rise of a eugenic approach [6] based on cause-oriented research.

Additionally, the mere concept of neurodiversity encounters resistance in the Autism community. Blogger and student Jake Crosby, who writes for Autisminvestigated.com, is an anti-neurodiversity activist. Being reportedly diagnosed with Asperger's himself, Crosby considers the NDM a movement for people who are not truly impaired (i.e., high functioning autism).

He and many of his followers view autism as a disability, an impairment that is in need of a cure. They also reject the political implications of the NDM: After Ari Ne'eman's nomination into the National Council of Disability, he wrote a blog entry called "Keeping Autism Neurodiversity out of the White House" [8] in which he harshly criticized the concept of neurodiversity, ASAN, and the whole NDM for being not representative of autistic individuals as himself who struggle with their disability in everyday situations.

While the NDM has a great support base and has already made quite some change in how autism is regarded in our society, the autism community remains divided. This is also apparent in the workplace problem: a disabled individual is going to face different barriers compared to an individual that is just considered different—but there will also be less lenience for mistakes or special needs and necessities.

3. From between sides: autism, neurodiversity and the workplace

One of the most relevant and challenging problems in the everyday life of individuals with Autism is finding and keeping work [9]. According to UN General Secretary Ban Ki-moon's message regarding the World Autism Awareness Day, around 80% of adults with autism are unemployed [10], in spite of existing evidence that the desire to work is just the same as in neurotypicals [11]. Individuals with autism, however, have to face different, and probably more challenges in the process of finding, and later maintaining, employment [12].

The NDM calls for employers to be open minded and more approachable [13]. Still, for individuals with autism who want to work, there are two options: try to gain employment in a nonspecific workplace that might not be accommodating enough, or find work in an autism-specific job environment [11].

For those who take the first route, even entering the job market is still rather difficult. Barriers such as various communication problems or confusing application processes have to be overcome before employment is possible [12]. When those barriers are mastered, numerous others usually follow: Of course, due to the misinformation on the topic of autism as well as to communication issues, workplace discrimination and, in the worst case, workplace bullying are common [14]. Literature targeted at adult employees with autism and their employers usually mention how to counteract bullying in the office [14]. It should also be noted that disclosure of a diagnosis to superiors, and colleagues is often avoided. Autistic individuals fear negative reactions, being stereotyped or held up to old prejudices [15, 16], which is exactly what autism advocates such as ASAN are fighting against.

This problem is amplified by the fact that autistic individuals react differently to leading styles than neurotypical individuals: Parr, Hunter, and Ligon [17] report that while neurotypicals are inspired and motivated by transformational leadership measures, autistic individuals reported increased anxiety and overall distress, thereby worsening both their job experience and their productivity.

Those difficulties in understanding verbal nuances or implicit subtext in team meetings or casual conversations, coupled with a certain rule affinity that many autistic individuals are prone to, make for a less than optimal relationship with colleagues, subordinates, and superiors alike [16].

On top of this, not all challenges that autistic individuals have to face in the workplace are interpersonal: the work environment also plays an important role [16]. The common open plan cubicle offices offer various distractions (noises from other people or electronic devices, flickering lights, air circulation, etc.). Neurotypicals usually are able to block them out, but for autistic individuals they can easily become overwhelming [9]. To cope with the sensory overload, autistic individuals develop strategies like wearing headphones and listening to music while working or avoiding the perceived superabundance of social interaction by taking breaks alone [9]. Of course, those are behaviors that seem weird to many neurotypical people, thus increasing the social difficulties in regular office settings.

Autistic individuals who take the second route, that is choosing to work in an autism-specific, supported work setting, usually report less communication and environmental problems than those who work in regular jobs [16]. Autism-specific job environments usually feature support in form of job coaches, specific training programs, and matching the employee's skills to the job requirements [18]. The following list provides an overview of companies that currently offer supported job environments.

Danish company Specialisterne ("The Specialists") does business consulting, for example, programming, software testing, and data entry. The IT firm strongly supports the NDM: Their logo is a Dandelion seed, paired with the slogan "Weed or herb? You decide. The value of what you see depends on who you are", which reflects the NDM's idea that society's point of view has to shift in order to recognize the value of neurodiverse individuals.

Specialisterne claim on their website that a majority of their workers is neurodiverse, diagnosed with autism, ADHD, Tourette's, or similar conditions. They use the tagline "Passion for

http://dx.doi.org/10.5772/65409

Details" and explain that it stands both for the company's work values and for the characteristic strengths of individuals with autism.

Founded in 2004, they are now internationally successful with offices all over Europe and, since 2013, even the US; the foundation's goal is to offer one million jobs for individuals with autism and to ultimately form a society where everyone has equal chances on the job market. In 2009, partnered with Lego Foundation and the Danish Ministry of Education, Specialisterne Foundation opened an education program for young people (aged 16–25) with autism, with a focus on developing social and personal skills. At the moment, there are 29 students attending the program.

Partnered with Specialisterne is software giant SAP. Established in 1975 in Weinheim, Germany, SAP reportedly had around 75,000 employees in 2015, of which 100 are individuals with autism, divided between eight countries. This was made possible through the campaign "Autism at Work" in 2015. The hiring process was conducted by Specialisterne. SAP, who claims to value diversity as highly as quality, even announced their goal to have 1% of employees to be autistic individuals.

Also based in Germany is Auticon, an IT company that employs only autistic individuals as consultants. Their slogan "Auticon—Querdenker mit System" (approximately "systematically thinking outside the box") highlights how autistic individuals are often able to work more detailed, concentrated, and systematic than neurotypicals and have different ways of looking at problems. To counteract social problems that might occur, Auticon successfully uses job coaches as a link between the consultants and the customers—although only when necessary and specifically needed. Around 2/3 of Auticon's employees are diagnosed with Autism Spectrum Condition.

In Singapore, the United Overseas Bank Group has, together with the Autism Resource Centre, started an initiative to include autistic individuals. In their department for handling costumer documents (checking, digitalization, and archiving), about a third of the 50 employees are diagnosed with autism.

In a press release from 2015, the head office noted that the sense for detail and the systematical approach that individuals with autism often possess make them very qualified for this particular work. The UOB has also successfully implemented job coaches and reported an overall increase of work productivity since the start of the initiative.

Meticulon is a Canadian IT startup company that, just as Auticon in Germany, employs only autistic individuals as IT consultants. The name is a play on "meticulous", referencing again the unusual abilities of their employees. They advertise their services with "Not your average anything!" and have been quite successful since their establishment in 2013.

As of lately, the Israeli military has become aware of the strengths of autistic individuals. In their Special Intelligence Unit 9900, young autistic adults use their above-average visual perception skills for various geography-related tasks, for example,. mapping or analyzing satellite images for the smallest changes. To ensure their abilities match the military's requirements (both perception skills and social abilities), young autistic adults who want to join the

Israeli Defense Forces have to participate in the Ro'im Rachok training program ("looking forward"). In three training intervals (3 months each), they are prepared for their job with a mixture of therapy sessions and military courses.

Looking at this surely not exhaustive list, it might seem that there are plenty of options to find supported work as an autistic individual. However, all of those companies together make for only a few hundred jobs, and even that is a rather optimistic estimate. With an estimated prevalence of Autism of 74 in 10,000 children [19], this obviously is insufficient.

It is also striking that nearly all of these supported jobs (excluding the UOB and the Israeli military) are in IT. This certainly matches the prevailing opinion that autistic individuals somehow naturally have an interest in computer sciences [20]. While it is true that autistic individuals have a distinct job strengths profile that is compatible with, but not limited to IT, the job interests of autistic individuals in non-supported jobs are rather broad [15].

Still, IT, finance, and military are currently the only occupational sectors that offer supported jobs for autistic individuals.

4. From the outside: academia and autism

Since its first characterization in 1943 by Leo Kanner, autism has been of great interest for the scientific community [3]. Still, it took fifty more years until the idea of an autism spectrum was developed, varying between lower than average IQ, often times nonverbal individuals, and so-called high functioning individuals with average to above-average IQ and the above stated characteristic abilities [21]. Current research still has a rather rigid view on autism. This is for example mirrored by the fact that, although the autism community and the NDM themselves prefer the use of the term condition [3], the official, scientific name still remains Autism Spectrum Disorder.

Academia seems to have acknowledged that many autistic individuals have a certain talent and interest in IT, math, and science as a whole [22, 23]. There also appears to be general consensus that autistic individuals have difficulties in social situations [1]. On the other hand, there have been debates on the topic of intelligence, since autistic children tend to perform badly on verbal-based intelligence tests like the Wechsler Intelligence Scale for Children (WISC), and since the WISC is one of the most popular intelligence tests for children, many autistic children were diagnosed as "mentally retarded" [24]. Following Temple Grandin's Thinking in Pictures—theory [25], there have recently been findings that in intelligence tests which do not use verbal communication (e.g., Raven's Matrices), autistic individuals score significantly higher (with a significantly bigger difference to the verbal-based results than their neurotypical peers; [24]). Those results also show that, while autistic individuals do score low on verbal-based tests as well as on spatial testings, they often show better than average results on rule-based tasks, memory tests, and embedded figure tests. Those results can even be replicated using the WISC, as some of its subtests (figure embedding, block design) test exactly those abilities [26].

Intelligence testing is, of course, an old and important tool for psychological diagnostics: Intelligence is a good predictor for success and job performance [27]. It is, however, important to ensure the instrument of choice actually measures what it intends to measure [28], which is not always the case. When scientists produce results that fit their expectations by using the same instruments or tasks that have produced the same or similar results in the past, they conduct biased, neurotypically centered research. This is apparent in the fact that the WISC is still used to test autistic children, even though its ineptitude is known [29]. It also explains the findings that indicate autistic individuals are less employable than neurotypicals, thereby giving lowest priority to actual, specific work-related skills, and focusing on categories like "independent use of public transportation" or "preferring routine" [30]: if researchers are fully convinced of an alleged fact, their results are likely to confirm this fact [31].

Another problem is addressed in a paper by Stevenson et al. [32]: The authors call out the scientific community on infantilizing autism. This ranges from media and the general public assuming that autism is a condition that mostly concerns children [32], to a neurotypically centered way of promoting neurodiversity: namely the idea of using neurodiversity as a tool to help autistic individuals feel better in group therapy settings, instead of actually believing in the neurodiversity concept, and implementing it in a clinical setting, thereby promoting equality between scientists and patients [23]. While self-advocacies like ASAN are trying to transfer their slogan Nothing About Us Without Us into public awareness, there still is no real dialogue between most researchers and autism communities, even though it is necessary in order to improve toward a productive and inclusive research, instead of researching "on Autism" [33].

5. Future perspectives

With this chapter, we wanted to offer a slightly different, more critical perspective on the current situation regarding autism, employment, and its social relevance. We found that while there are, in fact, employment possibilities for autistic individuals, they are scarce and rather specific in terms of occupational fields—aside from IT and finance, there is not much variety. Conventional, non-supported competitive employment offers more sectors to choose from; however, autistic individuals experience those jobs as stressful and report problems with bullying [9, 14].

This overall situation has consequences: autistic individuals as a whole report considerably lower self-efficacy than their neurotypical peers, both occupational and general [15]. This does not come as a surprise, given the fact that self-efficacy and employment status are correlated [15]. Self-efficacy is also known to be correlated to life satisfaction [34] and to be helpful in overcoming job-related barriers [35]. Curiously, neurotypical individuals do not show differences in general and occupational self-efficacy, while autistic individuals only show an increase in occupational self-efficacy when successfully employed [15]. This suggests a stricter division between work life and social or personal life for autistic individuals than for neurotypicals. Whether this has developmental causes, and whether work-specific self-efficacy training might be effective in helping autistic individuals overcome job barriers in different job settings obviously needs thorough research.

Considering the currently estimated prevalence for autism (as noted above, 74 in 10,000 children; [19]), the situation concerning autism and work is socially relevant. We, therefore, propose some changes that allow for a more open-minded interaction between employers and autistic individuals. First of all, there needs to be more education on the actual symptoms and distinctive behavioral features of autism for employers' associations. At the moment, clichés and prejudices still run rampant, coloring autistic individuals as a mixture of pop culture products like Rain Man and Sheldon Cooper. Educational campaigns specifically addressing the work market should help with that. With those prejudices out of the way, the stigma of autism should gradually fade, meaning that autistic individuals might have less fear to disclose their diagnosis to superiors and colleagues. Less social exclusion, as well as a more understanding environment would improve the work experience at nonsupported jobs.

Accompanying this is the currently prevailing deficit policy in the job market. Neurodiversity as a concept promotes a strengths-based approach instead. By focusing on workers' abilities instead of deficits, employers and employees could both profit.

However, we do not want to praise the neurodiversity concept as a cure-all without fault. We are aware of the criticism against it; the NDM does in fact skew toward economical topics more than necessary. Of the whole Autism Spectrum, the high functioning autistic individuals profit the most from the concept, as they are the most marketable, and probably easier to include in the job world than their so-called low-functioning peers. Those who do not fit the criteria of being high-functional for being nonverbal, more prone to repetitive movements, or similar symptoms, are in danger of being forgotten by the NDM. In order to avoid this, we propose to carefully evaluate economic and social motives while promoting the neurodiversity concept.

We believe that creating a triad of community, work, and research, connected through reciprocal communication, will help enormously to overcome prejudices and to establish realistic expectations for all parties. Adopting a different point of view is the first step toward a neurodiverse society.

Appendix

Resources for further information on autism-supporting employment:

Companies:

- www.specialisterne.com
- www.go.sap.com
- www.auticon.de
- www.uobgroup.com
- www.meticulon.com

http://dx.doi.org/10.5772/65409

- www.idfblog.com/blog/2014/04/10/autism-idf-meet-soldiers-intelligence-unit-9900

Advocacies:

- www.autisticadvocacy.org
- www.autismdigest.com
- www.the-art-of-autism.com

Author details

Timo Lorenz*, Nomi Reznik and Kathrin Heinitz

*Address all correspondence to: timo.lorenz@fu-berlin.de

Department of Education and Psychology, Freie Universität Berlin, Berlin, Germany

References

[1] Chown N, Beavan N. Intellectually capable but socially excluded? A review of the literature and research on students with autism in further education. Journal of Further and Higher Education. 2012;36(4):477–493

[2] Armstrong T. Neurodiversity: Discovering the extraordinary gifts of autism, ADHD, dyslexia, and other brain differences. 1st ed. Cambridge: Da Capo Press; 2010.

[3] Jaarsma P, Welin S. (2012). Autism as a natural human variation: Reflections on the claims of the neurodiversity movement. Health Care Analysis. 2012;20(1):20–30.

[4] Sparks BF, Friedman SD, Shaw DW, Aylward, EH, Echelard D, Artru AA, Maravilla KR, Giedd JN, Munson J, Dawson G, Dager SR. Brain structural abnormalities in young children with autism spectrum disorder. Neurology. 2002;59(2):184–192

[5] Brownlow C, Bertilsdotter RH, O'Dell L. Exploring the potential for social networking among people with autism: Challenging dominant ideas of 'friendship'. Scandinavian Journal of Disability Research. 2015;17(2):188–193.

[6] Kapp SK, Gillespie-Lynch K, Sherman LE, Hutman T. Deficit, difference, or both? Autism and neurodiversity. Developmental Psychology. 2013;49(1):59.

[7] Leiner BM, Cerf VG, Clark DD, Kahn RE, Kleinrock L, Lynch DC, Postel J, Roberts LG, Wolff S. A brief history of the Internet. ACM SIGCOM Computer Communication Review. 2009;39(5):22–31.

[8] Keeping Autism Neurodiversity out of The White House [Internet]. 2009. Available from: http://www.ageofautism.com/2009/12/keeping-autism-neurodiversity-out-of-the-white-house.html [Accessed: 2016-07-27]

[9] Hurlbutt K, Chalmers L. (2004). Employment and adults with Asperger syndrome. Focus on Autism and Other Developmental Disabilities. 2004;19(4):215–222

[10] Secretary-General's Message for 2015 [Internet]. 2015. Available from: http://www.un.org/en/events/autismday/2015/sgmessage.shtml [Accessed: 2016-08-18]

[11] Hendricks D. Employment and adults with autism spectrum disorders: Challenges and strategies for success. Journal of Vocational Rehabilitation. 2010;32(2):125–134.

[12] Lorenz T, Frischling C, Cuadros R, Heinitz K. Autism and overcoming job barriers: Comparing job-related barriers and possible solutions in and outside of Autism-specific emsployment. PLoS One. 2016;11(1) doi:10.1371/journal.pone.0147040

[13] Neurodiversity: A Balanced Opinion [Internet]. 2009. Available from: http://autismdigest.com/neurodiversity/ [Accessed: 2016-08-09]

[14] Simone R, Grandin T. Asperger's on the job: Must-have advice for people with Asperger's or High Functioning Autism, and their employers, educators, and advocates. Arlington, TX: Future Horizons; 2010.

[15] Lorenz T, Heinitz K. Aspergers–different, not less: occupational strengths and job interests of individuals with Asperger's syndrome. PLoS One. 2014;9(6). doi:10.1371/journal.pone.0100358

[16] Morris MR, Begel A, Wiedermann B. Understanding the challenges faced by neurodiverse software engineering employees: Towards a more inclusive and productive technical workforce. In: Proceedings of the 17th International ACM SIGACCESS Conference on Computers & Accessibility ACM; 26-28 October 2015; Lisbon. New York, NY: ACM; 2015. p. 173–184

[17] Parr AD, Hunter ST, Ligon GS. Questioning universal applicability of transformational leadership: Examining employees with autism spectrum disorder. The Leadership Quarterly. 2013;24(4);608–622.

[18] Capo LC. (2001). Autism, employment, and the role of occupational therapy. Work. 2001;16(3):201–207.

[19] French LR, Bertone A, Hyde KL, Fombonne E. Epidemiology of autism spectrum disorders. In: The neuroscience of autism spectrum disorders. 1st ed. Oxford: Elsevier; 2013. p. 3–24.

[20] Mazurek MO, Shattuck PT, Wagner M, Cooper BP. Prevalence and correlates of screen-based media use among youths with autism spectrum disorders. Journal of Autism and Developmental Disorders. 2012;42(8):1757–1767.

[21] Wing L. The autistic spectrum. The Lancet. 1997;350:1761–1766.

[22] James I. Autism and mathematical talent. The Mathematical Intelligencer. 2010;32(1): 56–58.

[23] Barnhart GS. Clinician perspectives of adult high-functioning autism support groups' use of neurodiversity concept [Thesis]. Minneapolis: Walden University; 2016.

[24] Kunda M, Goel, AK. How thinking in pictures can explain many characteristic behaviors of autism. In: Proceedings of the 7th IEEE International Conference on Development and Learning (IEEE '08); 09-12 August 2008; Monterey. New York, NY: IEEE; 2008. p. 304–309.

[25] Grandin T. Thinking in pictures: and other reports from my life with autism. 2nd ed. New York, NY: Vintage; 2006.

[26] Dawson M, Soulières I, Gernsbacher MA, Mottron L.The level and nature of autistic intelligence. Psychological Science. 2007;18(8):657–662.

[27] Schmidt FL, Hunter JE. The validity and utility of selection methods in personnel psychology: Practical and theoretical implications of 85 years of research findings. Psychological Bulletin. 1998;124(2):262.

[28] Cronbach LJ, Meehl PE. Construct validity in psychological tests. Psychological Bulletin. 1955;52(4):281.

[29] Nader AM, Courchesne V, Dawson M, Soulières I. Does WISC-IV underestimate the intelligence of autistic children? Journal of Autism and Developmental Disorders. 2016;46(5):1582–1589.

[30] Gal E, Landes E, Katz N. Work performance skills in adults with and without high functioning autism spectrum disorders (HFASD). Research in Autism Spectrum Disorders. 2015;10;71–77.

[31] Mynatt CR, Doherty ME, Tweney RD. Confirmation bias in a simulated research environment: An experimental study of scientific inference. The Quarterly Journal of Experimental Psychology. 1977;29(1):85–95.

[32] Stevenson JL, Harp B, Gernsbacher MA. Infantilizing autism. Disability Studies Quarterly. 2011;31(3).

[33] Lorenz T. The two towers [Thesis]. Berlin: Freie Universität Berlin; 2016.

[34] Weber M, Ruch W, Littman-Ovadia H, Lavy S, Gai O. Relationships among higher-order strengths factors, subjective well-being, and general self-efficacy–The case of Israeli adolescents. Personality and Individual Differences. 2013;55(3):322–327.

[35] Pinquart M, Juang LP, Silbereisen RK. Self-efficacy and successful school-to-work transition: A longitudinal study. Journal of Vocational Behavior. 2003;63(3);329–346.

Chapter 2

The Clinical Gestalts of Autism: Over 40 years of Clinical Experience with Autism

Michael Fitzgerald

Additional information is available at the end of the chapter

http://dx.doi.org/10.5772/65906

Abstract

The clinical gestalts of autism are very broad and much more heterogeneous than people realise. DSM V [1] gives a more narrow and condensed description of what autism is in the twentieth century. DSM focuses on problems with socioemotional reciprocity, non-verbal communication and difficult interpersonal relationships, restricted, repetitive patterns of behaviour, early onset and functional impairment. First, I want to flesh out the autism spectrum disorder gestalts as it presents to experienced clinical practitioners. It is the opposite of the "tick box" approach to diagnosis so common today. It focuses on the phenomena as they would have been focused on in the late nineteenth and early twentieth century, an approach that has faded into the background in the late twentieth and early twenty-first century. It is critical at this point of the twenty-first century that we re-engage with phenomenology and with the clinical gestalt of psychiatric conditions which show a great deal of overlap with much mixed phenomenology. We will start by examining social relations in autism spectrum disorders. Clearly, this is central to autism.

Keywords: clinical gestalts of autism, evolving concepts of autism

1. Introduction

There has been a very considerable evolution of the concept of autism since the Kanner 1943 paper [2]. The move has been from a very narrow concept of autism with Kanner to a much broader concept of autism today, which was foreshadowed by Hans Asperger in 1938 [3] and 1944 [4]. I will describe the characteristics of the broader autism phenotype as I have observed them over the past 40 years.

2. Social deficits

When professionals meet families with autism, they often very quickly become aware of how very clingy to one parent the child with autism is, with a fear of groups but being less anxious in a one-to-one situation, particularly with adults or having one "friend". In groups only relating to one person is common, often to the point of fixation, making inappropriate comments is extremely common to peers and adults, for example, saying to a doctor, "you are very trendy". Hiding behind mother when they are in consultation with the doctor and the doctor asks them questions is extremely common. When they come in to a doctor or examiner's officer, they will often sit on the "parent's chair" or alternatively sit away at the furthest point from the examiner, in the room. Extreme positions are very common.

They often will hold mother's face roughly to get her to look straight at them. In communication, they will often look past people and have reduced eye contact in consultation and elsewhere.

One parent often describes themselves as loners and good mixers at the very same time. They mean that sometimes they are loners and sometimes they are good mixers, but do not and cannot come down on either side. Ambivalence and inability to make up their minds on emotional matters are extremely common. One parent often emphasises their private time, while saying they are sociable. Children with autism can engage in extreme interpersonal aggression, but less degrees of interpersonal aggression are very common. Children, when they engage in rough play, will cause considerable upset at school and home and can include attempts to choke other children. These children with autism experience a great deal of suspicion and paranoid thoughts of people and feel people are against them, talking about them, and not liking them. They are extremely sensitive to highly expressed emotion.

In the marital situation, you often find a change in roles where the wife will go out to work and the husband will become a house-husband. The house-husbands will very often have autistic traits, if not autism. Being unemployed will not be rare in persons with autism or Asperger's syndrome. This is the default position from the stress of work and interpersonal relationships at work.

Girls (and to a lesser extent boys) with autism may live their lives one second after others around them and will copy the behaviour of people around them one second later and then hide their autism. The paradox is that persons with autism can be profoundly observant. This can lead to "as if" or chameleon-like personalities "hide" and "hide" their autism in this way.

3. School and college years

For young children, biting and kicking is fairly common in preschool and at home. They often show disrespect to teachers and other pupils in the school. They will speak to a teacher as a "mini-adult" and as if they are on the "same level" as the teacher. They will terminate

http://dx.doi.org/10.5772/65906

friendships if the friend does not do exactly what they want them to do. They have huge difficulty allowing other peers to have autonomy and to take control of interactions. Pinching and biting is common in preschool. They may make up their own social rules in school. Going under the desk at school is very common as a sensory avoidance, as is putting their head on the school desk. Because of their lack of social skills, they commonly, as children or adolescents, show oppositional defiant behaviour, which at times can be the biggest challenge for parents and teachers with them often losing temper, often arguing with adults, often being defiant, often being angry with adults, often being touchy and easily annoyed and being spiteful and vindictive, with a comorbid diagnosis for oppositional defiant disorder. This is often because of their empathy deficits and theory of mind deficits. They are often very controlling and dominating, which causes major problems at home and school. They always have to win. They have great difficulty in understanding the rules of a social game and particularly difficulty in engaging in group sports, which they do very rarely anyhow. Sports have formal rules, but also unwritten rules, that is, what they can get away with. This is why referees are necessary. They may be over-rigid in following the rules, and this causes major difficulties in social behaviour.

They often have very little sense of danger about roads, or strangers, or in school and particularly dangerous social situations. As they get older, they will often engage in school refusal and isolate themselves in their room on their computers. While some may only want to play with the opposite sex, or get on better with the opposite sex, others have a hatred of the opposite sex. They can sometimes relate reasonably well to siblings or family members or survive in school when looked after by a sibling, but others can be vicious and dangerous to their siblings. When they describe someone that they would call their friend or a bully, they will often describe the same person. Excessive and inappropriate sharing of their thoughts about self and others is common and can cause them to be bullied. They are often the "class clown" as a way of getting attention, and this can be very disruptive in school. In the school class, they will often shout out answers and have difficulty with timing, because of their social communication difficulties. Sometimes they will want to answer every question in the classroom, which causes problems in the classroom and for teachers. Children with autism can control their abnormal social behaviour in school with massive and exhausting effort, but only to "explode" at home with temper tantrums and oppositional defiant behaviour later in the evening. Some with very high IQs may find some other cognitive strategies to help them survive at school.

4. Transitional object and autism

Comfort blankets, teddy bears, etc., are very commonly carried around by children with autism. Winnicott [5] mistakenly called these transitional objects. They have nothing to do with child development in the Winnicottian sense, but everything to do with comfort, anxiety reduction, preservation of sameness and sensory issues. This is an example of psychoanalysis over-complicating simple and obvious phenomena.

5. Emotional and cognitive problems

Problems understanding their own and others' emotions are very common and probably universal. They often do not understand depression and ask, "What is the depression?" When asked whether they are happy or sad, they will say, "both happy and sad" or "I don't know". They often have low capacity for emotional expression and great difficulty in expressing emotions, including feelings and thoughts. Sometimes they want to give the absolutely correct answer, and there is therefore a great delay in answering a question. In a public intervention situation, they can therefore give the impression of not cooperating. They are often either fearless, show evidence of serious risk taking, or the opposite, huge fear, anxiety and panic. Autistic novelty seeking can also be seen [6]. They often also showed generalised anxiety.

6. Language

They will commonly be delayed in language, but will begin to speak in full sentences when they do begin to speak. Imitating accents is very common, particularly accents the child with autism will hear on television. They will often imitate these extremely accurately, and this will be noted as being different from neuro-typical children. Irish children will often be described as having an American accent, or a posh English accent, or an unusual tone to their accent. Small children often have a soulful or plaintive cry, which can be a most disturbing cry to listen to and it can go on for many hours. They often use a "babyish" immature voice at any age. Older persons with autism can have marvellous sense of verbal humour [7], playing on words, etc. They will often change their accent to suit their situation or copy the accent of the person they are talking to. They engage in a great deal of talking to themselves–self-talk. This is an effort to sort out emotionally cognitive puzzles and experience. Some children will often speak like adults, another reversal. They may engage in repetitive questioning and always want the questions answered exactly the same way. Some of the children will have a very high-pitch tone of voice, others low-pitched, other a monotonous tone.

They will sometimes pronounce every word accurately. They mostly have difficulty doing personal, emotional writing in the social sense. The autistic narrative will not give people a sense of social context. This is being called autistic narrative [8], seen in autobiographies of persons with autism. They are often obsessed with words, language and numbers. They will express too much, which is inappropriate sharing of personal thoughts. There will often engage in sub-vocal talking and singing. They pick up accents very rapidly. They very commonly answer questions with "I don't know". They will be very hesitant in answering questions, and it will take a long time for them to answer the questions. Loss of language or babble and words in the first 2 years does occur, not uncommonly. Sometimes the loss can even occur into the third year.

While most are extremely truthful and indeed, inappropriately truthful in social areas, a number can make up stories have a fantastic imagination and can fabricate false stories about parents. This is due to the difficulty of separating fact from fiction in their minds. Often their conversation is not very coherent, difficult to understand, which leads to misdiagnosis of thought disorder and schizophrenia. They often ask, "What's going to happen next?" They often make up words or their own language … neologisms. If something is spoken about as going to happen, then it must happen at exactly the time it was spoken about.

Parents with autism and very high IQ can use language to camouflage their symptoms, which leads to later diagnosis.

7. Identity

Identity diffusion is central to autism, and this will include their sexual and other identities. This is probably due to the neural connectivity problems in the brain [9]. Contradictory identities can exist side by side in their mind. They can switch to another and opposite identity very rapidly. This can be confused with so-called multiple personalities. This identity diffusion can cause stress in making decisions and in employment, and despite intelligence and good education, they may withdraw and cease to seek employment. They can confuse people with these contradictory identities. They do not have a clear sense of themselves and people find it difficult to understand them. This makes it very difficult for them to have a clear sense of other people. This increases interpersonal stress. They are often mistaken for the opposite sex and come across as being androgynous. Males can appear to have a soft female facies and females with a somewhat harder male facies. They may dress more like the opposite sex, which always causes confusion and shows signs of gender dysphoria. A small number will have transgender problems. Sometimes they feel unreal and de-personalised as living in a film and having an "as if" personality. Older adolescents with autism or Asperger's syndrome often appear to be "asexual". This can be very deceptive as the very same people can get involved in perverse, dangerous sexual activities.

8. Sensory problems in autism are almost universal

The sounds that cause major difficulties include the sound of a hoover or babies crying. This can be extremely upsetting and on rare occasions, put the crying baby at risk of violence from the persons with ASD. There were always contradictory findings in the sense that I have seen a child with ASD who loved the sound of hoovers. They often smell everything, are extremely sensitive to the texture of food and do not want different foods touching on the plate. They often find haircuts extremely upsetting and will wear their clothes inside out, because of sensory issues, to avoid clothes tags on their skin. Others will put everything in their mouth for sensory reasons, including towels. They often chew their clothes. Often they are not bothered by their own noise but bothered by the same noise created by someone else, which is contradictory.

They can overeat because of difficulty knowing when they have eaten enough/satiety. This may be due to the sensory issues in the gut, which doesn't tell them that they have sufficient food eaten. This requires empirical research. They often find the visual very stimulating and are fascinated by lights, by pictures and by spinning objects. Some are the opposite and are hyposensitive in relation to pain or hypersensitive, another contradiction.

9. Narrow interests

They are often very interested in nature, with gardens, with dogs, animals, sharks, horses, bugs, etc. Other and possibly the most common of all interests now are computers, iPhones, iPads, computer games and technology in general. They love to take things apart and work out how things work. No wonder so many are attracted to engineering work. Making lists is very common. This probably gives them some kind of control or order to their life. Some are massive collectors. The younger children love turning pages of books, per se. Older children love reading them, particularly novels on science fiction, history, encyclopaedias, books of facts, or Egyptology, palaeontology, physics, science, cosmology, etc. Being talented at music or being interested in music is quite common. Some are fascinated by younger children. They are often preoccupied with just one person. Others are obsessed with time, and of course Albert Einstein had autism [10] and was obsessed with time. At Christmas time, they can be fascinated with Christmas trees. Other fascinations include guns [11], ammunition, horror movies, violent movies and the topic of death. They are often preoccupied with their own and their parents' death. In rare cases, they can be very interested in serial killers [11] and a tiny number can engage in so-called mindless violence.

They are very easily led and can easily be led into criminal activities. They often love to push buttons, switch on and off lights, open and close doors.

Sometimes they will not change their clothes and wear the same clothes every day. They may fixate on a television character or a teacher. Girls will often have no interest in dolls. Boys and girls often will have no interest in toys and be more interested in everyday objects and can find small things missing, where others would miss them, with their massive attention to detail.

10. Physical issues

They often have low immune system and are highly prone to infections, particularly ear infections. Delayed toilet training is very common. Parents will often tell you the child had pyloric stenosis, hiatus hernia, difficulties feeding (poor eating, fussy eating), and swallowing, "was a colicky baby", or had eczema. Hypermobility of the joints and muscles is very common. They often somatise their problems and present with unexplained physical illness, or Alexithymia [12], which often occurs with Asperger's syndrome. Cerebral palsy and a vast number of chromosomal abnormalities occur. Many brain abnormalities can be presented, including agenesis of the corpus callosum or optic nerve hypoplasia. Clearly, these last two conditions would be extremely rare. A large head has been shown to be associated, but I have often seen a large head at birth. It would be interesting to measure the head circumference in utero. These children are often very tall for their age, and indeed, I have also noticed parents being equally tall. They can be confused with Marfan's syndrome.

11. Motor issues

It was an error in DSM V [1] to leave out motor issues from the main criteria and only mention them as associated features. The most common features that a parent of an autistic child will mention are motor issues including tippy-toe walking and "bum-shuffling". They often describe the "combat crawl". They will talk about the child having never rolled over. Other mothers describe a "crabby crawl" and "walking on their knees". Other features include the child having "one leg out and one leg under him". Sometimes you see a stiff gait with the hands rigidly by the side of the body and a rigid tense body. There is hugely reduced non-verbal expression. Moving sideways through a door has also been a feature. Other parents say the autistic child never crawled, but just stood up. Some mothers describe their child as walking very carefully, while more commonly they describe their children as walking awkwardly. Another feature can be "crawling on the abdomen", as described by parents. Other features can be unusual motor movements with legs crossed and jumping up and down. Sometimes severe clenching of teeth is noted. In lower functioning children with autism, head-banging is not uncommon. There are parents describing their children as having clumsy walk or walking like a "monkey". Another description by a mother was of "frog-like crawling" or crawling backwards. Asymmetric movements of the body, pulling of one leg after the other, can be seen. Clinicians need to be much more attentive to motor issues in the broader autism phenotype.

12. Non-verbal behaviour

Late smiling is noted or biting hands and rocking are common. The rocking can occur at any age. There is a huge amount of imitation and copying of others' non-verbal behaviour. Children and adults with autism can be brilliant at mimicking and very good at non-verbal humour, for example, slapstick humour [7]. Some will often stare inappropriately for a very long time or come excessively close and look at the other person in the face. They will often adopt the other person's attributes in an extreme way. Their dress can often lead to them being mistaken for a person of the opposite sex, which is probably due to their identity diffusion. Sleep problems are extremely common. They are often very tall, and this is one reason why a minority are therefore not bullied. They often wear, "rabbit type" uniforms, dress in a teddy bear outfit or of course nowadays, they will often have headphones to cut out noise. They can show a mixture of crying and laughing at the same time. Contradictory verbal and non-verbal behaviour is not uncommon. Clapping the hands when excited, flapping the hands and looking at things through the corner of their eyes are not uncommon.

13. Repetitive behaviour

They will often prefer to play with cups or other objects, rather than toys. They often particularly put things in and out of boxes repetitively. They love switching on and off lights. Indeed, Sigmund Freud's (who had Asperger's Syndrome) grandson, Ernest Freud played with a reel and this could be seen as a repetitive autistic play. He threw the reel out and pulled it back in, in a repetitive way. Of course one feature does not give a diagnosis. They often love to calculate repetitively and can have massive memories.

14. Pregnancy and labour

Extremely, commonly here are some complications in pregnancy and delivery which are very difficult to interpret and whether this has some special meaning or is just coincidence has to be resolved. Long labour and assistance with delivery are common. Emergency caesarean section, because of foetal distress, is very common. Other reasons for caesarean section can be a failure to go into labour or labour stopping in mid-point. Other causes can be a failure to dilate. Prolonged labour, cessation of labour or extremely quick labour are not uncommon. There seems to be increased rates of autism, when there is assisted reproduction. Other factors which include reduced amniotic fluid, placenta previa, breech or face presentation, shoulder presentation or other abnormal presentations are not uncommon. Multiple pregnancies can be associated. Other issues can be very stressful pregnancy, various drugs in pregnancy, or hyperemesis and pre-eclamptic toxaemia in mother. Of course, many of these features could be just coincidental.

15. Parents

In terms of occupations, it's very common for one or both parents to be accountants, engineers, computer specialists, policemen, landscape gardeners, lorry drivers, mathematicians, scientists, engineers, butchers, soldiers, taxi drivers, stonemasons and painters. In more recent years, I've noticed fathers being unemployed as a more common feature. This may be due to them having autistic features and withdrawing from the work situation. "House-husbands" is becoming much more common as an occupation for fathers of children with autism.

16. Conclusion

The concept of the autism spectrum disorder is now almost universally accepted. This chapter outlines the broader autism phenotype. The National Institute of Clinical Excellence (NICE) guidelines [13] recommend no specific instrument in the diagnosis of autism. Unfortunately, it is widely believed that there is one gold standard instrument for the diagnosis of autism, and this leads to many children on the spectrum being excluded from autism and from the autistic diagnosis, with great distress to the children themselves, to their families and the schools that they attend. This then excludes them from the specific autism services, and unfortunately, this happens in many parts of the world. The great array of autism instruments can be useful for information gathering, for new mental health professionals in the field. They do not give you a DSM diagnosis as outlined by the National Institute of Clinical Excellence guidelines. One of the instruments which are widely used in clinical practice which is quite appropriate for use in research is the ADI-R [14]. This has been widely criticised, for example, by the most experienced and distinguished professionals. An example is Professor Dorothy Bishop, Professor of Developmental Neuropsychology, University of Cambridge [15]. Professor Dorothy Bishop [15] states that, "the main problem with the ADI-R is not just the financial cost (although that is certainly prohibitive for many), but also the cost in time; time for training, time for administration and time for scoring and consensus coding", and "if it could be shown that there were real benefits in accuracy of diagnosis from adopting this lengthy procedure, then I'd be happy to say: "Ok, this is the best way forward and we just have to find a way to do it", but the originators of the instrument have never demonstrated that you actually need such a long process–it is really more an article of faith with them", and that, "part of the problem is that criteria for autism keep changing, and cut-offs are entirely arbitrary. I personally think we'd be better off with a dimensional, rather than categorical, conceptualisation of autism–that is, one with a measure that gave a quantitative index of level of autism symptoms on different dimensions" [15].

Professor Bishop points out that there are "plenty of children who come out as meeting criteria on one instrument only, and there seem no sensible guidelines as to how you then proceed, other than to seek expert clinical opinion". The bottom line, she told me [Adam Feinstein], was that those devising the diagnostic instruments for autism "should be doing studies to see what is the minimum set of items you can have to get reasonable diagnostic accuracy". I doubt that we really need a three-hour interview for each case.

The International Meeting for Autism Research (IMFAR) was held in London in May 2008 [16] "where many of the most experienced and distinguished Autism Researchers in the world lambasted the tool for missing many cases of Autism".

This creates a public health problem, the missing of these persons with autism. This is especially so in countries that put excessive emphasis on clinical use of the ADI-R [14] for the diagnosis and particularly where the prevalence of autism as we know now is much greater than in the past. The Centres for Disease Control, (USA) 2016, put the prevalence of autism at 1 in 68, that is, 1 in 42 for boys and 1 in 189 for girls.

From a clinical perspective, the most serious problem facing the autism field is missing the diagnosis of autism in many situations. Unfortunately, the NICE guidelines are so often ignored.

Dr. Lorna Wing [17] used the concept of the autism spectrum disorder or the broader autism phenotype which is accepted by clinicians in most parts of the world today and forms the basis of autism in the DSM V and also in the proposed criteria for ICD XI to be published in the next few years. Unfortunately, a few practitioners are still using very narrow criteria. This is a problem as I've shown myself that when you use criteria like Kanner and Eisenberg [18] for autism, one gets very low rates. Fitzgerald showed that using the same patients, the prevalence of autism varied in a total sample of possible autism patients of 309, with 85%, (256), meeting the DSM III/R criteria to 8% using Kanner and Eisenberg's criteria [18]. Professor G. Baird's study from the Lancet [19] gave a prevalence of 116.1 per 10,000 [20], and Professor Simon Baron-Cohen's study from Cambridge in the British Journal of Psychiatry (BJP) put the prevalence at 157 per 10,000.

I hope that this chapter will make the reader aware of the dangers of a narrow concept of autism and the severely negative consequences for children being excluded from a diagnosis of autism, which means they are excluded from services. Everyone in the field agrees the critical importance of early diagnosis and early treatment, and these children have a better outcome. Children deserve nothing less.

Author details

Michael Fitzgerald

Address all correspondence to: prof.m.fitzgerald@gmail.com

Clinical Psychiatry, Trinity College Dublin, Ireland

References

[1] Diagnostic and Statistical Manual of Mental Disorders (2013): DSM V. Washington: American Psychiatric Association.

[2] Kanner L. (1943): Autistic disturbances of affective contact. Nervous Child 2, 217–250.

[3] Asperger H. (1938): Das Psychisch Abnormale Kind. Wiener Klinischen Wochenzeitschrift 51, 1314–1317.

[4] Asperger H. (1944): Die "Autischen Psychopathen" Im Kindesalter. Archiv. Fur Psychietrie und Nervenkrankheiten 17, 76–136 (Autistic Psychopathy in Childhood. Trans. Uta Frith. In Frith U. (1991) Autism and Asperger's Syndrome), Cambridge: Cambridge University Press.

[5] Winnicott D.W. (1958): Collected papers through paediatrics to psychoanalysis. London: Tavistock.

[6] Fitzgerald M. (2008): ADHD, creativity, novelty seeking & risk. New York: Nova Science.

[7] Lyons V., Fitzgerald M. (2004): Humour in Asperger's syndrome. Journal of Autism Developmental Disorders 34(5), 521–531.

[8] Fitzgerald M. (2004): Autism & creativity. New York: Routledgey.

[9] Casanova M., Switla A., Trippe J., Fitzgerald M. (2007): Comparative mini columnar morphometry of three distinguished scientists. Autism 11(6), 557–569.

[10] Fitzgerald M. (2000): Einstein: brain and behaviour. Journal of Autism Developmental Disorder 6, 620–621.

[11] Fitzgerald M. (2000): Young, violent and dangerous to know. New York: Nova Science.

http://dx.doi.org/10.5772/65906

[12] Fitzgerald M., Belgrove M. (2006): The overlap between alexithymia and Asperger's syndrome. Journal of Autism & Developmental Disorders 36(4), 575–576.

[13] National Institute for Health & Clinical Excellence (2011): Autism: recognition, referral & diagnosis of children and young people on autism spectrum. Clinical Guidelines 128, London: British Psychological Society & Royal College of Psychiatrists.

[14] Lord C., Rutter M. (1994): Autism diagnostic interview revised. Journal of Autism & Developmental Disorders 25(5), 659–686.

[15] Bishop D. (2010): Definition, diagnosis & assessment in a history of autism by A. Feinstein. Chichester: Wiley-Blackwell.

[16] Feinstein A. (2010): A history of autism. Chichester: Wiley-Blackwell.

[17] Fitzgerald M., Matthews P., Birbeck G., O'Connor J. (1996): Irish families under stress, Vol. 7, A Prevalence and Psychosocial Study in the EHB area of Dublin. Dublin: EHB.

[18] Kanner L., Eisenberg L. (1956) Early infantile autism American. Journal of Orthopsychiatry 26(3), 556–566.

[19] Baird G., Simonoff E., Charman T., et al. (2006): Prevalence of disorders of the autism spectrum in a population cohort of children in South Thames: the special needs and autism project. Lancet 368, 210–215.

[20] Baron-Cohen S., Scott F., Allison C., Williams J., Bolton P., Matthews F., Brayne C., et al. (2009): Prevalence of autism spectrum conditions: UK school-based population study. British Journal of Psychiatry 194, 500–509.

Section 2

Correlates of Autism Disorder

Chapter 3

Sex Bias in Autism

Felwah S. Al-Zaid

Additional information is available at the end of the chapter

http://dx.doi.org/10.5772/67402

Abstract

Autism is a neurodevelopmental disorder with unknown exact etiology. Interestingly, it affects males more than females in a striking ratio (4:1), respectively. This biased ratio served as a clue to search about the factors that are sex linked and hence sex hormones and X chromosomes were good candidates. Although understanding the basic sex dimorphism in male and female brains is essential to understand autism pathology. Theories regarding the biased sex ratio in autism have been raised, and some have been supported by evidence from human studies. Furthermore, sex-linked genetic dysregulation has also been reported in autism. In this chapter, an overview of what is known about sex bias in autism is reviewed, emphasizing the importance of carrying on in uncoding the sex bias in autism.

Keywords: autism, androgens, digit ratio, RORA gene, X chromosome

1. Introduction

The exact etiology of autism is unknown and no single cause has been identified yet, but the disease is highly heritable and the heterogeneity in clinical presentation is thought to be due to different etiologies, complicates genetic and molecular analysis [1]. The studies strongly suggest a genetic basis of the disease with a complex mode of inheritance. However, autism occurs more in boys than girls in a 4:1 male to female ratio [2]. This bias toward the male gender caught the scientist's attention to search about the factors that are sex linked or gender specific.

2. Sex differences in the brain

Although there is an individual variation in human brain morphometry, it is known that male and female brains are different, both anatomically and physiologically. Male brain has a larger cerebrum than female brain, and more white matter than gray matter, respectively [3, 4]. Despite the larger total volume of white matter in men, the ratio of corpus callosum to total cerebral volume is smaller in them [4]. This ratio is consistent with the finding that the increased size of the brain predicts decreased interhemispheric connectivity [5] and that larger brain comes with smaller corpus callosum [6]. Moreover, the male amygdala experiences an extended period of growth during childhood and men have a larger amygdala compared to women.

At micro-architectural level, male cerebral cortex has more neurons than that of female's and those neurons are densely packed with the exception of some areas of the brain [7]. This dense packing of neurons in male brain is associated with more intrahemispheric white matter projecting from these neurons suggesting, indirectly, a pattern of increased local connectivity and decreased interhemispheric connectivity in the male brain [8, 9].

Physiologically, and consistent with the above-mentioned observations, the language-related activation in female brain is more bilateral, suggesting a greater interhemispheric connectivity in females than males [10–12]. This sexual dimorphism of brain structure maybe related to sex chromosomes, hormonal effects, and environmental factors or as a result of a combination of all these factors. These morphological differences have a profound effect on brain physiology and substantiate one of the main hypotheses for etiology of autism as it will be discussed later.

3. Role of sex hormones in developing brain

Androgens including testosterone act on the developing brain to produce sex differences at the level of neuroanatomy and brain function. For more understanding of the role of sex hormones in brain development, scientists have divided its actions into prenatal and postnatal effects and described it via two main distinct mechanisms.

In the prenatal period, a very critical period of brain development especially in the first trimester, sex hormones have a permanent organizational effect. The organization mechanism is defined as a developmental mechanism in which steroids act on the brain during critical periods of brain development to mediate permanent sexually dimorphic differentiation of brain morphology, giving rise to male and female sexual behaviors and physiology in adulthood. On the other hand, in the postnatal period, sex hormones have a transient activational effect. Activation mechanism is defined as the acute effect of gonadal hormones on the fully developed nervous system, and it is responsible for maintaining sex specific behaviors in adulthood; it is not permanent and is associated with changes in sex hormones levels, for example, hormonal changes during menstrual cycle [13, 14]. Most studies about organizational effect of sex steroids focused on the role played by androgens in masculinization of the brain, while little is known about the feminization of the brain, which was though initially to be a passive process that occurs in the absence of high levels of androgens. However, a growing recognition that it might be induced through early postnatal estrogens, although the exact mechanisms remain unclear [14].

http://dx.doi.org/10.5772/67402

4. Androgens

Androgens are steroid hormones, principally testosterone and 5α-dihydrotestosterone, synthesized and secreted into the blood stream in the form of testosterone. Once testosterone reaches its target tissues, it is either metabolized by an aromatase into estradiol, which performs its action by binding to estrogen receptors (ERα, ERβ or GPER) or metabolized by 5α-reductase into dihydrotestosterone (DHT) in majority of the male sexual organs. Testosterone can perform direct actions prior to any metabolic processing via binding to androgen receptors (ARs), a member of nuclear receptor super family. Once it binds to its receptors, AR enters the nucleus, binds the DNA and affects the transcription. Binding of estradiol to its receptors affects the transcription similarly.

During the male life, testosterone has three surges; the first is mediated via fetal testosterone (fT) between 4 and 6 weeks of gestation, which can almost reach pubertal levels. This early surge results in genitalia masculinization and sex dimorphic brain development in the mean of cell proliferation, death, migration, and synaptic formation [15]. The second surge occurs soon after birth called neonatal testosterone (nT) and drops by 4–6 months, during this surge, testosterone reaches pubertal levels and was found to be linked to gender-related typical and atypical behaviors and also contributes to normal growth of male-external genitalia [16]. The third surge is the pubertal one.

Testosterone is essential for the development of male secondary sexual characteristics, for general well-being, prevention of osteoporosis, and it has a direct effect on muscle development. It can easily cross the blood brain barrier and bind to AR, which are expressed in the cerebral cortex, cerebellum, mediobasal hypothalamus, amygdala, corpus callosum, and cingulate cortex [17, 18].

Testosterone in the brain was shown to affect the development of neurons as it prevents apoptosis, influences the neuronal connectivity, and alters the neurochemical profile. Both estradiol and testosterone modulate seretonergic and γ-aminobutyric acid neurotransmission. They increase the dendritic spines through the brain derived neurotropic factor-5 [18].

DHEA and its DHEA-S are known as neurosteroids as they can undergo *de novo* synthesis in the CNS [19], but in humans, the blood represents the main source of DHEA and DHEA-S in the brain. Brain DHEA-S potentiates the action of glutamate and enhances the depolarization and calcium ion entry [20]. Interestingly, DHEA-S acts as antiglucocorticoid as it antagonizes the immunosuppressant and lympholytic actions of cortisol [21]. Subsequently, DHEA protects the hippocampus from the neurotoxic effect of glutamate analog and corticoids [22].

5. Sex-related theories of autism

Autism is a disease of male gender as the male to female ratio is 4:1 [23]. This bias toward the males served as a clue to search for a link between the gender and etiology of autism.

The clinical manifestation of the disease created many hypotheses that support this sex-linked relationship. The theories focusing on the sex ratio include the extreme male brain theory (EMB) of autism, which is an extension of the empathizing systemizing theory (E-S) and it links autism to prenatal exposure to high fetal testosterone [24]. The other theory is the X-linked imprinting theory of autism, which proposes the vulnerability of male to autism based on the fact that males have a single X chromosome [25].

6. The extreme male brain theory (EMB) of autism

Autism is a disease of male gender as the male to female ratio is 4:1 [23]. This bias toward the males served as a clue to search for a link between the gender and etiology of autism. The clinical manifestation of the disease created many hypotheses that support this sex-linked relationship.

E-S theory supported the clinical presentation of the disease and its strong association with the male gender. This theory proposed that females have stronger empathizing, which reflects the ability to identify the other mental status and respond to it with appropriate emotions. On the other hand, systemizing that is stronger in males reflects the drive to analyze a system in term of rules that govern the system [17]. A further extension of the E-S theory of autism is the EMB, which was proposed by Hans Asperger more than 60 years ago. EMB encodes that based on the E-S theory, females are stronger in sympathizing and males are stronger in systemizing, and thus, autism can be considered as an extreme of the normal male profile [24]. This psychological difference is a result of sex differences in the brain structure. Changes in normal brain anatomy have been established in children with autism. They have a larger than average head, which contains abnormally large brain. Cerebral cortex is enlarged with more white matter than the gray matter in autistics. Moreover, they have a greater growth of amygdala. All these changes reflect an exaggeration of normal male brain growth and describe the autistic brain as hypermasculinized brain, which goes along with extreme male brain theory of autism [26]. Studies in humans showed that prenatal exposure to high levels of fetal testosterone resulted in masculinization of the brain. This was first observed in girls with congenital adrenal hyperplasia (CAH), a congenital condition associated with abnormally high level of testosterone. Those girls showed autistic behavioral manifestations [27]. This observation led scientists to hypothesize that one cause of autism is a prenatal exposure to high levels of fetal testosterone.

Consistently, the Cambridge Fetal Testosterone project, in which a correlation between prenatal testosterone exposure and the development of behaviors related to autism was directly investigated, demonstrated an association between fetal testosterone, measured in women who had amniocentesis for other reasons, and the development of autistic traits in their children. Baron-Cohen and his colleagues had recently provided the first direct evidence of elevated fetal steroidogenic activity in autism through their longitudinal study [27, 28]. Moreover, this relationship was observed in both boys and girls denoting that this effect is due to the fetal testosterone rather than the sex of the child per se.

http://dx.doi.org/10.5772/67402

7. The X-linked imprinting theory of autism

Many clinical observations related to autism epidemiology raised the interest in finding a link between disease etiology and genetic mechanism. Strong familiarlity and the higher incidence in siblings with a 3–5% recurrence rate (which accounts for 50–100-fold increase in autism risk compared to the general population) are among the main factors that suggested genetic basis for autism [29]. Moreover, the incidence of autism was found to be increased in monozygotic twins (60%), which indicate a strong genetic influence [30]. Epidemiological studies also found male relatives to male and female autistics to be affected more than female relatives. Accordingly, are females protected by a genetic mechanism? The X-linked imprinted hypothesis, hypothesize that, "the threshold for phenotypic expression of many autism related characteristics is influenced by an imprinted X-linked gene(s) that is protective in nature [25]. Imprinted genes are genes that are exclusively expressed from one parent (one allele only is expressed) [31]. They are known to play an important role in growth and development. Moreover, they affect neurodevelopment, brain function, and behavior [32, 33]. In case of the X-linked imprinted gene theory, the gene is expressed only on the X chromosome that is inherited from the father. Subsequently, as only females can carry paternal X chromosome, the threshold for phenotypic expression is higher in them compared to male [25].

8. Hyperandrogenism in autism

In the light of EMB theory of autism, numerous studies were conducted to investigate postnatal testosterone levels in autistic children. Although it has been demonstrated by some studies that children with autism have significantly elevated androgen levels [34, 35], other studies by Tordjman et al. [36] and Lutchmaya et al. [37] have not found significant differences in testosterone levels in autism. Moreover, postpubertal androgen levels were found to be lower than controls in autistic children [38]. We investigated the role of androgens in Saudi autistic children and our findings demonstrated a significant elevation of both total testosterone, which was increased by 53% in autism and free testosterone, which was 238% higher in autistic children, without significant differences in the sex hormone binding globulin (SHBG) levels between autistic group and control group. The significant increase of free testosterone in a magnitude higher than that of total testosterone is explained by the lack of concomitant increase in SHBG. Both total testosterone and free testosterone were positively and strongly correlated with each other and both of which had a positive strong correlation with DHEA, which was also significantly elevated in autistic children by 50% suggesting an adrenal source of the elevated androgens [35]. Significant elevation of those androgens has been reported in American autistic children in comparison with laboratory reference values by Geier's study, which reported 158% increase in total testosterone, 214% increase in serum free testosterone, and 192% increase in DHEA [34]. On the other hand, Croonenberghs and his colleagues reported a significantly lower testosterone levels in autistic children (12–18 years of age) compared to their age matched controls. This report does not conflict with the results of Geier's and Al-Zaid study for two reasons, first, the age group included in Croonenberghs's study was postpubertal, and second, the decrease in testosterone level in this age group was explained by a greater negative feedback at the hypothalamic level. The preoptic region in the hypothalamic nucleus is androgen sensitive, and it is 2.5 times larger in males. The prenatal growth of this region is strongly determined by the presence of testosterone. Subsequently, too much testosterone early in life could influence androgen receptors or its sensitivity in this region. At a later age, namely during puberty, this could cause a negative feedback resulting in lower testosterone concentrations [38]. On the other hand, Tordjman et al. [36] and Lutchmaya et al. [37] reported a non-significant difference in testosterone level between autism group and their age matched control. However, it is important to note a significant limitation in the Tordjman's study, which was the remarkable heterogeneity in subjects involved in the study as it included prepubertal and postpubertal subjects.

In addition, high testosterone level in children was found to be associated with moodiness, low attachment, and low sociability in prepubertal ages [39], which are common observations in autistic children [40]. Interestingly, the main source of the elevated intrauterine fetal testosterone is not from maternal source, but it is from the fetus itself [14]; this suggests a genetic underlying problem in the fetus and also suggests that it is a lifelong condition. Moreover, the reported observation of low 2nd:4th digit ratio is not only in autistic children, but it is in their siblings and parents [41] suggesting also a genetic connection with autism. The genetic involvement of androgen dysregulation in autism has been reported, in a recent study, which linked a polymorphism in androgen receptor gene (SRD5A2) to autism in Slovak autistic children [42]. More recently, the discovered dysregulation of RORA gene in autism and its influence on the aromatase enzyme, a key regulator for sex hormone biosynthesis pathway, provides a possible broader explanation for the link between autism and hyperandrogenism [2]. Another explanation for the elevated androgens in autistic children was suggested by Geier and his colleagues who reported a significant abnormality in the DHEA synthesis pathway in autistic children. Normally, DHEA can either be converted into the storage molecule, dehydroepiandrosterone sulfate (DHEA-S), or into testosterone. In patients with autism, a decrease in transsulfuration metabolites was observed, resulting in a marked shift toward DHEA with a decrease in DHEA-S production and subsequent increase in testosterone [34] (**Figure 1**).

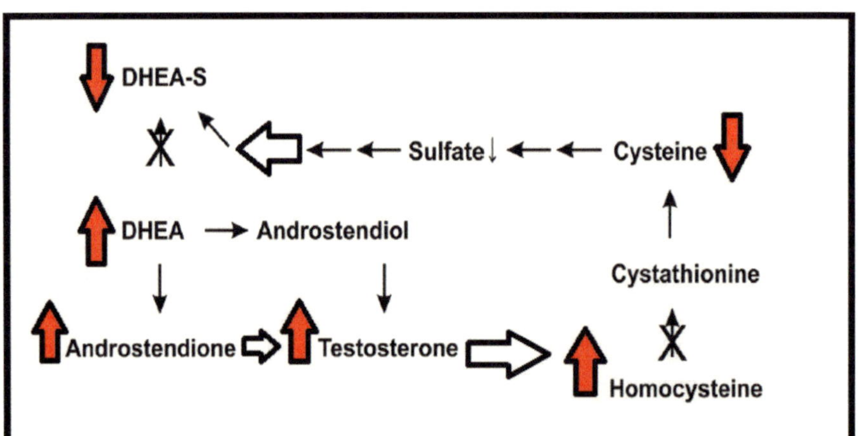

Figure 1. The potential interactions between the transsulfuration and androgen pathway in autism [34].

9. The 2nd:4th digit ratio as a promising screening tool in autism

The levels of androgens are not routinely assayed during pregnancy and direct measures of fetal testosterone concentrations are not usually available. To test the prenatal androgen theory of autism, indirect measures have been used in an attempt to investigate the consequences of fetal testosterone exposure. In 2001, Manning has proposed the 2nd:4th digit ratio as an indirect proxy to the prenatal androgen exposure. They studied the 2nd:4th digit ratio in 95 families with children diagnosed with autism and compared them to families with no autistic children. This study concluded that the highest 2nd:4th digit ratio was found in children without ASDs (autism spectrum disorders), lower in children with asperger syndrome and significantly lowest in children with autism [41]. We recently investigated the 2nd:4th digit in Saudi boys with autism and found it to be significantly lower in them compared to sex and age matched controls (**Figure 2**), and we concluded that 2nd:4th digit ratio could serve as a potential screening tool for autism [43]. This suggests that low 2nd:4th digit ratio is associated with an increased risk of autism. This finding is consistent with several other studies, which reported a lower ratio in British autistic patients [41], Thai patients [44] and Slovak patients [45]. A lower 2nd:4th digit ratio indicates the exposure of Saudi autistic children to high levels of fetal testosterone, as was substantiated by large amount of correlational evidence in both animal and human studies [46, 47]. Several theoretical observations may substantiate the connection between a lower 2nd:4th digit ratio and the increased fetal testosterone levels. First, the ratio is sexually dimorphic with males having a lower ratio compared to the females [48]. Second, the ratio is determined before birth, most probably by the 14th week of pregnancy, and it is not affected by later testosterone concentrations or fluctuations [46]. Third, the ratio was reported to correlate negatively with testosterone and positively with estradiol levels in adults [48]. Overall, this finding implicates increased fetal testosterone levels in the pathophysiology of autism.

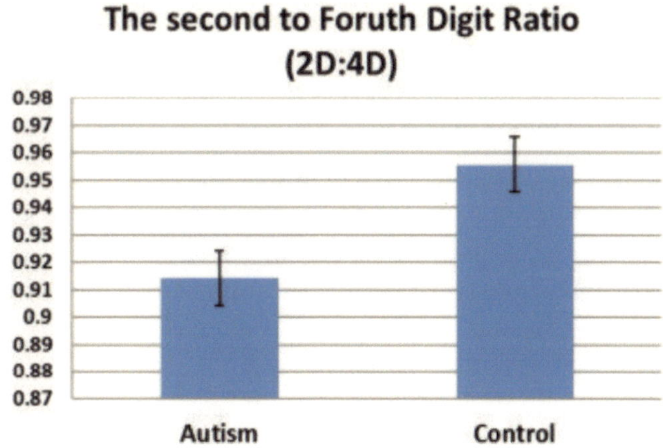

Figure 2. Bar chart demonstrating the second to fourth digit ratio (2D:4D) in the Saudi boys with autism and age and sex matched controls [43].

The significantly elevated levels of androgens in Saudi autistic children together with the significantly lower 2nd:4th digit ratio are consistent with the fetal androgen and extreme male brain theories of autism [24].

10. Sibling sex ratio in autism

It was hypothesized that the parental hormonal levels around the time of conception influence the sex ratios at birth [49]. Accordingly, high parental level of testosterone was suspected to be associated with the production of male offsprings.

In 2010, Mouridsen and his group showed that the sibling sex ratio in a group of 326 individuals with ASDs (245 males, 81 females) at the Danish university clinic was 0.585, which was significantly higher than that in the Danish live birth sex ratio over the same period. However, in autism childhood subclass of ASDs, the result reflected a non-significant difference in male proportion among siblings of autism than that in the Danish live birth sex ratio over the same period of time. Based on the published evidence, which indicates that the human sex ratio at birth is strikingly stable and it is controlled by the parental hormone levels around the time of conception [49], significantly higher male sex ratio was observed in the siblings of Danish autistic patients [50]. These findings indirectly support the EMB theory of autism. However, recently in 2015, Cheslack-Postava and his colleagues failed to find a link between autism and the number of sibling males in a large population-based study [51]. Thus, further studies of sibling sex ratio in autism need to be conducted on a large population scale in order to reach a clear conclusion.

11. The retinoic acid-related orphan receptor-alpha (RORA) gene and sex hormones in autism

A novel autism candidate gene has been identified, a hormone dependent transcription factor, which is the retinoic acid-related orphan receptor-alpha (RORA) [52]. The RORA gene was found to be differentially and reciprocally regulated by androgens and estrogens [2]. Both estradiol and dihydrotestosterone (DHT) enhance the binding of ER and AR, respectively, to the RORA gene promoter regions.

While the estrogen was found to enhance the RORA gene expression, the DHT had a reciprocal effect as it represses the expression of RORA gene. The target of the RORA gene expression is the aromatase enzyme responsible for estradiol biosynthesis. As aromatase is the key hydroxylating enzyme that converts androstenedione into estrone and testosterone into estradiol, it is therefore considered as a crucial protein in the regulation of the sex hormones levels in various tissues including the brain (**Figure 3**).

A deregulation of the RORA gene was found in autism and it was linked to an increase in androgen biosynthesis and to the higher levels of androgens in the lymphoblastoid cells observed in autistic children. The abnormality in the RORA gene in autism includes reduced expression and increased methylation in lymphoblastoid cell lines and decreased expression of RORA gene in the brain of autistic children [52]. The reduction in the brain RORA gene in autistic children negatively impacts many physiological process regulated by the RORA gene, which includes differentiation of Purkinje cells [53], cerebral development [54, 55], neuronal protection against oxidative stress [56], suppression of inflammation [57], and regulation of circadian rhythm [58].

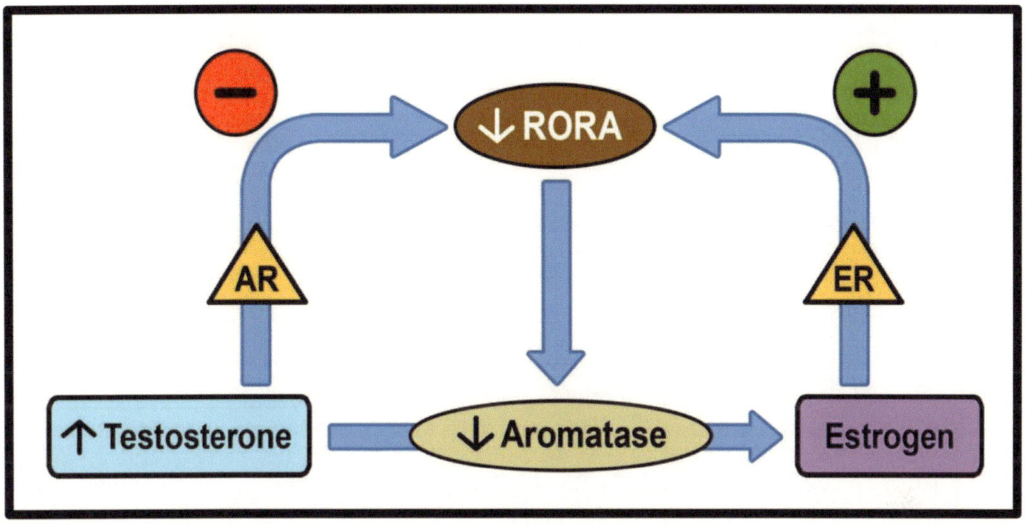

Figure 3. A model for the reciprocal hormonal effects on RORA gene [2].

The other aspect related to the abnormality in RORA gene in autism is its influence on the sex hormones level. Postmortem studies on autistic brains showed reduction in both RORA gene expression and aromatase in the frontal cortex and the cerebellum [52]. This reduction is exacerbated by negative feedback mechanisms as a result of decreased aromatase level with the subsequent accumulation of its substrate testosterone and reduced production of its product estradiol. The end result is a vicious cycle of increased testosterone and reduced estradiol [2]. This deregulation of the RORA gene in autism and its subsequent influence on the brain and the sex hormone levels in autistic children could provide a molecular explanation for the observed hyperandrogenism in children with autism.

12. Conclusion

In conclusion, autism has a striking male to female ratio, which acts as a code for autism etiology. Uncoding the sex bias in autism would aid dramatically in understanding the underlying mechanisms. Subsequently, early screening, treatment, and prevention measures could be conducted. Furthermore, sex-linked genetic and hormonal factors have been hypothesized in autism, and some evidences have been found. However, further direct investigations should be carried on.

Author details

Felwah S. Al-Zaid

Address all correspondence to: D_fl329@hotmail.com; f.al-zaid14@imperial.ac.uk

1 Department of Physiology, College of Medicine, King Saud University, Riyadh, KSA

2 Division of Brain Sciences, Department of Medicine, Imperial College London, UK

References

[1] Levy S, Mandell D, Schultz R. Autism. *Lancet*. 2009; 374:1627–38.

[2] Sarachana T, Xu M, Wu RC, Hu VW. Sex hormones in autism: Androgens and estrogens differentially and reciprocally regulate RORA, a novel candidate gene for autism. *PLoS One*. 2011; 6(2): 17116.

[3] Giedd GN. Quantitative MRI of the temporal lobe, amygdala, and hippocampus in normal human development: Ages 4–18 years. *J Comp Neurol*. 1996 Mar 4;366(2):223–30.

[4] Allen JS, Damasio H, Grabowski TJ, Bruss J, Zhang W. Sexual dimorphism and asymmetries in the gray-white composition of the human cerebrum. *Neuroimage*. 2003 Apr;18(4):880–94.

[5] Ringo JL, Doty RW, Demeter S, Simard PY. A proof of the need for a spatial clustering of interneuronal connections to enhance cortical computation. *Cereb Cortex*. 1994; 4: 331.

[6] Jancke L, Staiger JF, Schlaug G, Huang Y, Steinmetz H. The relationship between corpus callosum size and forebrain volume. *Cereb Cortex*, 1997 Jan–Feb;7(1):48–56.

[7] Pakkenberg B and Gunderson HJ. Neocortical neuron number in humans: Effect of sex and age. *J Comp Neurol*. 1997 Jul 28; 384(2):312–20.

[8] Rabinowicz MD et al. Structure of the cerebral cortex in men and women. *J Neuropathol Exp Neurol*. 2002; 61: 46.

[9] Witelson SF, Glazer II, Kigar DL. Women have greater density of neurons in posterior temporal cortex. *J Neurosci*; 1995 May;15(5 Pt 1):3418–28.

[10] Shaywitz et al. Sex differences in the functional organization of the brain for language. *Nature*. 1995; 373: 607.

[11] Schulkin J. Autism and the amygdale: An endocrine hypothesis. *Brain Cogn*, 2007; 65: 99.

[12] Baxter LC et al. Sex differences in semantic language processing: A functional MRI study. *Brain Lang*; 2003 Feb;84(2):264–72.

[13] Breedlove SM, Hampson E. Sexual differentiation of the brain and behavior. *Behav Endocrinol*; 2nd edition. 2002. Cambridge, MA: Massachusetts Institute of Technology Press. pp. 30–74.

[14] Cohen-Bendahan, C. C., et al. (Prenatal sex hormone effects on child and adult sex-typed behavior: Methods and findings. *Neurosci Biobehav Rev*. 2005; 29(2): 353–84.

[15] MacLusky NJ, Bowlby DA, Brown TJ, Peterson RE, Hochberg RB. Sex and the developing brain: Suppression of neuronal estrogen sensitivity by developmental androgen exposure. *Neurochem Res*. 1997;22:1395–414.

[16] Alexander GM. Postnatal testosterone concentrations and male social development. *Front Endocrinol*. 2014;5:15.

[17] Baron-Cohen S, Knickmeyer R, Belmonte M. Sex differences in the brain: Implications for explaining autism. *Science*. 2005; 310: 819–22.

[18] Jordan C, Doncarlos L. Androgen in health and disease: An overview. *Horm Behav*. 2008; 53(5): 589–95.

[19] Baulieu E. Neurosteroides: A novel function of the brain. *Psychoneuroendocrinology*. 1998; 23: 963–87.

[20] Irwin RP, Margakis NJ, Rogawski MA et al. Pregnenolone sulfate augment NMDA receptor mediated increase in intracellular Ca^{2+} in cultured rat hippocampal neurons. *Neurosci Lett*. 1992; 141: 30–4.

[21] Blauer KL, Poth M, Rogers WM. Dehydroepiandrosterone antagonizes the suppressive effects of dexamethasone on lymphocyte proliferation. *Endocrinology*. 1991; 129: 3174–9.

[22] Mao X and Barger S. Neuroprotection by dehydroepinadrosterone-sulfate: Role of NFkappaB-like factor. *Neuroreport*. 1998; 9: 759–63.

[23] Chakrabarti, S & Fombonne E. Pervasive developmental disorders in preschool children: Confirmation of high prevalence. *Am J Psychiatry*. 2005; 162: 1113–41.

[24] Baron-Cohen S. Trends cognition. The extreme male brain theory of autism. *Trends Cogn Sci*. 2002 Jun 1; 6(6):248–54.

[25] Skuse, D. H. (2000). Imprinting, the X-chromosome, and the male brain: Explaining sex differences in the liability to autism. *Pediatr Res*. 47(1):9–16.

[26] Schulkin J. Autism and the amygdale: An endocrine hypothesis. *Brain Cogn*. 2007; 65: 99.

[27] Knickmeyer R, Baron-Cohen S, Fane B, Wheelwright S, Mathews G, Conway G. Androgens and autistic traits: A study of individuals with congenital adrenal hyperplasia. *Horm Behav*. 2006; 50(1): 148–53.

[28] Baron-Cohen S, Auyeung B, Nørgaard-Pedersen B, Hougaard D M, Abdallah MW, Melgaard L, Cohen AS, Chakrabarti B, Ruta L and Lombardo MV. Elevated fetal steroidogenic activity in autism. *Mol Psychiatry*. 2015; 20, 369–76.

[29] Szatmari, P, MacLean, JE, Jones, MB, Bryson, SE, Zwaigenbaum, L, Bartolucci, G, Mahoney, WJ and Tuff, L. The familial aggregation of the lesser variant in biological and nonbiological relatives of PDD probands: A family history study. *J Child Psychol Psychiatry*. 2000; 41: 579–86.

[30] Bailey, A, et al. Autism as a strongly genetic disorder: Evidence from a British twin study. *Psychol Med.* 1995; 25(1): 63–77.

[31] Lobo, I. Genomic imprinting and patterns of disease inheritance. *Nat Educ.* 2008; 1(1):66.

[32] Davies W, Isles AR, Wilkinson LS. Imprinted gene expression in the brain. *Neurosci Biobehav Rev.* 2005; 29:421–430.8.

[33] Isles AR, Wilkinson LS. Imprinted genes, cognition and behaviour. *Trends Cogn Sci.* 2000; 4:309–18.

[34] Geier DA, Geier MR. A prospective assessment of androgen levels in patients with autistic spectrum disorders: Biochemical underpinnings and suggested therapies. *Neuro Endocrinol Lett.* 2007; 28(5): 565–73.

[35] Al-Zaid FS, Alhader AA and Al-Ayadhi L . Altered Ghrelin levels in boys with autism: A novel finding associated with hormonal dysregulation. *Sci Rep.* 2014; 4, 6478.

[36] Tordjman S, Anderson GM, McBride PA, Hertzig ME, Snow ME, Hall LM, Ferrari P, Cohen DJ. Plasma androgen in autism. *J Aut Dev Disord.* 1995 Jun; 25(3): 296–304.

[37] Lutchmaya S, Baron-Cohen S, Raggat P, Kmickmeyer R, Manning J. 2nd to 4th digit ratios, foetal testosterone and estradiol. *Early Hum Dev.* 2004; 77(1–2): 23–8.

[38] Croonenberghs J, Van Grieken S, Wauters A, Van West D, Brouw L, Maes M, Deboutte D. Serum testosterone concentration in male autistic youngsters. *Neuro Endocrinol Lett.* 2010;31(4):483-8.

[39] Pennebaker J, Groom C, Loew D. Testosterone as a social inhibitor: Two case studies of the effect of testosterone treatment on language. *J Abnorm Psychol.* 2004; 113(1): 172–5.

[40] Brodkin ES. BALB/c mice: Low sociability and other phenotypes that may be relevant to autism. *Behav Brain Res,* 2007; 176(1): 53–65.

[41] Manning JT, Baron-Cohen S, Wheelwright S, Sanders G. The 2nd to 4th digit ratio and autism. *Dev Med Child Neurol.* 2001; 43: 160–4.

[42] Schmidtova E, Kelemenova S, Cele P, Ficek A, Osttnikova D. Polymosrphisms in genes involved in testosterone metabolism in Slovak autistic boys. *Endocrinologist.* 2010; 20(5): 245–9.

[43] Al-Zaid F S, Alhader A A and Al-Ayadhi L Y. The second to fourth digit ratio (2D:4D) in Saudi boys with autism: A potential screening tool. *Early Human Develop.* 2015; 91(7):413–41.

[44] Noipayak P. The ratio of 2nd and 4th digit length in autistic children. *J Med Assoc Thai.* 2009; 92(8):1040–5.

[45] Krajmer P, Spajdel M, Kubranska A, Ostatnikova D. 2D:4D finger ratio in Slovak autism spectrum population. *Bratisl Lek Listy.* 2011; 112(7): 377–9.

[46] Honekopp, J Bartholdt L, Beier L, Liebert A. Second to fourth digit length ratio (2D:4D) and adult sex hormone levels: New data and a meta-analytic review. *Psychoneuroendocrinology*. 2007; 32(4): 313–21.

[47] Breedlove SM. Minireview: Organizational hypothesis: Instances of the fingerpost. *Endocrinology*. 2010;151(9):4116–22.

[48] Manning JT, Scutt D, Wilson J, Lewis-Jones DI. The ratio of 2nd to 4th digit length: A predictor of sperm numbers and concentrations of testosterone, luteinizing hormone and oestrogen. *Human Reprod*. 1998. 13: 3000–4.

[49] James WH. Evidence that mammalian sex ratios at birth are partially controlled by parental hormone levels around the time of conception. *J Endocrinol*. 2008; 198: 3–15.

[50] Mouridsen S, Rich B, Isager T. Sibling sex ratio of individuals diagnosed with autism spectrum disorder as children. *Dev Med Child Neurol*. 2010; 52(3): 289.

[51] Cheslack-Postava K, Susser E, Liu K, Bearman PS. Can sibling sex ratios be used as a valid test for the prenatal androgen hypothesis of autism spectrum disorders? *PLoS One*. 2015; 10(10): e0141338. doi:10.1371/journal.pone.0141338.

[52] Nguyen A, Rauch TA, Pfeifer GP, Hu VW. Global methylation profiling of lymphoblastoid cell lines reveals epigenetic contributions to autism spectrum disorders and a novel autism candidate gene, *RORA*, whose protein product is reduced in autistic brain. *FASEB J*. 2010;24(8):3036–51.

[53] Hadj-Sahraoui N, Frederic F, Zanjani H, Delhaye-Bouchaud N, Herrup K, et al. Progressive atrophy of cerebellar Purkinje cell dendrites during aging of the heterozygous staggerer mouse (Rora+/sg). *Dev Brain Res*. 2001; 126(2): 201–9.

[54] Gold DA, Gent PM, Hamilton BA. RORa in genetic control of cerebellum development: 50 staggering years. *Brain Res*. 2007; 1140(1): 19–25.

[55] Harding HP, Atkins GB, Jaffe AB, Seo WJ, Lazar MA. Transcriptional activation and repression by RORa, an orphan nuclear receptor required for cerebellar development. *Mol Endocrinol*, 1997; 11(11): 1737–46.

[56] Boukhtouche F, Vodjdani G, Jarvis CI, Bakouche J, Staels B. Human retinoic acid receptor-related orphan receptor a1 overexpression protects neurones against oxidative stress-induced apoptosis. *J Neurochem*. 2006; 96(6): 1778–89.

[57] Delerive P, Monte D, Dubois G, Trottein F, Fruchart-Najib J. The orphan nuclear receptor RORa is a negative regulator of the inflammatory response. *EMBO Rep*. 2001; 2(1): 42–8.

[58] Sato, T., Fukue, Y., Teranishi, H., Yoshida, Y., Kojima, M. Molecular forms of hypothalamic ghrelin and its regulation by fasting and 2-deoxy-d-glucose administration. *Endocrinology*. 2005; 146:2510–6.

Chapter 4

Distribution of Month of Birth of Individuals with Autism Spectrum Disorder Differs from the General Population in the Netherlands

Anna Cieslinska, Jannicke Simmelink,
Gosia Teodorowicz, Hans Verhoef, Hilde Tobi and
Huub F. Savelkoul

Additional information is available at the end of the chapter

http://dx.doi.org/10.5772/67205

Abstract

The prevalence of autism spectrum disorders (ASDs) is causally dependent on genetic and environmental influences. We investigated whether autism spectrum disorders are associated with month of birth compared to the general population using a retrospective study, comparing ASD cases ($n = 3478$) with the general population ($n = 2{,}716{,}876$) born between 1995 and 2008. Associations were examined using χ^2 tests and Walter and Elwood's seasonality χ^2 tests for the total ASD group, and separately for autistic disorder and Asperger syndrome. For the total ASD group, the distribution of month of birth was different compared to the general population ($p < 0.0001$), with July as the highest contributor, and a season-of-birth effect was found for this group ($p = 0.02$). For the autistic disorder group, the months of birth distribution were different ($p = 0.01$), with July as the highest contributor. No season-of-birth effect over the year was found ($p = 0.09$). No association was found for the months of birth of individuals with Asperger syndrome ($p = 0.06$), with no seasonal trend over the year ($p = 0.60$). In conclusion, a drop in sun exposure during the first trimester of pregnancy might explain the peak in July births and the associated risk for ASD development.

Keywords: autism spectrum disorder, month of birth, seasonality, periodicity, sunlight exposure

INTECH
open science | open minds

1. Introduction

The study of associations between season of birth or conception and the occurrence of neurodevelopmental disorders such as autism can provide important clues about causes of such a disease with unknown etiology. Such associations would then suggest periodicity of an environmental etiologic agent acting during the prenatal, perinatal, or early postnatal phase of development. One such environmental factor with seasonal recurrence originally suspected to increase the risk for the development of autism was a viral infection, for example, rubella [1]. Other potentially relevant factors that frequently vary by season include variations in nutrient intake by (pregnant) mother and deficiencies in nutritional factors such as vitamin D [2], maternal allergies during pregnancies [3], and exposure to pesticides (organophosphates and organochlorines) [4]. Previous studies have shown variable conclusions as to a specific month of birth that contributed to an enhanced risk of development of symptoms of autism within the first few years of life [5–12]. However, not all studies have found an association between month or season of birth and autism [13–15]. These apparent discrepancies might be based on methodological differences among the studies reviewed, including the use of diverse diagnostic criteria, and the statistical analysis employed.

Although genetic factors are strongly suspected to be a cause of autism spectrum disorders (ASDs), concordance in monozygotic twins is 40–90% and the phenotypic expression of the disorder varies widely, even within monozygotic twins [16, 17]. Thus, environmental factors also seem to play an important causal role. The number of people with ASD in the Netherlands increased to 190,000 in 2009 from 90,000 in 2001 [18]. Although there are many possible explanations, including more frequent diagnosis and reporting [19], this increase strikingly coincided with the medical advice to avoid sun exposure [20, 21]. This advice has probably lowered vitamin D activation in the skin resulting in lower levels of activated vitamin D (calcitriol, a fat-soluble steroid hormone) in developing brain of the fetus. These findings are particularly relevant in view of emerging evidence suggestive of a role for vitamin D in neuropsychological functioning, including a range of diseases from autism to Alzheimer's [22]. A study in which the prevalence of ASD was correlated to the season birth showed a variation that was linked to latitude of the home region [19]. This would be consistent with maternal vitamin D deficiency being a risk factor for development of autism, possibly by affecting fetal brain development as well as possibly by affecting maternal immune system status during pregnancy [19]. A study from Lee et al. aimed to determine whether the birth date distribution for individuals with autism spectrum disorders (ASD), including singletons and multiple births, differed from the general population. The presence of seasonal trends in ASD singletons and concordant multiple births suggests a role for non-heritable factors operating during the pre- or perinatal period, even among cases with a genetic susceptibility [17]. Although several studies have been conducted on this topic [11, 12], it is potentially of great public health importance in view of the burden of ASD, which in European countries and the USA affects 60–100 per 10,000 children [18, 20, 23, 24].

The current study aimed to test our hypothesis that month of birth and ASD are associated. This hypothesis was investigated separately for people with autistic disorder and Asperger syndrome. We also explored the association between the sun exposure during pregnancy and ASD.

2. Subjects and methods

2.1. Design and data acquisition

We compared cases with autism spectrum disorders with controls without such disorders regarding their date of birth. In this retrospective study, ASD cases were extracted from a registry held by Netherlands Society for Autism Spectrum Disorders (Dutch acronym: NVA), an interest group of people with autism and their relatives [25]. Approval to use from their database anonymous data on month of birth and type of autism according to DSM IV criteria was obtained from the chairman, F. Stekelenburg. As one of its activities, it distributes since 2007 a personalized pass that Dutch citizens with an ASD can use to avoid difficult situations, such as police arrest, queues at public facilities, or events. Such passes are issued only when the application form is accompanied by an affidavit, signed by a psychiatrist, psychologist, educationist, or a representative of an institution for ASD diagnosis to certify that the holder has an autistic disorder, Asperger syndrome, pervasive developmental disorder-not otherwise specified (PDD-NOS) as categorized by the DSM IV criteria that were valid at the time of diagnosis. Other diagnoses, including multiple complex developmental disorder (McDD)/ Rett syndrome, were not considered because the number of cases was too low for meaningful analysis. Based on the permission we obtained, we extracted information on date of birth, gender, autism diagnosis but no other personal information from persons in this registry who were born in the period 1995–2008. This period contained the largest number of patient entries with at least 150 per year, and for whom full information on all items was available. As controls, we used the general population of people born in the Netherlands in the same period, for whom the distribution of date of birth is publicly available in aggregated form from the Dutch Central Bureau of Statistics (Statistics Netherlands, http://www.cbs.nl/en-GB/) [26].

Data on the cumulative number of sun hours per month, averaged over the Netherlands for the period 1998 until 2008, were obtained from the Royal Netherlands Meteorological Institute [27]. These data were used to approximate the number of hours of sun during pregnancy for each trimester.

2.2. Statistical analysis

Data were analyzed using MS Excel and STATA version 10.1 (StataCorp, College Station, Texas, USA). Group differences were assessed by Pearson's χ^2 test, which evaluates a null hypothesis that the frequency distribution of the binary variable indicating cases and controls is equally distributed over the months of the year. This test treats all response variables as nominal, that is, it does not take the ordering of the months into account and makes no assumptions about seasonal variation. An alternative method of data analysis is to test birth data against a sinusoidal function. Thus, in addition, we used Walter and Elwood's seasonality test [28, 29], which evaluates the adequacy of a sinusoidal curve over time, with one maximum and one minimum for the frequency of births per year, using a goodness-of-fit χ^2 statistic. Compared to the Pearson's χ^2 test, the Walter and Elwood's seasonality test has greater power for detecting seasonal trends that follow a sinusoidal pattern, but it has the limitation that it may have limited power for seasonal trends that follow a non-sinusoidal pattern [30].

We then explored what time period during pregnancy is critical for being associated with ASD. For each person, we calculated maternal sun exposure, expressed as the cumulative number of sun hours per month, during the first plus second pregnancy trimester, the second plus third trimester, and the total duration of pregnancy, under the presumption that all pregnancies were carried to term and lasted 9 months. Thus, it became possible to assess the association between ASD and maternal sun exposure during pregnancy. As an example of such a calculation of the average sun exposure in hours per month: when born in January, sun hours in the last 3 months were calculated as ((0.5*sun hours in January) + sun hours in December + sun hours in November + (0.5* sun hours in October)). This value divided by 3 is the mean sun exposure in hours per month for the last 3 months of pregnancy.

Goodness-of-fit χ^2 tests can be difficult to interpret because of the arbitrary designation of months to season and their lack of power relative to other statistical tests. Bolton et al. discuss these limitations and point out that any one method of data analysis will likely be insufficient if used alone [15].

3. Results

In this retrospective study, we compared month of birth between a convenience sample of individuals with ASD registered with the Netherlands Society for Autism Spectrum Disorders and born between and including 1995 and 2008 (n = 3478) and persons born in the Netherlands in the same period (n = 2,716,876). **Table 1** shows the total number of cases and controls, and the number of individuals for each ASD disorder, broken down by sex.

	Cases				Controls	
	Total	Male	Female	Unknown	Male	Female
ASD	3478	2895	554	29	1,392,415	1,324,461
Autistic disorder	911	775	131	5	NI	
Asperger syndrome	627	547	75	5	NI	
PDD-NOS	1718	1407	293	18	NI	
Other*	297	227	67	3	NI	

Total numbers of autism cases (3478) and control population (2,716,876) births in the period 1995–2008 in the Netherlands. Unknown: The gender of these individuals was not included in the forms, but these individuals are included in the analysis. ASD: Autism spectrum disorders; NI: Not indicated; PDD-NOS: Pervasive developmental disorder not otherwise specified.

*Not analyzed further.

Table 1. Number of ASD cases and controls from the general population, by disorder and sex.

3.1. ASD versus general population

The distribution of month of birth for individuals with ASD was different from that of the general population ($p < 0.0001$; χ^2-test), with the strongest divergence occurring in the period July–September (**Figure 1**). The month of birth distribution for the total group of individuals with ASD was associated with a sinusoidal curve, indicating the presence of a season-of-birth effect ($p = 0.02$; Walter and Elwood's χ^2-test).

3.2. Autism disorder versus general population

The distribution of month of birth for individuals with autistic disorder differed from that of the general Dutch population ($p = 0.01$; χ^2 test), with a peak in July (**Figure 2**). There seemed to be an excess of births in individuals with autistic disorder in the period from May to October, and a decline during November–April, with a nadir in February. However, there was no strong statistical support for sinusoidal trends over the year ($p = 0.09$; Walter and Elwood's χ^2).

3.3. Asperger syndrome versus general population

There was evidence, albeit limited, that the distribution of month of birth of individuals with Asperger was differently distributed than the distribution of the general population (**Figure 3**; $p = 0.06$; Pearson's χ^2 test). Births among individuals with Asperger syndrome seemed to peak in September and were relatively infrequent in June, while being approximately equally distributed over the remaining months of the year. In agreement with a visual inspection of the

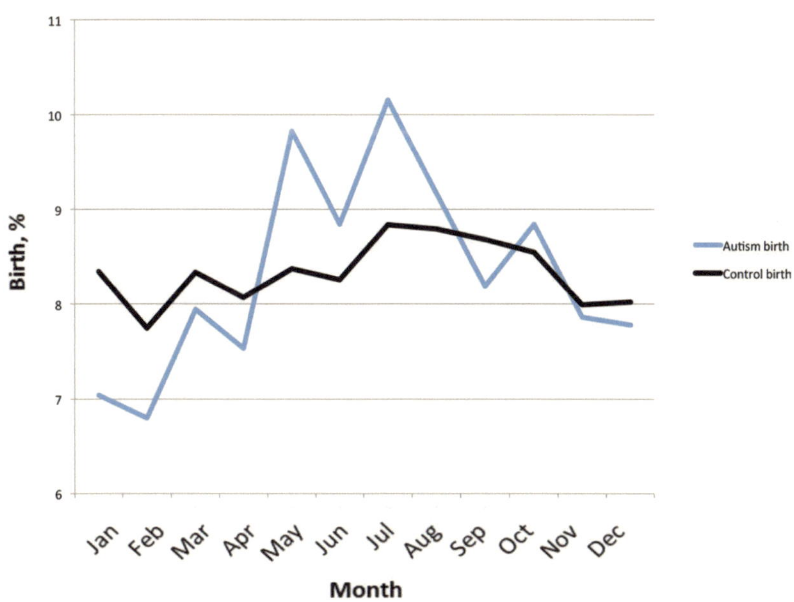

Figure 1. Relative distribution of births per month in ASD and the general population births born between 1995 and 2008. ASD birth reflect autism (blue line) and control birth reflect general population (black line).

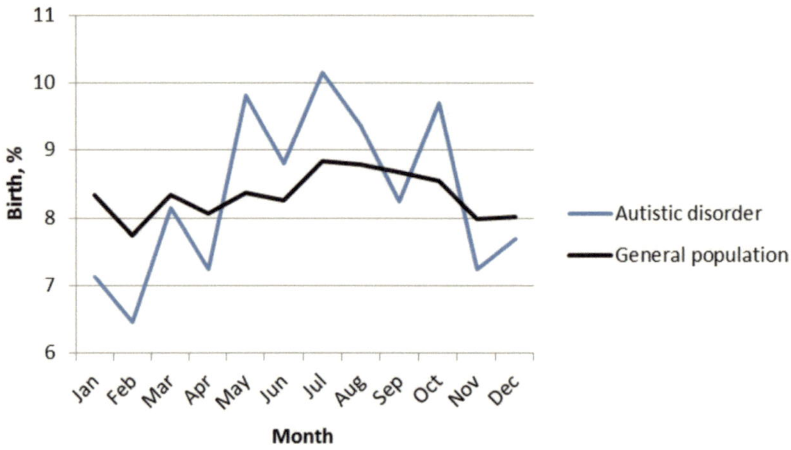

Figure 2. Relative distribution of births per month in autistic disorder and the general population births born between 1995 and 2008. Autistic disorder birth with blue line and general population with black line.

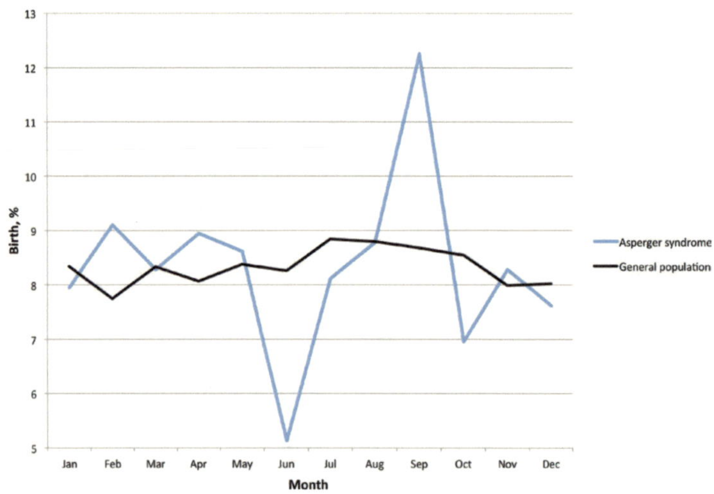

Figure 3. Relative distribution of births per month in Asperger and the general population births born between 1995 and 2008. Asperger syndrome birth with blue line and general population birth with black line.

data (**Figure 3**), there was no evidence that the birth distribution of the Asperger cases over the year was distributed as a sinusoid curve ($p = 0.60$; Walter and Elwood's χ^2).

3.4. Cumulative hours of sun in the Netherlands

Figure 4 shows the raw meteorological data of the mean number of hours of sun per month, averaged over the period 1998–2008 and averaged over the Netherlands. This number peaked in May and June and was lowest in November–January. From these data we calculated sun exposure, that is, the mean hours of sun during a period (trimester) in pregnancy (**Figure 5**).

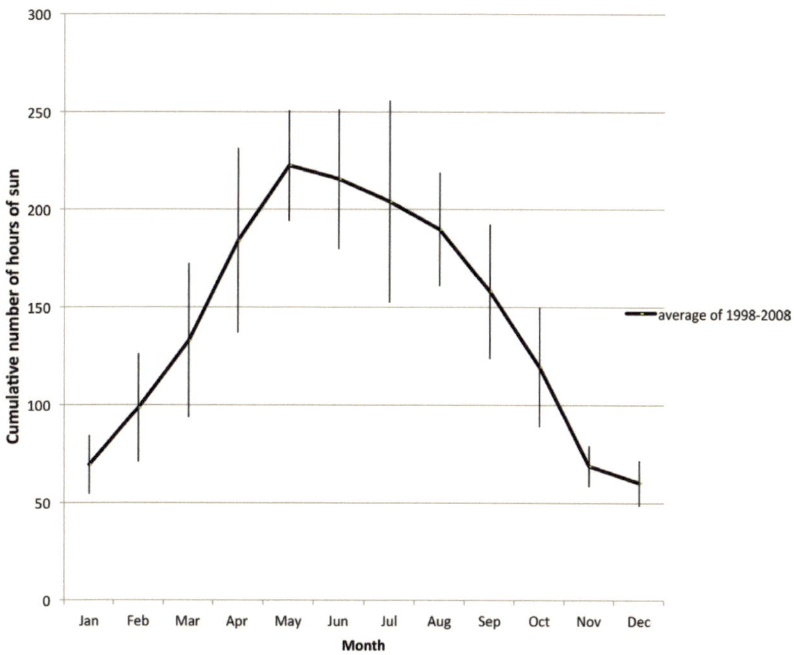

Figure 4. Mean monthly number of hours of sun (average ± 1SD) over the years 1998–2008, averaged over the Netherlands.

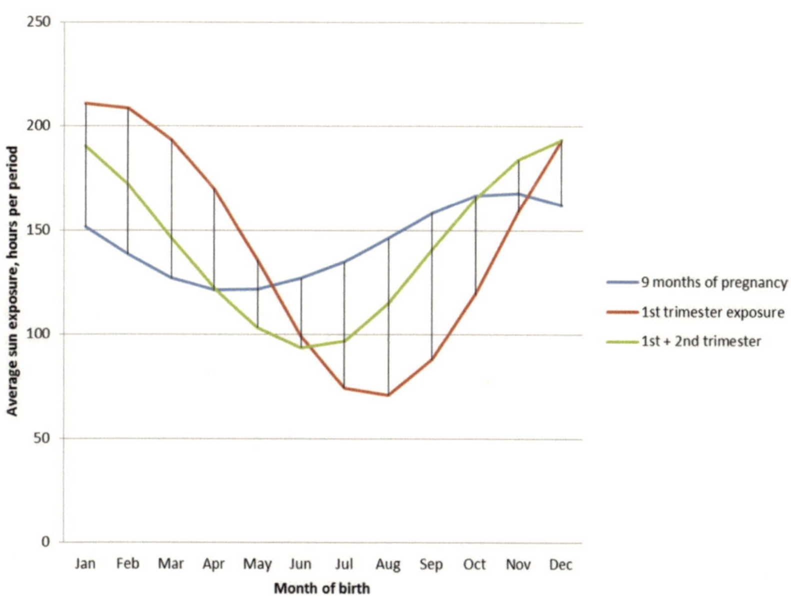

Figure 5. Trends of distribution of sun exposure during a given period in pregnancy, by month of birth. Data from the complete 9 months of pregnancy reflected in blue line, data from only the first trimester of pregnancy in red line, and data from first plus second trimester of pregnancy reflected with green line. For example, the mother of a person born in August had increasing exposure to sunlight in the first, second and third trimesters of the pregnancy that led to the birth of that person. Data from aggregated trimesters are effectively averaged estimates of individual trimesters.

Comparing these data to the complete 9 months pregnancy period, it became clear that the drop in sun exposure during the first trimester, more than the combination of first and second trimester, might explain the peak in July births of ASD. Such a relation was not observed when analyzing the second and third trimester or when combining the sun exposure of other combinations of trimesters (data not shown). These data support that sun exposure might be a risk factor for ASD.

4. Discussion

This retrospective study showed a difference in the distribution of months of birth for individuals with ASD compared to the general Dutch population, using a dataset several times larger than the largest autism study to date. For autistic disorder, an increased ASD births in July contributes to this difference. The birth data of ASD are distributed as a sinusoidal curve, implying seasonality over the year. This distribution of births per month for individuals with autistic disorder did differ from the distribution in the general Dutch population. In contrast, the distribution of births per month of individuals with Asperger was different from the general population and did not show a seasonal birth effect.

As the children included in this analysis were all diagnosed at the time when the DSM IV criteria were still valid and widely used we adopted this original classification [31]. The characteristic heterogeneity in disease expression was captured through the different categorical diagnoses, including autism, Asperger's syndrome, and pervasive developmental disorder not otherwise specified (PDD-NOS), as well as other regressive neurodevelopmental disorders of early childhood frequently associated with autistic symptoms (Rett's syndrome and childhood disintegrative disorder). With successive research the PDD-NOS group appeared increasingly doubtful, and all categories were eventually dropped in the current DSM V criteria [32]. Because of the large degree of heterogeneity also observed in our PDD-NOS group, we did not further analyze this group in the current study.

The ratio male versus female cases in this study was approximately 4:1, similar as that known in the general ASD population [17]. The χ^2 test with 11 df data for male and female ASD was not shown, but this test was significant for male ASD births, while not for female ASD births. This implies a difference in distribution of month of birth of male individuals with ASD compared to the general population. A study on singleton and multiple ASD births described birth peaks in April, July, and October for singleton ASD births [8]. Our study confirmed the birth peak in July for the ASD births, but not for October, while April showed the lowest number of ASD births in this study. Hebert et al. studied the association of ASD with season of birth in the UK and described an association between ASD and spring births, but the analysis was weak due to the small sample size (86 children with ASD) [9]. This study differs with our findings, as April had the smallest number of ASD births. The study of Hebert used a cohort that recruited pregnant women resident in Avon, UK, while we studied the total Dutch population of ASD. A Dutch study in 2000 compared mentally retarded autistic disorder patients and mentally retarded individuals with PDD-NOS, with each other and with birth data of the general Dutch national population [18]. No difference was observed in birth distribution of the patients with autistic disorder compared to the general Dutch population, contrary to our findings. This difference might be explained by the difference in case numbers, (540 vs. 911) and the variation in years of birth of the case between 1932 and 1992, while in our study the year of birth span was 14 years only.

An association was suggested based on the According to the Centers for Diseases Control and Prevention, February is the month with the highest percentage of influenza cases (nearly 50% of all cases). This research identifies environmental factors that are possibly relating to autistic disorder. Early life history reveals increased prevalence of viral insult and manifestation of neurological signs in the early development of the ASD children that also reach statistical significance. Several of these, stiffness upon delivery, generalized seizures and infantile spasms, and sleep disturbance might be further investigated as early risk signs.

Our study contained a large sample size (3478 ASD children) with a large number of cases and controls per month, strengthening our analysis. However, our test would even be more valid when instead of births in the general Dutch population, the date of birth of relatives of the case group (for example, siblings of the individuals with ASD) would be used as controls. This study included only Dutch ASD so confounding from inter-country-specific factors was not applicable for this study. In this study, there was no recall bias, because the date of birth is fixed information that does not interfere with the detection of ASD. Sun exposure was also not a confounding factor, as it has no influence on the date of birth. Interfering genetic factors cannot count for a 100% risk while environmental factors also contribute to the risk of developing ASD. This study is an initial step to generating hypotheses and data of cumulative hours of sun per month can be used for an explorative analysis to find an association. The distribution of month of birth within the ASD group showed that the birth in July coincided with almost the lowest sun exposure in the first trimester and first plus second trimester of pregnancy. This also counted for the peak in July births for autistic disorder. Comparing the distribution of month of birth for autistic disorder with the sun exposure, we observed a decrease in September with an associated highest sun exposure in the first and second trimester for the trimesters separately.

A previous study [11] showed that the birth date distribution for individuals with autism spectrum disorders (ASD), including singletons and multiple births, differed from the general population. The presence of seasonal trends in ASD singletons and concordant multiple births suggested a role for non-heritable factors operating during the pre- or perinatal period, even among cases with a genetic susceptibility [8]. When analyzing the variation in season of birth and the ASD prevalence a correlation was found with the effective latitude and this is consistent with maternal vitamin D being a risk factor for development of autistic disorder. Maternal vitamin D affects fetal brain development and the maternal immune system status during pregnancy [11]. Support for the maternal vitamin D deficiency theory has been reported based on rat studies, but specifically for multiple sclerosis and schizophrenia [19, 20]. However, rat study by Féron et al. showed that vitamin D deficiency reduces the expression of a number of genes involved in neuronal structure [21]. The fetus is during development entirely dependent on the mother for its supply of 25-hydroxyvitamin D(25(OH)D [25], which is a product of the vitamin D metabolism after the metabolizing step in the skin by exposure to ultraviolet light. From 4 weeks of gestation to birth, 25(OH)D diffuses across the placenta [26], of which 1,25(OH)2 vitamin D is produced by the fetal kidneys and the placenta [23, 27]. 1,25(OH)2D does not readily cross the placenta [27]. It is also known that cord blood 25(OH)D concentrations in infants, as in maternal blood, vary seasonally [28, 29]. The brain develops mostly in the later stages of pregnancy [22]. Maternal infectious diseases during pregnancy can be an indicator for a vitamin D deficiency, and thus maternal infectious diseases can adversely affect brain development [11]. Maternal serum level of 1,25-dihydroxyvitamin D more than doubles early in the first trimester in human pregnancy [23, 24], indicating a high need for vitamin D during pregnancy and supports that a low sun exposure is a risk factor for ASD.

In conclusion, a drop in sun exposure in the first trimester of pregnancy might explain the peak in July births with an associated risk for ASD development. As a result, a deficiency of vitamin D in the first trimester of pregnancy is a risk factor for ASD as vitamin D deficiency in the developing brain of a fetus may disturb the development of the brain and therefore causes functional defects [10, 19]. The action of UV rays in sunlight on the skin is the most powerful natural source of vitamin D generation, and factors that reduce the amount and intensity of sunlight significantly increase the risk of vitamin D deficiency [30]. These results support the need for future study of autistic birth dates with detailed pre- and perinatal information that may lead to discovering specific risk factors for autism in select groups.

Acknowledgements

This work was supported by a senior scientist WIAS Wageningen graduate school scholarship (AC). We thank Mr F. Stekelenburg as the former chairman of the Netherlands Association for Autism Spectrum Disorders (NVA; De Bilt, The Netherlands) for permission to use their database.

Author details

Anna Cieslinska[1,2], Jannicke Simmelink[1], Gosia Teodorowicz[1], Hans Verhoef[1,3], Hilde Tobi[4] and Huub F. Savelkoul[1]*

*Address all correspondence to: huub.savelkoul@wur.nl

1 Cell Biology and Immunology Group, Wageningen University, Wageningen, The Netherlands

2 Faculty of Biology and Biotechnology, University of Warmia and Mazury, Olsztyn, Poland

3 School of Hygiene and Tropical Medicine, MRC International Nutrition Group, London, UK

4 Education and Competence Studies Group, Wageningen University, Wageningen, The Netherlands

References

[1] Chess S. Autism in children with congenital rubella. J Autism Child Schizophr 1971;1:33–47.

[2] Cannell JJ. Autism and vitamin D. Med Hypotheses 2008;70:750–759.

[3] Croen LA, Grether JK, Yoshida CK, Odouli R, Van de Water J. Maternal autoimmune diseases, asthma and allergies, and childhood autism spectrum disorders: a case-control study. Arch Pediatr Adolesc Med 2005;159:151–157.

[4] Roberts EM, English PB, Grether JK, Windham GC, Somberg L, Wolff C. Maternal residence near agricultural pesticide applications and autism spectrum disorders among children in the California Central Valley. Environ Health Perspect 2007;115:1482–1489.

[5] Bartlik BD. Monthly variation in births of autistic children in North Carolina. J Am Med Womens Assoc 1981;36:363–368.

[6] Barak Y, Ring A, Sulkes J, Gabbay U, Elizur A. Season of birth and autistic disorder in Israel. Am J Psychiatry 1995;152:798–800.

[7] Gillberg C. Do children with autism have March birthdays? Acta Psychiatr Scand 1990;82:152–156.

[8] Mouridsen SE, Nielsen S, Rich B, Isager T. Season of birth in infantile autism and other types of childhood psychoses. Child Psychiatry Hum Dev 1994;25:31–43.

[9] Konstantareas MM, Hauser P, Lennox C, Homatidis S. Season of birth in infantile autism. Child Psychiatry Hum Dev 1986;17:53–65.

[10] Tanoue Y, Oda S, Asano F, Kawashima K. Epidemiology of infantile autism in southern Ibaraki, Japan: differences in prevalence in birth cohorts. J Autism Dev Disord 1988;18:155–166.

[11] Lee LC, Newschaffer CJ, Lessler JT, Lee BK, Shah R, Zimmerman AW. Variation in season of birth in singleton and multiple births concordant for autism spectrum disorders. Paediatr Perinat Epidemiol 2008;22:172–179.

[12] Hebert KJ, Miller LL, Joinson CJ. Association of autistic spectrum disorder with season of birth and conception in a UK cohort. Autism Res 2010;3:185–190.

[13] Kolevzon A, Weiser M, Gross R, et al. Effects of season of birth on autism spectrum disorders: fact or fiction? Am J Psychiatry 2006;163:1288–1290.

[14] Landau EC, Cicchetti DV, Klin A, Volkmar FR. Season of birth in autism: a fiction revisited. J Autism Dev Disord 1999;29:385–393.

[15] Bolton P, Pickles A, Harrington R, Macdonald H, Rutter M. Season of birth: issues, approaches and findings for autism. J Child Psychol Psychiatry 1992;33:509–530.

[16] Baird G, Simonoff E, Pickles A, Chandler S, Loucas T, Meldrum D, Charman T. Prevalence of disorders of the autism spectrum in a population cohort of children in South Thames: the Special Needs and Autism Project (SNAP). Lancet 2006;368:210–215.

[17] Muhle R, Trentacoste SV, Rapin I. The genetics of autism. Pediatrics 2004;113:e472–e486.

[18] Autism Spectrum Disorders: a lifetime of difference. The Hague: Health Council of the Netherlands. Nr. 2009/09; ISBN: 978-90-5549-760-7.

[19] Grant WB, Soles CM. Epidemiologic evidence supporting the role of maternal vitamin D deficiency as a risk factor for the development of infantile autism. Dermato-Endocrinology 2009;1(4):223–228.

[20] Fombonne E. Epidemiology of autistic disorder and other pervasive developmental disorders. J Clin Psychiatry 2005;66(suppl 10):3–8.

[21] Cannell JJ. Autism and vitamin D. Med Hypotheses 2008;70(4):750–759.

[22] Ross AC, Taylor CL, Yaktine AL, Del Valle HB, Eds. Dietary Reference Intakes Calcium and Vitamin D. Institute of Medicine, The national Academies Press, Washington DC, US; 2011, pp. 75–124.

[23] Fombonne E. Epidemiology of pervasive developmental disorders. Pediatr Res 2009; 65(6):591–598.

[24] https://www.cdc.gov/ncbddd/autism/documents/addm-fact-sheet---comp508.pdf

[25] http://www.autisme.nl/media/48545/engelse_vertaling.pdf

[26] van der Ven E, Termorshuizen F, Laan W, Breetvelt EJ, van Os J, Selten JP. An incidence study of diagnosed autism-spectrum disorders among immigrants to the Netherlands. Acta Psychiatr Scand. 2013;128(1):54–60.

[27] http://www.knmi.nl/nederland-nu/klimatologie/maand-en-seizoensoverzichten

[28] Walter SD, Eldwood JM. A test for seasonality of events with a variable population at risk. Br J Prev Soc Med 1975;29:18–21.

[29] Disanto G, Handel AE, Para AE, Ramagopalan SV, Handunnetthi L. Season of birth and anorexia nervosa. Br J Psychiatry 2011;198(5):404–405.

[30] Walter SD. Seasonality of mania: a reappraisal. Br J Psychiatry 1977;131(10):345–350.

[31] http://dsm.psychiatryonline.org/doi/pdf/10.1176/appi.books.9780890420249.dsm-iv-tr

[32] http://dsm.psychiatryonline.org/doi/book/10.1176/appi.books.9780890425596

Chapter 5

Migration and Autism Diagnosis

Daina Crafa

Additional information is available at the end of the chapter

http://dx.doi.org/10.5772/65981

Abstract

Clinicians in many countries are increasingly working with children from migrant families. Although autism is diagnosed at an approximately equal rate in children in developed countries internationally (estimated 1% of the population), many studies report that children in migrant communities are at relatively higher risk for autism. Risk factors as well as symptom rates appear to vary across cultures. This chapter reviews the current state of the science and outlines conceptual considerations for clinicians assessing foreign, migrant, and minority children for diagnosis of autism. Possible reasons for higher rates among migrant children are discussed and suggestions for clinical evaluation are made.

Keywords: autism, migration, rates, risk factors, diagnosis, clinical assessment, culture, cross-cultural, heterogeneity, maternal migration, epigenetics, gene-environment interaction, symptom distribution, clinical measurements

1. Culture hidden in plain sight

For many people, the word *autism* evokes images of Claire Danes or Dustin Hoffman portraying highly gifted, albeit socially affected, individuals. In reality autism spectrum disorder can be severely disabling, and are considered among the most common childhood psychiatric disorders affecting millions of children internationally each year [1]. They are a spectrum frequently marked by social impairment. Perhaps because of this characterization, the influences of the social world are not always included in discussions of autism diagnosis, although they may play a crucial role for determining whether a child is on the autism spectrum. Migration and cultural influences on social behavior in particular appear to impact autism diagnosis in critical ways, and may increase risk for developing autism as well as the potential for misdiagnosis. Moreover, children do not need to have migrated themselves to be affected, and can therefore be difficult to identify. This chapter will discuss the population and risk factors in detail and issue considerations and precautions for diagnosis.

2. Who is at risk?

Global migration rates have hit an all-time high within the current decade according to estimates made by the United Nations [2–4]. In several Middle Eastern countries, including the U.A.E. and Qatar, and Kuwait, more than 70% of residents are migrants. Among English-speaking countries, Canada and Australia have the highest percentages of foreign-born residents by population at more than 20% [5, 6]. Global rates of autism in migrants are not well documented. However, increasing migration rates may leave clinicians in many countries working with increasing numbers of children from migrant families.

Although autism spectrum disorder is diagnosed at an approximately equal rate in children internationally, numerous studies report that children of migrant communities are diagnosed with autism at higher rates than nonmigrant children [7]. Arguably the most famous and still-cited of these studies involved epidemiological surveys conducted by Christopher Gillberg's research group at the University of Göteborg in Sweden, each of which found higher rates of autism in migrant children [8–10]. The earliest of these studies identified higher rates of autism in urban children whose parents were born in "exotic" countries compared to children with parents born in Sweden. A population survey that examined cases specifically of autistic disorder that emerged across a decade of births also reported higher rates in migrant children. Likewise, their third study identified higher rates specifically in children who were born in Sweden to Ugandan parents. This study of Ugandan-Swedish children arguably contributed to a new research trend: studying autism rates in children born locally whose parents (usually mothers) had migrated.

A series of studies performed in the U.K., which also emerged around the same time as the publications by Gillberg's group, provided supporting evidence for the emerging theory that autism was higher in children born to migrant families whether or not the children were born locally [11, 12]. The study by Goodman and Richards specifically found that first- and second-generation African-Caribbean children were diagnosed with autism at disproportionately higher rates [11], while Wing found higher rates of autism when the father's country of origin was outside the U.K. [12]. A study from Japan reported that migrants from one region of the country who moved to another region of the country also showed higher rates of autism, even though they had not crossed national boarders [13].

The migration theory of autism that emerged from these studies was initially crude—some authors proposed that genetic disorders or viral infections had been brought from the parent's homeland. One author famously later argued that no reasonable biological reason that autism would emerge after migration has been given [14]. The bulk of the findings supporting the migration theory of autism are from studies that are now decades old, and recent literature has suggested that the story may be more complicated. A few studies published within recent memory found no evidence that the child's immigration status played a role in rates of diagnosis [15].

Although a dearth of literature provides contemporary evidence for the migration theory of autism, a number of recent studies from around the world continue to report higher rates in locally born children whose parents have migrated [16–23]. The vast majority of these studies have relied on national medical registries in countries such as Sweden or the Netherlands that record autism incidents along with family history, while several studies have additionally relied on census or survey reports.

Crafa and Warfa [24] compared autism rates of children born after their mothers migrated into predominantly Caucasian countries, and reported autism rates that were much higher than average compared to children whose parents were born locally. This review article examined population-wide rates in an effort to control for sample heterogeneity reported in by other similar articles.

One study considered whether maternal versus paternal migration status mattered, and only maternal status emerged as statistically significant [19].

Some of these studies have additionally provided possible biological explanations that are arguably well reasoned. Perhaps the most convincing reason is that stress caused by act of migration itself could increase autism risk by producing epigenetic changes in mothers who give birth after migrating to a new country or location, which echoes the state-of-the-art among the neurosciences as well [24]. This biological explanation will be detailed in the next section.

There are, of course, several contentions and caveats surrounding the maternal migration theory of autism. Different rates of autism appear to be prevalent in niche groups within a country. For example, Somali refugees in the U.S. state of Minnesota comprise a small community of refugees whose children have alarmingly high rates of autism (an estimated 1:28 children compared to the 1:68 estimated global average [25, 26]).

Something known as the Latina paradox defines one of the main ostensible challengers to the maternal migration theory of autism. Although most of the literature shows higher rates of autism in children with even one parent who migrated before their birth, several studies in the U.S. report lower rates of autism in children born in the U.S. with Hispanic parents who have migrated from Mexico [27, 28]. One review of maternal migration prior to birth likewise reported that children of all races and ethnicities who were born after maternal migration (including non-Hispanic Caucasian children) were more likely to have autism compared to children of their same race with locally born mothers, except for Hispanic children who were significantly *less* likely to have autism compared with their ethnic counterparts [24]. These findings suggest that there may be social or biological explanations, which will be explored in the next sections.

Few other research findings contradict the maternal migration theory of autism. One meta-analysis (commonly cited as potentially refuting the maternal theory of autism) reports that pregnancy complications increase risk of autism. This study reports specifically that "the elevated risk of autism among the offspring of women born abroad was just shy of statistical significance" [29]. However, it does not consider the role of ethnicity and includes some of the Hispanic studies mentioned above in its calculations. Although institutional racism and other obstacles to care could explain different diagnosis rates of certain minority communities, multiple epidemiological studies have reported that race does not appear to be a risk factor for autism among children from local families [29, 30].

3. Biological theories of autism and migration

The biological relationship between autism and migration is currently somewhat of a mystery, and only a few contemporary theories have been proposed. Each of the proposed theories rely on the concept of a gene-environment interaction, which is exactly as it sounds—environmental factors interact with the genes of a fetus, child, or mother in some way that influences whether the autistic symptoms are expressed. Current theories disagree about the mechanisms of these interactions.

The example of HOXA-1 and rubella. Perhaps among the most famous recent attempts to explain the biological effects of maternal migration was made by Dyches et al. [31]. Echoing the earliest studies of migration and autism, which suggested that viral infections like rubella coming from the mother's home country could potentially increase autism risk [8–10], Dyches and her colleagues proposed that an interaction between viral infections and genetic susceptibility could potentially increase autism risk. They proposed as an example that an interaction between rubella and the widely studied HOXA1 gene may potentially explain higher autism rates in children born after their mothers' migrations. At the time the HOXA1 gene was considered a key potential candidate for causing autism, although continued study has failed to support a strong link to the disorder [32–34]. HOXA1 plays a role in early neural development and an allele variant on this gene was believed to be a possible precursor to autism. Dyches et al. proposed that having a genetic precursor, like a HOXA1 allele variant, alongside an environmental trigger might cause these mothers to have autistic children. They offer intrauterine rubella as an example of one potential environmental trigger that could affect children of migrant mothers [31]. Intrauterine rubella is believed to cause autism after an epidemic outbreak in the 1960s in the U.S. [31, 35]. Dyches et al. suggested that mothers might be at risk for having an autistic child if the HOXA1 variant is present and they are coming from countries where rubella is present or receive the vaccine for rubella during early pregnancy [31].

The scientific knowledge of autism has grown exponentially since the publication of their article in 2004. The take-away messages from their article withstand modern advancements. However, their example of HOXA1 and rubella no longer reflects the state of the art.

Although many promising studies of HOXA1 emerged from early studies, it appears to be rare and not the penultimate explanation initially thought [32, 36, 37]. While intrauterine rubella does affect central nervous system development and has been linked to autism [36, 38], there is no scientific evidence that rubella vaccines cause autism [39, 40]. Data reporting a link between vaccines and autism were determined to be falsified in 2011 [41].

Dyches et al. appear to have been onto something when they suggested that intrauterine changes caused by a gene-environment interaction could explain the emergence of autism after maternal migration. Although this was not their main point, findings over the past decade have accumulated demonstrating that poor intrauterine and pregnancy conditions increase the risk for autism.

The epigenetics of pregnancy and migration. Neuroscientist Daina Crafa and colleagues proposed that poor intrauterine and pregnancy conditions could be brought about by stressors related to migration [24]. They proposed that epigenetic processes explain the relationship between these changes. *Epigenetic processes* refer to biological regulation of genes—while the genes a person has are fixed across their lifespan, epigenetic processes determine whether the properties of genes are expressed by turning them "on" and "off." Gene expression may change across a person's lifespan, and methylation is a primary mechanism of epigenetic changes to gene expression. Numerous studies have linked physiological stress with higher methylation during maternal imprinting (i.e., when genes are transferred from mother to fetus), poor intrauterine and pregnancy conditions, and autism [18, 21, 22, 29, 42–52].

Crafa and Warfa argue that circumstances surrounding the act of migration often produce substantial stress that could theoretically induce these epigenetic changes [24, 53]. Stressors potentially occur before or after migration, and may be quite varied. These could include war or trauma in the mother's home country or discrimination or acculturative stressors.

Their theory claims to account for the Latina paradox [24, 53]. Hispanic women included in several U.S. studies were significantly less likely to experience certain poor pregnancy or birth conditions compared with other ethnic groups, and this literature is where the term *Latina paradox* was originally born [54–56]. Some researchers have suggested that having a positive social network after migration could lower stress and therefore stress-related consequences, including autism [57–59]. Like the previous theory described in this section, it is based on careful literature review and has not been experimentally tested.

The possible role of vitamin D. Vitamin D (25-hydroxyvitamin D) is linked to cellular function and has frequently been investigated as a possible determinant for autism. Numerous studies have demonstrated that low vitamin D levels in a mother during pregnancy or her offspring during early childhood may predict autism risk; however, it is generally agreed that further research is necessary [60–63]. Several researchers studying maternal migration have hypothesized that mothers migrating from certain regions may carry lower levels of vitamin D and have higher rates of children with autism. While some studies have reported promising results, no study has yet demonstrated a link between vitamin D, maternal migration, and autism. Fernell et al. found that Somali mothers had lower levels of vitamin D compared with Swedish mothers whether or not they had an autistic child. They reported nonsignificant findings that Somali mothers with autistic children appear to have the lowest levels of vitamin D [64]. In a review of autism rates in the U.S., Dealberto reported higher rates of autism in "black" participants living in the U.S. as well as those who had migrated from Africa or the Caribbean, and hypothesized that this could be due to vitamin D levels, though the hypothesis was not directly tested [65].

4. Cultural considerations for correct diagnosis

The clinical science surrounding autism and migration is still in its infancy. However, one message is becoming clear: children from diverse backgrounds are at greater risk for misdiagnosis. This section will review the current knowledge.

Although characterized by social impairments, autism spectrum disorder is robustly intertwined with the social world. The social cultures of both patient and clinician can influence who is diagnosed with autism, perhaps due to the heterogeneous nature of the disorder [66, 67]. Dr. Stephen Shore, professor and spokesperson on the autism spectrum, famously said, "If you've met one person with autism, you've met one person with autism" because the appearance of the disorder can be tremendously varied. The diverse nature of autism can sometimes be confused with other types of diversity to an untrained eye, and sometimes culture can look like autism and autism can look like culture. Both types of confusion disservice children of migrant families.

Children from foreign or minority families are sometimes diagnosed with autism later in childhood than their locally born counterparts [66]. There are multiple reasons for this, and confusing symptoms with cultural differences is one of them. In the absence of pronounced stereotype, social or communication deficits are sometimes mistaken for cultural differences. For example, a quiet child whose mother tongue is a foreign language may hesitate to speak because of language differences or because of poor language development. A child who avoids eye contact may not want to appear rude or may be showing signs of an undiagnosed malady. Social traits that are considered signs of autism in some countries may serve other social functions for foreign children.

In many "Western" countries, reduced eye contact is considered as one of the trademarks of autism. It is the earliest symptoms of autism to emerge during childhood, and clinicians in the U.S. and Western Europe often rely on it for diagnosis. It has been theorized that children with autism have "weak central coherence" which means that they look to the contextual information rather than the center of a scene and has been used to describe why children with autism avoid eye contact [68, 69].

However, in many Asian cultures, eye contact is considered rude and children are taught to avoid making eye contact [70]. Healthy children in multiple Asian countries have been found to exhibit "weak central coherence" (also called field-dependence) and some authors have asked whether Asian children can truly meet the criteria for autism that is used for diagnosis in the U.S. [71, 72]. Other studies reported that behaviors associated with autism were reported more often in healthy participants in Japan, India, and Malaysia compared with the U.K. [73]. However, a study of Korean children reported that similar social behaviors, including eye contact, were observed [72, 74]. A second study, which compared children from Israel, South Korea, U.K., and U.S., found that behaviors in the social domain remained stable across cultures although verbal and nonverbal behaviors and other symptoms varied by culture [75].

Although Asian studies seem to demonstrate similarities in the social domain, the international literature is more varied. German children showed lower social responsiveness and higher hyperactivity and conduct disorder compared to U.S. children [76]. Several studies report that children from Saudi Arabia display more externalizing behaviors compared to children from Jordan or the U.A.E. [77–79]. The few reviews of research in African children reports that symptoms may be comparable on the continent to "Western" diagnosis schemas, but the prevalence and distribution of these symptoms across children is uncertain [80, 81].

Diverse clinical presentations may lead to misdiagnosis in the clinic, and awareness of such cultural differences may help ensure diagnostic accuracy. Several studies have demonstrated that using clinical diagnostic tools, such as the ADOS, may help reduce misdiagnosis in ethnic minorities and would potentially benefit children from diverse backgrounds, although these tools may not be universally optimal [82, 83].

5. Other obstacles to obtaining diagnosis

In addition to cultural differences in the presentations of autism, several other factors may delay diagnosis for children from diverse backgrounds. In many countries, children from migrant families face obstacles to healthcare access. For example, healthcare may not be accessible or affordable. Parents may not be able to speak the local language and may not have access to or be aware of translation services [84–86]. A country's immigration policy may influence whether a family with an autistic child can seek help [87]. Moreover, vast arrays of medical models exist globally. Parents may be skeptical of autism or of the local approach to clinical practice. Some cultures may stigmatize autism or attribute it to incest [88]. The clinician is tasked with the difficult challenge of identifying these circumstances and assisting children in need.

6. Closing remarks

Autism is a complex disorder that appears to traverse continents, although the symptoms of autism may vary in prevalence from one location to the next. Clinicians working with children from migrant families or who have been raised in rich cultural communities may need to utilize extra care when diagnosing.

Standardized clinical measures may facilitate the task of diagnosis. Additionally, clinical tools designed broadly for working with diverse patient groups may also be useful. The McGill Illness Narrative Interview, for example, is designed to act as an interview guide for clinicians who want to understand the cultural backgrounds of patients or their families [89]. Available in more than 10 languages, it may provide a framework that can be useful when talking to parents to understand the cultural background of a child from a migrant family.

As long as global migration rates remain high, in many countries clinicians are likely to encounter autistic children from migrant families. This chapter has aimed to provide an overview of the state of the art to help equip clinicians for these modern challenges.

Author details

Daina Crafa

Address all correspondence to: daina.crafa@mail.mcgill.ca

Integrated Program in Neuroscience (IPN), Douglas Mental Health Institute, McGill University, Montreal, Canada

References

[1] United Nations Population Division. (2013). The number of international migrants worldwide reaches 232 million. Population Facts, 2, 1–4.

[2] Buescher, A. V., Cidav, Z., Knapp, M., & Mandell, D. S. (2014). Costs of autism spectrum disorders in the United Kingdom and the United States. JAMA Pediatrics, 168(8), 721–728.

[3] Center for Disease Control. (2016). Data and statistics. Retrieved Aug 20, 2016, from http://www.cdc.gov/ncbddd/autism/data.html

[4] Horlin, C., Falkmer, M., Parsons, R., Albrecht, M. A., & Falkmer, T. (2014). The cost of autism spectrum disorders. PLoS One, 9(9), e106552.

[5] United Nations. (2016). International Migration Report. United Nations, New York.

[6] Statistics Canada. (2013). Foreign-born population as a proportion of total population, G8 countries and Australia. Retrieved Aug 20, 2016, from: http://www12.statcan.gc.ca/nhs-enm/2011/as-sa/99-010-x/2011001/c-g/c-g01-eng.cfm

[7] Elsabbagh, M., Divan, G., Koh, Y. J., Kim, Y. S., Kauchali, S., Marcín, C., Montiel-Nava, C., Patel, V., Paula, C. S., Wang, C., Yasamy, M. T., & Fombonne, E. (2012). Global prevalence of autism and other pervasive developmental disorders. Autism Research, 5, 160–179.

[8] Gillberg, C., Steffenburg, G., Börjesson, B., & Andersson, L. (1987). Infantile autism in children with immigrant parents: a population based study from Göteborg, Sweden. British Journal of Psychiatry, 150, 856–858.

[9] Gillberg, C., Steffenburg, S., & Schuman, H. (1991). Is autism more common now than ten years ago? British Journal of Psychiatry, 158, 403–409.

[10] Gillberg, C., Schaumann, H., & Gillberg, I. C. (1995). Autism in immigrants: children born in Sweden to mothers born in Uganda. Journal of Intellectual Disability Research, 39(2), 141–144.

[11] Goodman, R., & Richards, H. (1995). Child and adolescent psychiatric presentations of second-generation Afro-Caribbeans in Britain. The British Journal of Psychiatry, 167(3), 362–369.

[12] Wing, L. (1980). Childhood autism and social class: a question of selection?. The British Journal of Psychiatry, 137(5), 410–417.

[13] Tanoue, Y., Oda, S., Asano, F., & Kawashima, K. (1988). Epidemiology of infantile autism in southern Ibaraki, Japan: differences in prevalence in birth cohorts. Journal of Autism and Developmental Disorders, 18(2), 155–166.

[14] Fombonne, E. (2005). Epidemiological studies of pervasive developmental disorders. In F. R. Volkmar, R. Paul, A. Klin, & D. Cohen (Eds.), Handbook of Autism and Pervasive Developmental Disorders, Wiley, Hoboken, NJ, pp. 42–69.

[15] Powell, J. E., Edwards, A., Edwards, M., Pandit, B. S., Sungum-Paliwal, S. R., & Whitehouse, W. (2000). Changes in the incidence of childhood autism and other autistic spectrum disorders in preschool children from two areas of the West Midlands, UK. Developmental Medicine & Child Neurology, 42(9), 624–628.

[16] Haglund, N. G., & Källén, K. B. (2011). Risk factors for autism and Asperger syndrome: perinatal factors and migration. Autism, 15, 163–183.

[17] Hultman, C. M., Sparén, P., & Cnattingius, S. (2002). Perinatal risk factors for infantile autism. Epidemiology, 13, 417–423.

[18] Keen, D. V., Reid, F. D., & Arnone, D. (2010). Autism, ethnicity and maternal immigration. British Journal of Psychiatry, 196, 274–281.

[19] Lauritsen, M. B., Pedersen, C. B., & Mortensen, P. B. (2005). Effects of familial risk factors and place of birth on the risk of autism: a nationwide register-based study. Journal of Child Psychological Psychiatry, 46, 963–971.

[20] Lin, S. C., Yu, S. M., & Harwood, R. L. (2012). Autism spectrum disorders and developmental disabilities in children from immigrant families in the United States. Pediatrics, 130, S191–S197.

[21] Magnusson, C., Rai, D., Goodman, A., Lundberg, M., Idring, S., Svensson, A., Koupil, I., Serlachius, E., & Dalman, C. (2012). Migration and autism spectrum disorder: a population-based study. British Journal of Psychiatry, 201, 109–115.

[22] Van der Ven, E., Termorshuizen, F., Laan, W., Breetvelt, E. J., van Os, J., & Selten, J. P. (2013). An incidence study of diagnosed autism-spectrum disorders among immigrants to the Netherlands. Acta Psychiatrica Scandinavica, 128, 54–60.

[23] Williams, K., Helmer, M., Duncan, G. W., Peat, J. K., & Mellis, C. M. (2008). Perinatal and maternal risk factors for autism spectrum disorders in New South Wales, Australia. Child Care and Health Development, 34, 249–256.

[24] Crafa, D., & Warfa, N. (2015). Maternal migration and autism risk: systematic analysis. International Review of Psychiatry, 27(1), 64–71.

[25] Hassan, M. (2012). Predicting the prevalence of autism among ethnic groups. Archives of Disease in Childhood, 97, A95–A96.

[26] Minnesota Department of Health. (2012). Autism spectrum disorders and the Somali community. Retrieved from http://www.health.state.mn.us/divs/cfh/topic/autism/somali.cfm on April 28, 2013.

[27] Croen, L. A., Grether, J. K., & Selvin, S. (2002). Descriptive epidemiology of autism in a California population: who is at risk? Journal of Autism and Developmental Disorders, 32, 217–224.

[28] Schieve, L. A., Boulet, S. L., Blumberg, S. J., Kogan, M. D., Yeargin-Allsopp, M., Boyle, C. A., Visser, S. N., & Rice, C. (2012). Association between parental nativity and autism

spectrum disorder among US-born non-Hispanic white and Hispanic children, 2007 National Survey of Children's Health. Disability and Health Journal, 5, 18–25.

[29] Gardener, H., Spiegelman, D., & Buka, S. L. (2009). Prenatal risk factors for autism: comprehensive meta-analysis. The British Journal of Psychiatry, 195(1), 7–14.

[30] Fombonne, E., Simmons, H., Ford, T., Meltzer, H., & Goodman, R. (2001). Prevalence of pervasive developmental disorders in the British nationwide survey of child mental health. Journal of the American Academy of Child & Adolescent Psychiatry, 40(7), 820–827.

[31] Dyches, T. T., Wilder, L. K., Sudweeks, R. R., Obiakor, F. E., & Algozzine, B. (2004). Multicultural issues in autism. Journal of Autism and Developmental Disorders, 34, 211–222.

[32] Freitag, C. M. (2007). The genetics of autistic disorders and its clinical relevance: a review of the literature. Molecular Psychiatry, 12(1), 2–22.

[33] Ingram, J. L., Stodgell, C. J., Hyman, S. L., Figlewicz, D. A., Weitkamp, L. R., & Rodier, P. M. (2000). Discovery of allelic variants of HOXA1 and HOXB1: genetic susceptibility to autism spectrum disorders. Teratology, 62(6), 393–405.

[34] Li, J., Tabor, H. K., Nguyen, L., Gleason, C., Lotspeich, L. J., Spiker, D., Risch, N., & Myers, R. M. (2002). Lack of association between HoxA1 and HoxB1 gene variants and autism in 110 multiplex families. American Journal of Medical Genetics, 114(1), 24–30.

[35] Chess, S. (1971). Autism in children with congenital rubella. Journal of Autism and Childhood Schizophrenia, 1(1), 33–47.

[36] Persico, A. M., & Napolioni, V. (2013). Autism genetics. Behavioural Brain Research, 251, 95–112.

[37] Warrier, V., Chee, V., Smith, P., Chakrabarti, B., & Baron-Cohen, S. (2015). A comprehensive meta-analysis of common genetic variants in autism spectrum conditions. Molecular Autism, 6(1), 1.

[38] Rapin, I., & Tuchman, R. F. (2008). Autism: definition, neurobiology, screening, diagnosis. Pediatric Clinics of North America, 55(5), 1129–1146.

[39] Fombonne, E. (2008). Thimerosal disappears but autism remains. Archives of General Psychiatry, 65(1), 15–16.

[40] Parker, S., Todd, J., Schwartz, B., et al. Thimerosal-containing vaccines and autistic spectrum disorder: a critical review of published original data. Pediatrics 2005; 115(1):200. 26.

[41] Godlee, F., Smith, J., & Marcovitch, H. (2011). Wakefield's article linking MMR vaccine and autism was fraudulent. BMJ, 342, c7452.

[42] Houtepen, L. C., Vinkers, C. H., Carrillo-Roa, T., Hiemstra, M., van Lier, P. A., Meeus, W., Branje, S., Heim, C. M., Nemeroff, C., Mill, J., Schalkwyk, L. C., Creyghton, M. P., Kahn, R. S., Joëls, M., Binder, E. B., & Boks, M. P. (2016). Genome–wide DNA methylation levels and altered cortisol stress reactivity following childhood trauma in humans. Nature Communications, 7, 19067.

http://dx.doi.org/10.5772/65981

[43] Kinney, D. K., Munir, K. M., Crowley, D. J., & Miller, A. M. (2008). Prenatal stress and risk for autism. Neuroscience and Biobehavioral Reviews, 32, 1519–1532.

[44] Nelissen, E. C., van Montfoort, A. P., Dumoulin, J. C., & Evers, J. L. (2011). Epigenetics and the placenta. Human Reproduction Update, 17(3), 397–417.

[45] Rangasamy, S., D'Mello, S. R., & Narayanan, V. (2013). Epigenetics, autism spectrum, and neurodevelopmental disorders. Neurotherapeutics, 10(4), 742–756.

[46] Rodrigues, G. M., Toffoli, L. V., Manfredo, M. H., Francis-Oliveira, J., Silva, A. S., Raquel, H. A., Martins–Pinge, M. C., Moreira, E. G., Fernandes, K. B., Pelosi, G. G., & Gomes, M. V. (2015). Acute stress affects the global DNA methylation profile in rat brain: modulation by physical exercise. Behavioural brain research, 279, 123–128.

[47] Romens, S. E., McDonald, J., Svaren, J., & Pollak, S. D. (2015). Associations between early life stress and gene methylation in children. Child Development, 86(1), 303–309.

[48] Schanen, N. C. (2006). Epigenetics of autism spectrum disorders. Human Molecular Genetics, 15, R138–R150.

[49] Shapiro, G. D., Fraser, W. D., Frasch, M. G., & Séguin, J. R. (2013). Psychosocial stress in pregnancy and preterm birth: associations and mechanisms. Journal of Perinatal Medicine, 41(6), 631–645.

[50] Tordjman, S., Somogyi, E., Coulon, N., Kermarrec, S., Cohen, D., Bronsard, G., Bonnot, O., Weismann–Arcache, C., Botbol, M., Lauth, B., Ginchat, V., Roubertoux, P., Barburoth, M., Kovess, V., Geoffray, M. M., & Xavier, J. (2014). Gene× Environment interactions in autism spectrum disorders: role of epigenetic mechanisms. Frontiers in psychiatry, 5, 53.

[51] Walker, C. K., Anderson, K. W., Milano, K. M., Ye, S., Tancredi, D. J., Pessah, I. N., et al. (2013). Trophoblast inclusions are significantly increased in the placentas of children in families at risk for autism. Biological Psychiatry, 74, 204–211.

[52] Zoladz, P. R., & Diamond, D. (2016). Psychosocial predator stress model of PTSD based on clinically relevant risk factors for trauma-induced psychopathology. Posttraumatic Stress Disorder: From Neurobiology to Treatment, 125, 125–143.

[53] Crafa, D. (2013). Do maternal ethnicity and pre-birth migration increase risk for autism? Unpublished Master's Thesis, Queen Mary University of London, London, England, Centre for Psychiatry.

[54] Acevedo-Garcia, D., Soobader, M. J., & Berkman, L. F. (2005). The differential effect of foreign-born status on low birth weight by race/ethnicity and education. Pediatrics, 115, e20–e30.

[55] Collins, J. W., Jr., & Shay, D. K. (1994). Prevalence of low birth weight among Hispanic infants with United States–born and foreign–born mothers: The effect of urban poverty. American Journal of Epidemiology, 139, 184–192.

[56] Fuentes-Afflick, E., & Lurie, P. (1997). Low birth weight and Latino ethnicity. Examining the epidemiologic paradox. Archives of Pediatric and Adolescent Medicine, 151, 665–674.

[57] Dyer, J. M., Hunter, R., & Murphy, P. A. (2011). Relationship of social network size to infant birth weight in Hispanic and non-Hispanic women. Journal of Immigration and Minority Health, 13, 487–493.

[58] Lueck, K., & Wilson, M. (2011). Acculturative stress in Latino immigrants: the impact of social, socio-psychological and migration-related factors. International Journal of Intercultural Relations, 35(2), 186–195.

[59] Palmer, R. F., Walker, T., Mandell, D., Bayles, B., & Miller, C. S. (2010). Explaining low rates of autism among Hispanic schoolchildren in Texas. American Journal of Public Health, 100, 270–272.

[60] Cannell, J. J. (2013). Autism, will vitamin D treat core symptoms?. Medical Hypotheses, 81(2), 195–198.

[61] Eyles, D. W., Burne, T. H., & McGrath, J. J. (2013). Vitamin D, effects on brain development, adult brain function and the links between low levels of vitamin D and neuropsychiatric disease. Frontiers in Neuroendocrinology, 34(1), 47–64.

[62] Mazahery, H., Camargo, C. A., Conlon, C., Beck, K. L., Kruger, M. C., & von Hurst, P. R. (2016). Vitamin D and autism spectrum disorder: a literature review. Nutrients, 8(4), 236.

[63] Whitehouse, A. J., Holt, B. J., Serralha, M., Holt, P. G., Hart, P. H., & Kusel, M. M. (2013). Maternal vitamin D levels and the autism phenotype among offspring. Journal of Autism and Developmental Disorders, 43(7), 1495–1504.

[64] Fernell, E., Bejerot, S., Westerlund, J., Miniscalco, C., Simila, H., Eyles, D., Gillberg, C., & Humble, M. B. (2015). Autism spectrum disorder and low vitamin D at birth: a sibling control study. Molecular Autism, 6(1), 1.

[65] Dealberto, M. J. (2011). Prevalence of autism according to maternal immigrant status and ethnic origin. Acta Psychiatrica Scandinavica, 123, 339–348.

[66] Twyman, K. A., Maxim, R. A., Leet, T. L., & Ultmann, M. H. (2009). Parents' developmental concerns and age variance at diagnosis of children with autism spectrum disorder. Research in Autism Spectrum Disorders, 3, 489–495.

[67] Wilkinson, L. A. (2011). How many doctors does it take to diagnose an autism spectrum disorder? Autism, 1, e101.

[68] Happé, F., Briskman, J., & Frith, U. (2001). Exploring the cognitive phenotype of autism: weak "central coherence" in parents and siblings of children with autism: I. Experimental tests. Journal of Child Psychology and Psychiatry, 42(3), 299–307.

[69] Happé, F., & Frith, U. (2006). The weak coherence account: detail-focused cognitive style in autism spectrum disorders. Journal of Autism and Developmental Disorders, 36(1), 5–25.

[70] Lian, M. J. (1996). Teaching Asian American children. In E. Duran (Ed.), Teaching Students with Moderate/Severe Disabilities, Including Autism: Strategies for Second Language Learners in Inclusive Settings, Charles C. Thomas, Springfield, pp. 239–253.

http://dx.doi.org/10.5772/65981

[71] Koh, H. C., & Milne, E. (2012). Evidence for a cultural influence on field-independence in autism spectrum disorder. Journal of Autism and Developmental Disorders, 42(2), 181–190.

[72] Kim, S. H., Kim, Y. S., Koh, Y. J., Lim, E. C., Kim, S. J., & Leventhal, B. L. (2016). Often asked but rarely answered: can Asians meet DSM-5/ICD-10 autism spectrum disorder criteria? Journal of Child and Adolescent Psychopharmacology, 26, 835–842.

[73] Freeth, M., Sheppard, E., Ramachandran, R., & Milne, E. (2013). A cross-cultural comparison of autistic traits in the UK, India and Malaysia. Journal of Autism and Developmental Disorders, 43(11), 2569–2583.

[74] Wakabayashi, A., Tojo, Y., Baron-Cohen, S., & Wheelwright, S. (2004). The Autism-Spectrum Quotient (AQ) Japanese version: evidence from high-functioning clinical group and normal adults. Shinrigaku kenkyu: The Japanese Journal of Psychology, 75(1), 78–84.

[75] 75. Matson, J. L., Worley, J. A., Fodstad, J. C., Chung, K. M., Suh, D., Jhin, H. K., Ben–Itzchak, E., Zachor, D.A., & Furniss, F. (2011). A multinational study examining the cross cultural differences in reported symptoms of autism spectrum disorders: Israel, South Korea, the United Kingdom, and the United States of America. Research in Autism Spectrum Disorders, 5(4), 1598–1604.

[76] Bölte, S., Poustka, F., & Constantino, J. N. (2008). Assessing autistic traits: cross-cultural validation of the social responsiveness scale (SRS). Autism Research, 1(6), 354–363.

[77] Al-Salehi, S. M., Al-Hifthy, E. H., & Ghaziuddin, M. (2009). Autism in Saudi Arabia: presentation, clinical correlates and comorbidity. Transcultural Psychiatry, 46(2), 340–347.

[78] Amr, M., Ali, W. B., Hablas, H., Raddad, D., El-Mehesh, F., El-Gilany, A. H., & Al-Shamy, H. (2012). Sociodemographic factors in Arab children with autism spectrum disorders. Pan African Medical Journal, 13(1), 65.

[79] Eapen, V., Mabrouk, A. A., Zoubeidi, T., & Yunis, F. (2007). Prevalence of pervasive developmental disorders in preschool children in the UAE. Journal of Tropical Pediatrics, 53(3), 202–205.

[80] Ametepee, L. K., & Chitiyo, M. (2009). What we know about autism in Africa: a brief research synthesis. The Journal of the International Association of Special Education, 10(1), 11–13.

[81] Bakare, M. O., & Munir, K. M. (2011). Autism spectrum disorders (ASD) in Africa: a perspective. African Journal of Psychiatry, 14(3), 208–210.

[82] Begeer, S., El Bouk, S., Boussaid, W., Terwogt, M. M., & Koot, H. M. (2009). Underdiagnosis and referral bias of autism in ethnic minorities. Journal of Autism and Developmental Disorders, 39(1), 142–148.

[83] Zaroff, C. M., & Uhm, S. Y. (2012). Prevalence of autism spectrum disorders and influence of country of measurement and ethnicity. Social Psychiatry and Psychiatric Epidemiology, 47(3), 395–398.

[84] Fiscella, K., Franks, P., Doescher, M. P., & Saver, B. G. (2002). Disparities in health care by race, ethnicity, and language among the insured: findings from a national sample. Medical Care, 40(1), 52–59.

[85] Lin, S. C., Stella, M. Y., & Harwood, R. L. (2012). Autism spectrum disorders and developmental disabilities in children from immigrant families in the United States. Pediatrics, 130(Supplement 2), S191–S197.

[86] Lin, S. C., & Stella, M. Y. (2015). Disparities in healthcare access and utilization among children with autism spectrum disorder from immigrant non-English primary language households in the United States. International Journal of MCH and AIDS (IJMA), 3(2), 159–167.

[87] Martinez, O., Wu, E., Sandfort, T., Dodge, B., Carballo-Dieguez, A., Pinto, R., Rhodes, S. D., Moya, E., & Chavez-Baray, S. (2015). Evaluating the impact of immigration policies on health status among undocumented immigrants: a systematic review. Journal of Immigrant and Minority Health, 17(3), 947–970.

[88] Walli, R. R., Attaib, N. M., & Sufya, N. M. Evaluation some risk factors of Libyan children with autism spectrum disorders in Tripoli. Libyan Journal of Medical Research, 8, 50–58.

[89] Groleau, D., Young, A., & Kirmayer, L. J. (2006). The McGill Illness Narrative Interview (MINI): an interview schedule to elicit meanings and modes of reasoning related to illness experience. Transcultural Psychiatry, 43(4), 671–691.

Chapter 6

Impact of Infant Feeding Methods on the Development of Autism Spectrum Disorder

Touraj Shafai, Monika Mustafa, Jeffrey Mulari and Antonio Curtis

Additional information is available at the end of the chapter

http://dx.doi.org/10.5772/67624

Abstract

There is strong and convincing evidence that infant's sensory stimulation, which is associated with breastfeeding, contributes significantly to the infant's neurodevelopment. Our study compared the prevalence of autism spectrum disorder (ASD) in children who were breastfed, given breast milk through a bottle (breast-milk fed), or formula-fed. We reported significant association of ASD in children who were formula-fed from birth or weaned early from the breast. The statistical data revealed that increasing the duration of breastfeeding resulted in a decrease in prevalence of ASD. The odds ratio of a child not having autism was 0.27, 0.93, and 6.67 for breastfeeding for less than 6, 6–12, or longer than 12 months, respectively. There is significant evidence that this association is mediated by the ingredients of the breast milk and infant's endogenous oxytocin. Oxytocin is a neurotransmitter and neuromodulator and we postulate that oxytocin may increase neuroplasticity, synaptic connections, and alter ASD genes' expression. Animal experiments and imaging studies demonstrate the central role of oxytocin in maternal love and bonding. Currently, there are no specific treatments for patients diagnosed with autism; therefore, it is imperative to identify the risk factors that contribute to the development of ASD. In this communication, we demonstrate that lack of breastfeeding is highly associated with ASD development in children with genetic susceptibility.

Keywords: autism, neuroplasticity, oxytocin, epigenetics, breastfeeding, enriched environment

1. Introduction

The short- and long-term benefits of breastfeeding for mother and baby have been well documented [1]. The short-term benefits of breastfeeding include a lower incidence of many childhood communicable diseases, childhood lymphocytic leukemia, inflammatory bowel disease, lower incidence of type 1 diabetes, and higher IQ [2]. The long-term benefits of breastfeeding include lower incidence of noncommunicable disorders (NCDs), obesity, diabetes type 2, and hypercholesterolemia resulting in cardiovascular diseases and hypertension [2–4]. Furthermore, breastfeeding results in improved maternal health by reducing the incidence of maternal premenopausal breast and ovarian cancer as well as lowering the incidence of maternal obesity and its complications [2].

World Health Organization (WHO) recommends exclusive breastfeeding for the first 6 months and to continue breastfeeding with addition of safe and nutritious complementary food up to 2 years of age and beyond.

In the past 10 years, the global exclusive breastfeeding rate improved only marginally from 33% in 1995 to 37% in 2014. Suboptimal breastfeeding results in higher health care expenses for pediatrics and maternal care, and global productivity-related economic losses of $302 billion or 0.49% of world gross income annually [4].

The impact of breastfeeding in lowering the incidence of mental health disorders has recently gained scrutiny. Neurodevelopmental disorders, especially autism and attention deficit disorder, are reported to be significantly associated with formula feeding [5–7]. The annual expenditure for the care of autistic children and adults in the United States is estimated to be in excess of $120 billion [8].

The short- and long-term benefits of breastfeeding for mother and baby have been well documented. In our study, we demonstrate the mental health benefits of breastfeeding and identify early weaning and formula feeding as possible risk factors for development of ASDs in genetically susceptible children.

2. What causes autism?

Autism was reported as a distinct entity by Leo Kanner, professor of psychiatry at Johns Hopkins University in 1943. In his article "Autistic Disturbances of Affective Contact" he described 11 cases, 3 girls and 8 boys as having infantile autism. He noted that the family members were intelligent but generally they were not warm-hearted, and that the parenting style might have contributed to the development of autism. Autism spectrum disorders consist of a group of neurodevelopmental disorders, characterized by a triad of impairments in social interaction, communications, and imagination, associated with narrow range of repetitive activities. Hans Asperger, a Viennese physician, also described a type of autism that he called autistic psychopathy in 1944, which later became to be known as Asperger syndrome. However, since the original article was written in German and was not translated into English until nearly 40 years later, there was no awareness until later when Asperger syndrome was included as a form of autism. However, a Russian neurologist, Grunya Sukharev, published an article in 1926 titled, the schzoid psychopathy in children with nearly identical description as Asperger syndrome.

The etiology of autism had been quite elusive, although there is common belief that autism has a genetic basis; however, the gene expression may be influenced by environmental factors. The genetic influence in development of autism has been shown by twin studies, where there is a high probability that monozygotic twins, who have identical genes, develop autism at a high rate. Heritability index, a measure of genetic transmission of neurobehavioral disorders, autism, hyperactivity, schizophrenia, and major depression are 0.95, 0.8, 0.8, and 0.75, respectively [9].

In the past 40 years, a number of environmental toxins were considered to be the main culprit in the development of autism. Prenatal factors, including maternal folate deficiency and short interpregnancy intervals, do not appear to be causal factors [10]. Perinatal factors, newborn jaundice, breech presentation, and prematurity do not seem to be responsible for autism development. Multiple gene theory and second hit theory which advocate ASD genes induce increased susceptibility to environmental toxins have also been refuted as a cause of autism.

The fraudulent report of finding measles viruses in the guts of 12 children with autism, published in Lancet in 1998, therefore linking autism to MMR vaccine was retracted by the coauthors in 2004 and by the journal's editor in 2010. Allegations that vaccine's ingredients (thimerosal, aluminum) are responsible for the epidemic of autism have been soundly refuted by epidemiological studies and there is no scientific basis that there is a causal association between vaccines and autism [11].

In the past 20 years, multidisciplinary research has resulted in better understanding of the complex nature of ASDs. The multicenter study reported by Sanders et al. on the association of copy number variations, characterized by submicroscopic deletions or duplications on chromosomes in the individuals with ASDs, demonstrate the genetic etiology of this disorder [12–14]. However, there is evidence that a number of individuals with CNV genotype have normal phenotypes, indicating incomplete gene penetrance and the influence of environmental factors [12].

3. The role of oxytocin in infant's brain development

There is significant evidence that oxytocin plays a major role in the development of the mammalian brain [1]. Oxytocin, a neuropeptide is secreted by the paraventricular (PVN) and supraventricular (SON) nuclei in the hypothalamus. Oxytocin was thought to be only a parturition hormone, which initiates the uterine contractions during childbirth and the myoepithelial cells in the breast, pushing breast milk from the alveoli through the milk ducts during breastfeeding. However, animal experiments have generated significant evidence that oxytocin plays a major role in the development of the mammalian's central nervous system. Oxytocin is implicated in both romantic and maternal love and all aspects of reproduction and breastfeeding. Romantic and maternal love are some of the most inspiring manifestations of human behavior and responsible for the survival of our species. Additionally, oxytocin is a neurotransmitter and neuromodulator and implicated in neuroplasticity of the infant's central nervous system. There are numerous oxytocin receptors in the central nervous system and the peripheral tissues. However, there are separate oxytocin receptors for romantic and maternal love [1].

Oxytocin is generated by the specialized neuroendocine cells in the hypothalamus, which are activated by the sensory nerves in the infants' oral mucosa and released during breastfeeding. Additionally, oxytocin is released during skin-to-skin contact with the mother due to sensory nerves responding to warmth, touch, and stroking by the mother [15]. The sensory nerves enter the spinal cord or brain stem and connect to the nucleus tractus solitarius (NTS). Furthermore, oxytocin release is triggered by the breast milk/food in the infant's stomach, which results in the release of cholecystokinine in the gut. Cholecystokinine stimulates the release of oxytocin by activating the sensory vagal nerve fibers, which results in central and peripheral oxytocin release [1, 15].

The endogenous release of oxytocin results in behavioral changes in both mother and baby, including bonding and attachment. Additionally, oxytocin stimulates the sense of well-being and suppresses the HPA axis [10, 15].

4. Environmental influence on the infant's brain development

Anthropological studies clearly demonstrate the necessity of the closeness of the mother-baby dyads. The statement by famous anthropologist, Sarah Blaffer Hrdy that "for species such as primates, the mother is the environment" holds very true. Primates such as monkeys, apes, and humans are referred to by scientists as the "carrying mammals" versus the "nested mammal" because of the difference in the sugar and the fat contents of their breast milk and feeding frequency. The human infant's central nervous system depends on the microenvironment that is similar to the maternal uterine environment, which is full of sensory exchanges involving warmth, sound, movement, transportation, feeling, touch, smell, and access to the nutrients in the mother's breast milk.

Anthropological studies indicate that the mammalian brain development requires an enriched environment with the mother providing breast milk, emotional and physical support and protection. This is in contrast to a mother who is formula-feeding her infant with little or no emotional and physical support. The infant is not held by the mother or the caretaker, she is frequently ignored and sometimes is physically or emotionally abused. This type of environment which we call a toxic environment frequently results in developmental delay, lower IQ, and neurodevelopmental disorders. The elegant experiments by Volkmar and Grenough demonstrate the effect of environmental enrichment in laboratory rats, which resulted in more complexity and dentritic branching of the visual cortex [16]. Furthermore, Weaver et al. [17] have shown that epigenetic factors can induce gene activation by histone acetylation without changing the DNA sequence. Therefore, histone acetylation results in gene activation in the offspring when they reach maturity.

Imaging studies (**Figure 1**) comparing the activation of oxytocin receptor sites in formula and breastfeeding mothers demonstrate significant enhancement of oxytocin receptors in breastfeeding

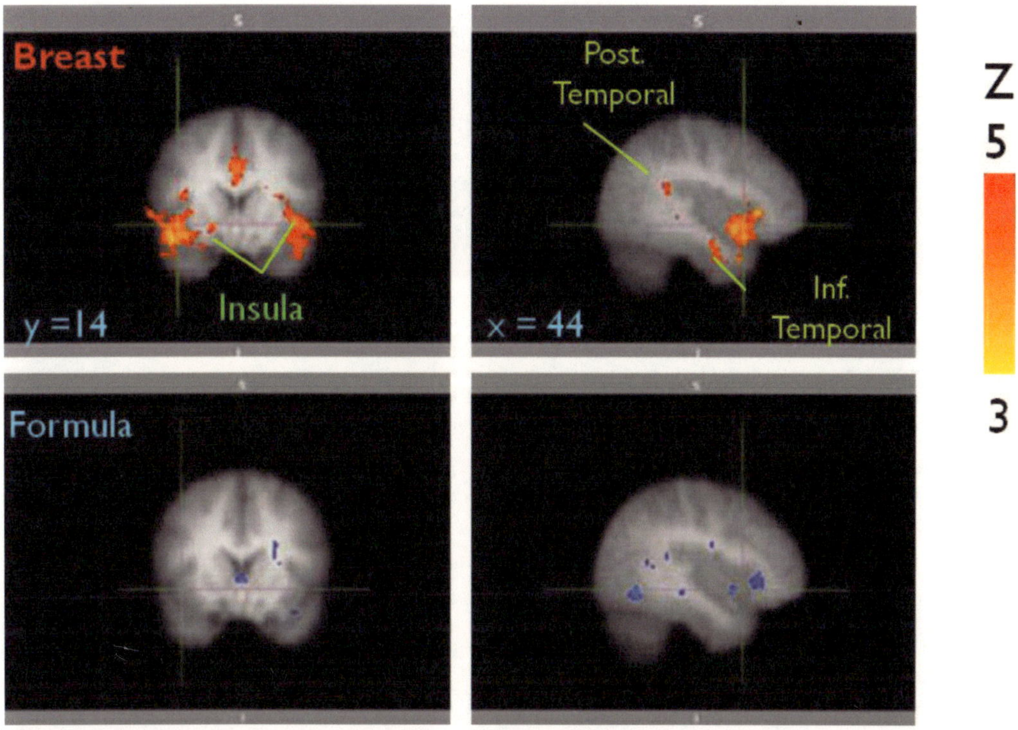

Figure 1. Comparison of the functional MRI studies of breastfeeding and formula feeding mothers after viewing the pictures of their own infants. Oxytocin receptors are significantly enhanced in breastfeeding mothers.

mothers, which correlates with greater neural response [1]. Furthermore, higher plasma and salivary oxytocin levels are reported in breastfeeding compared to formula feeding mothers, 36% in plasma and 23% in saliva, respectively [18]. We hypothesize that an increase in brain oxytocin level may improve learning, speech, cognition, parental attachment, and emotional ties. Additional support for the beneficial effect of oxytocin in premature infants is reported from the University of Chicago hospitals. Premature infants, who received sensory stimulations, including auditory, tactile, visual, and vestibular, gained more weight and were discharged home sooner than the control group who did not receive any sensory or only tactile stimulation. Measurements of salivary cortisol levels in the infants showed a decline in the infants associated with ATVV (auditory, tactile, visual, and vestibular) stimulation corresponding to the rise in blood oxytocin level (**Figure 2**).

In the past decade, there has been credible evidence that ASDs are associated with oxytocin dysfunction [19]. Modahl et al. [20] reported lower serum oxytocin in children with ASDs. Additionally, oxytocin infusion to adults with ASD resulted in temporary improvement in some of their symptoms [21, 22]. However, it is generally believed that oxytocin does not cross the blood-brain barrier. Therefore, trials of oxytocin nasal spray, which would bypass the blood-brain barrier was attempted for a period of 6 weeks to adults with ASD, which resulted only in temporary improvements in some of the autistic symptoms [23]. These findings indicate that oxytocin has a critical function during the first 5 years of life when the accelerated brain growth occurs.

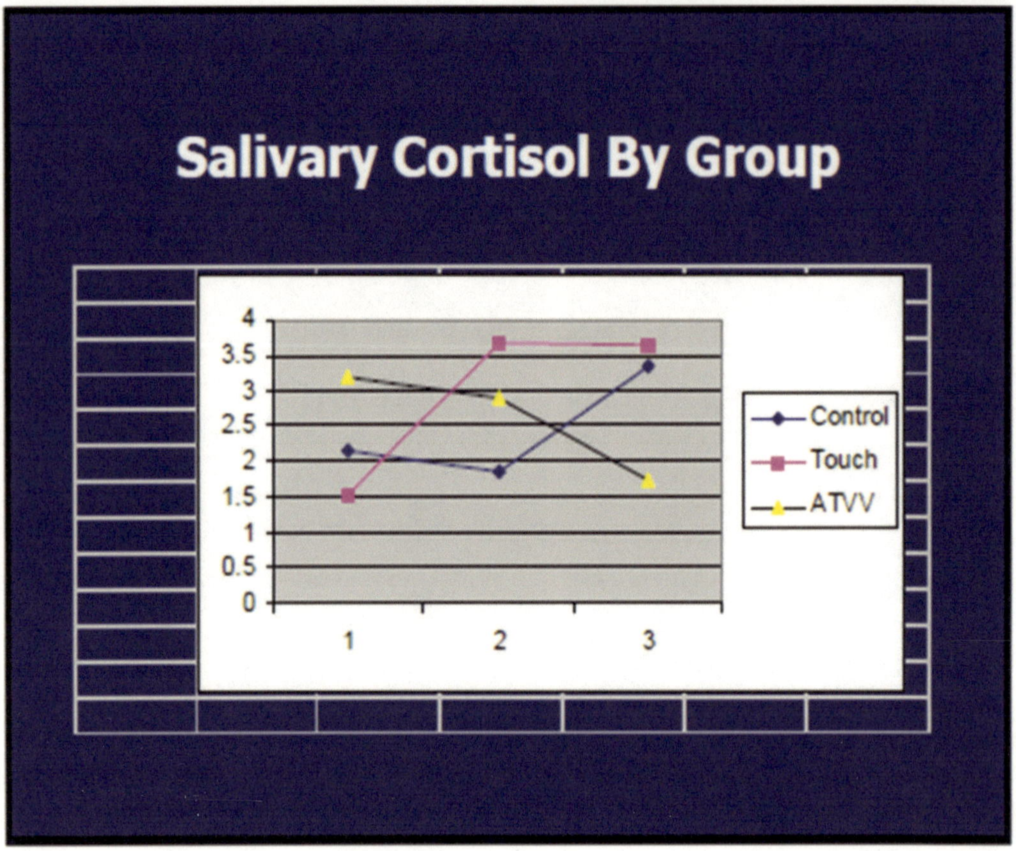

Figure 2. Salivary cortisol levels in three groups of premature infants, showing a decline associated with ATVV sensory stimulation, which corresponds to a rise in serum oxytocin.

Population genetic studies have shown that structural alteration of oxytocin are responsible for development of autism [24]. Finally, genetic alterations in oxytocin receptor protein are reported to be associated with ASDs [25].

5. Industrialization, global conflicts, the rise of formula feeding, and autism

It is commonly believed that the rate of breastfeeding in the industrialized nations sank to its lowest level after the 1950s and began to climb in the past 20–30 years. We assume that autism has always existed, but not recognized until the 1940s when it was described independently by Leo Kanner and Hans Asperger. However, it is clear that throughout our history, the prevalence of ASDs was quite low, due to the high rate of breastfeeding and sensory interaction between the mother and her infant. There is clear evidence that there is an increase in the prevalence of ASDs, especially in the United States that in recent years has reached alarming numbers. However, expansion of diagnostic criteria and diagnostic substitution may explain the increase in ASDs diagnosis in the United States. Furthermore, the prevalence of autism is lower in other industrialized nations because of higher rates of breastfeeding and paid maternity leave. In parts of Africa and the Middle East, infants are breastfed for 4 years and they report lower rates of autism.

Historically, the first description of autism was reported independently by three physicians, Grunya Sukharev from Russia, Leo Kanner from the United States, and Hans Asperger from Austria at about the same time. The authors do not describe possible cause(s) for autism and no mention of the type of feedings during infancy. However, we know of the desperate conditions of populace in Russia and Austria. In the United States, many women were working in the factories and the infants were fed cow's milk or powdered milk. There are no reliable statistics on the breastfeeding rates in the mid-twentieth century. However, cow's milk or powdered milk feeding became very popular in Europe and the United States. Many women chose injection of a prolactin inhibitor after childbirth to prevent producing any breast milk. In the 1980s, the formula companies began aggressive marketing of infant formulas directly to the consumers. This resulted in World Health Organization's campaign to counter the formula industry by the passage of the Code of Ethics of Marketing of Breast Milk Substitutes, followed by Baby-Friendly Hospital Initiative.

In the past 20 years, improved public awareness of many benefits of breastfeeding for mother-baby dyads has resulted in higher breastfeeding initiations [3]. This is especially true in college-educated mothers and middle-class families. The rates of breastfeeding in the United States vary greatly by race, ethnicity, parents' income, parents' education, and the community support. Many college-educated mothers elect to breastfeed their babies and exclusive breastfeeding rates in this population at 6 months stands at 16%. The rate of breastfeeding is inversely associated with families' income. Therefore the breastfeeding rates for the families at or above 6 times poverty line at 6 months is 21%, for those at 4.2 times poverty line is 20% and for those below the poverty line is 12%. Accordingly, the breastfeeding rates by mothers at six times above the poverty line, those between 4.2 times, and those below the poverty line are at 21, 20, and 12%, respectively [26]. Breastfeeding rates also vary greatly among the racial groups, whites are at 19%, Hispanics at 16%, and African Americans are at 9% at 6 months [26].

The United States WIC program, Women, Infants and Children, which funds nutrition program for pregnant mothers and children, who are below the 180% poverty level, began providing infant formulas beginning in 1974 to the WIC recipients. The WIC program was enacted in 1972 following a White House Conference on the ill-effects of poverty on pregnancy and the well-being of breastfed infants. During the first 2 years, the program was very successful in eliminating malnutrition in pregnant women and their babies.

However, for the past three generations the great majority of WIC recipients have received free formula for their infants for 1 year. The WIC population has the lowest breastfeeding rates in the United States and numerous interventions to improve breastfeeding rates in this population have not been effective.

There are numerous benefits of exclusive breastfeeding to both mother and her infant, which are attributed to the ingredients of breast milk [2]. However, recent research and genomic studies demonstrate that the infant's social environment may play a significant role in her brain development. The environmental factors may be positive, including high socioeconomic status (SES), high maternal IQ, breastfeeding, and mother-infant sensory interactions. Negative environmental factors include poverty, formula feeding, lack of high school and college education, absence of mother-baby sensory interaction, neglect, and abuse.

Fragile X syndrome is the most common inherited cause of intellectual disability and the focus of intense research on multiple levels from molecular to the cognitive functions and the IQ of the individuals. Fragile X syndrome is caused by CGC (dinucleotide) repeats on the X chromosome, replacing the FMRP (fragile X mental retardation protein) gene, which results in autism. However, environmental enrichment results in a favorable outcome in some of these children. The IQ of the boys with fragile X syndrome is known to be higher in association with parental responsiveness to the child, having educational material in the home and parental efforts to provide developmental enrichment [27]. The association of home environment with IQ is larger than any other variables, including the child's level of FMRP and mean parental IQ.

There is clear and convincing evidence that oxytocin has a major role in the development of oxytocin system, connecting the periaqueductal gray matter (PAG), the limbic system and the lateral orbitofrontal cortex, which are identified with maternal behavior [1]. Furthermore, the oxytocin system appears to include a number of pathways, especially in the limbic system, which are affected in various degrees in individuals with ASDs.

6. Association of early weaning and formula feeding with autism

Tanoue and Oda [28] first reported the association of early weaning and autism over 25 years ago. The authors also noted that in their study population, autism was more common in the lower socioeconomic class. The result of a survey comparing the rates of autism in three groups of children was reported by Schultz et al. [29]. The children who were breastfed for 6 months had a lower incidence of autism than the group who were fed formula without DHA&ARA supplementation. However, the group of children who were given formulas supplemented with DHA&ARA also had a lower rate of autism. We strongly believe that the study was flawed because it was conducted in 2004, only 2 years after DHA&ARA supplementation of infant formulas. The diagnosis of autism is usually confirmed in children who are older than 3–4 years old.

6.1. Methods

In this communication, we hypothesize that breastfeeding and nurturing result in a decrease in autism diagnosis. In order to explore this hypothesis, we conducted a confidential written survey of parents to ascertain the association of parent's reported ASD diagnosis with the duration of breastfeeding, breast milk, or formula feeding. The study focused on the children who were 2–8 years old at the time of the survey and to include only formulas supplemented with DHA and ARA. The survey did not include any questions regarding the brand of the formulas used, because of possible frequent formula changes as well as difficulty recalling the brand name of formulas. Our study was based on an anonymous written retrospective survey which was conducted from our offices. The survey forms were made available from our

http://dx.doi.org/10.5772/67624

offices. The completed survey forms were returned through fax to our office. Statistical analysis was performed using binary logistic regression analysis on the data of the children who were breastfed or formula-fed and those who received breast milk via a bottle. In each group there were a number of children who did not have autism. The children without ASD diagnosis were used as the "control group." The odds ratios, *P*-values, and confidence intervals were calculated in relation to the duration of breastfeeding, formula feeding, or breast milk feeding using binary regression analysis.

6.2. Results

One hundred and forty-five parents responded to our survey. Eighty-five parents reported no ASD diagnosis and 60 parents reported that their child had ASD diagnosis. The children were divided into three groups. The infants who were formula-fed from birth were placed in the formula-fed group. The infants who were breastfed from birth were placed in the group of breastfed children, regardless of the length of breastfeeding. Twelve of the 60 children who were formula-fed from birth had ASD diagnosis as shown in **Table 1**. Twenty-six were reported to have been breastfed from less than 2 weeks to greater than 2 years and reported to have a diagnosis of autism as shown in **Table 1**. The survey results demonstrate that increasing the duration of breastfeeding is associated with a decline in ASD diagnosis as shown in **Table 2**. The statistical data reveal that children who were breastfed longer than 12 months are 6.67 times less likely to have autism diagnosis than children who were breastfed less than 12 months as shown in **Table 3**. Breastfeeding of less than 6 months duration was significantly associated with autism diagnosis. Twenty-two out of 64 children who were fed breast milk through a bottle were reported to have ASD diagnosis as shown in **Table 4**. The odds ratio analysis of the association of breast milk feeding and ASD diagnosis is shown in **Table 5**. This survey indicates that increasing the duration of breast milk feeding was not associated with a significant decrease in autism diagnosis. We believe that the infants who are bottle-fed with breast milk or formula have little sensory interaction with the mother or caregiver during the feeding **Table 6**. We hypothesize that breast milk feeding is associated with lower oxytocin release and oxytocin receptors in the infant's central nervous system. Similarly, in children who were formula-fed and had ASD diagnosis, less sensory interaction between mother-baby during bottle feeding and absence of maternal hormones, especially estrogens, in the infant's feeding result in lower oxytocin and its

Children with ASD diagnosis	Children without ASD diagnosis	Total
Number of formula-fed children		
12	22	34
Number of breastfed children		
21	26	47
Number of breast milk fed children		
22	42	64
55	90	145

Table 1. Number of breastfed children with ASD diagnosis should be 21 and without ASD diagnosis should be 26 autism relative to the feeding methods, breastfeeding, breast milk, or formula feeding.

Duration of breastfeeding	Number of children with ASD diagnosis	Number of children without ASD diagnosis
<2 months	8	2
2–3.99 months	4	1
4–5.99 months	2	2
6–8.99 months	4	0
9–11.99 months	2	2
12–14.99 months	2	8
15–17.99 months	2	3
18–23.99 months	2	0
>24 months	0	3

Table 2. Number of children with and without ASD diagnosis relative to the duration of breastfeeding.

Months of breastfeeding	Odds ratio	P-value	95% confidence intervals
<6	0.27	0.04	(0.08–0.95)
6–11.99 months	0.93	0.94	(0.14–6-23)
>12 months	6.67	0.009	(1.61–26.47)

Table 3. Odds ratios of association of breastfeeding duration and ASD diagnosis.

Duration of breast milk feeding	With ASD diagnosis	Without ASD diagnosis
<2 months	4	8
2–3.99 months	4	6
4–5.99 months	4	4
6–8.99 months	4	8
9–11.99 months	4	5
12–14.99 months	0	5
15–23.99 months	2	2
>24 months	0	4

Table 4. Number of children with and without ASD relative to the duration of breast milk feeding.

receptors in the infant's brain [30]. The presence of estrogens as well as other maternal hormones in the breast milk has been well documented. Johnson et al. and Champagne et al. have reported that estrogens are transcriptional promoters of oxytocin and oxytocin receptor's gene in experimental animals [31, 32]. The absence of estrogens in the infant's feeding or the use of oxytocin blockers in experimental animals results in lower endogenous oxytocin and oxytocin receptors [30–32]. Oxytocin and estrogens have regulatory influence on the oxytocinergic system and have been shown to alter many aspects of cellular function and differentiation as well as potential to remodel the nervous system [33, 34]. Additionally, oxytocin is a neurotransmitter and

http://dx.doi.org/10.5772/67624

Months of breast milk feeding	Odds ratios	P-value	95% confidence interval
<6 months	0.67	0.37	(0.11–4.31)
6–11.99 months	1.08	0.08	(0.35–3.40)
>12 months	3.67	0.12	(0.69–19.56)

Table 5. Odds ratios of association of breast milk feeding duration and prevalence of ASD diagnosis.

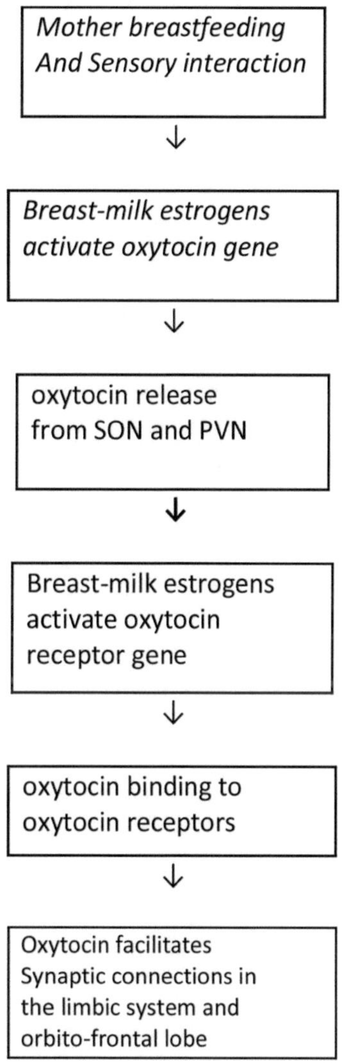

Table 6. Cascade of oxytocin system activation in the newborn infants.

neuromodulator and may increase neuroplasticity, synaptic connections, and alter ASD genes expression.

There is clear and convincing evidence that links the ingredients of breast milk and infant's sensory stimulation during breastfeeding to lowering the prevalence of autism. However, there are questions raised that infants who are later diagnosed to have autism may have dysregulated breastfeeding behavior [35]. A small retrospective study of the association of autism and dysregulated breastfeeding behavior revealed that the majority of infants in this study who developed autism were breastfeeding well and a few who were identified as having dysregulated breastfeeding behavior were breastfeeding more often and quite vigorously [35].

In this communication, we demonstrate the association between breastfeeding and decline in prevalence of ASD. We further believe that this effect is mediated by an increase in the endogenous oxytocin in the infant's central nervous system [1, 13, 15]. The elegant experiments by Krol et al. demonstrate the significance of breastfeeding and oxytocin increase in the central nervous system of infants with CD-38 gene variation. CD-38 gene encodes the enzyme system that releases the oxytocin from the hypothalamic neuroendocrine cells. The individuals who have two copies of the C allele of the enzyme release less oxytocin than the individuals with the A (normal) allele and therefore are at risk of developing ASD [36]. Furthermore, the infants with CC allele of the enzyme who were not breastfed showed less eye contact with their caregiver at 6 months, an early sign of autism, while the infants who were exclusively breastfed continued to maintain normal eye contact with their mother. The author state that oxytocin in the breast milk is absorbed in the infant's intestinal tract and cross the blood-brain barrier. However, this appears to be very unlikely because breast milk contains small amounts of oxytocin, 8 pg/ml in the first few days, and decreases with increased milk production. It is believed that oxytocin is digested in the infant's digestive tract and even if it is absorbed into the blood stream, it does not cross the blood-brain barrier [10]. We postulate that the rise of oxytocin in the infant's central nervous system is due to the presence of estrogens in the breast milk acting as transcriptional promoter of oxytocin gene. We believe that the finding is further indication that breastfeeding provides protection against autism development.

In this communication, we demonstrate the evidence supporting our hypothesis that breastfeeding for 1 year or more is highly associated with reduced prevalence of autism and identify the lack of breastfeeding as a risk factor for the development of ASD in genetically susceptible children.

Acknowledgements

The opinions stated in this communication are only the opinions of the authors. The authors declare no competing interest.

Author details

Touraj Shafai[1]*, Monika Mustafa[1], Jeffrey Mulari[2] and Antonio Curtis[2]

*Address all correspondence to: shafaidocs@yahoo.com

1 Department of Paediatrics, School of Medicine, University of California, Riverside, California

2 Department of Mathematics, Riverside City College, Riverside, California

References

[1] Bartel A, Zeki S, The neural correlates of maternal and romantic love, Elsevier, Neuroimage, 21;2004:1155–1165.

[2] Breastfeeding and Maternal and Infant Health Outcomes in Developed Countries, Evidence Report, Agency for Healthcare Research and Quality, U.S. Department of Health and Human Services, 2007, Rockville, MD.

[3] Infant and young child feeding, Fact Sheet, World Health Organization on global rates of breastfeeding Bulletin, February 2015.

[4] Victora C et al., Breastfeeding in 21st century, epidemiology, mechanism and lifelong effect, Lancet, 2016,387:10017;475–490.

[5] Shafai T, Mustafa M, Hild T, Mulari J, Curtis A, Influence of infant feeding methods: breastfeeding, breast milk or formula feeding on the prevalence of autism spectrum disorders, The Journal of Southern California Clinicians, 2013;7:1;33–38.

[6] Shafai T, Mustafa M, Hild T, Mulari J, Curtis A, Association of early weaning and formula feeding with autism spectrum disorders, Breastfeeding Medicine, 2014; 9:5;275–276.

[7] Sabuncuoglu O, Orengul C, Bikmazer A et al., Breastfeeding and parafunctional oral habits in children with and without attention deficit/hyperactivity disorder, Breastfeeding Medicine, 2014;9:244–250.

[8] Ganz ML, The life-time distribution of the incremental societal cost of autism, Archives of Pediatrics and Adolescent Medicine, 2007;61:343–349.

[9] McGuffin P, Riley B, Plomon R, Toward behavioural genomics, Science, 2001;291:1132–1249.

[10] Gardener H, Speigelman D, Buka L, Prenatal risk factors for autism: comprehensive meta-analysis, The British Journal of Psychiatry, 2009;195:7–14.

[11] Bulletin, Institute of Medicine, Immunization Safety Committee, Vaccines and Autism, Washington D.C., National Academic Press, 2004.

[12] Sanders JS, et al., Multiple recurrent de novo CNVs, including duplication of the 7q 11.23 Williams syndrome region, are strongly associated with autism, Neuron, 2011;70:863–885.

[13] Gilman SR, Iossifov, Levy D, Ronemus M, Vitkup D, Rare de novo variants associated with autism implicate a large functional network of genes involved in formation and function of synapses, Neuron, 2011;70:898–907.

[14] Levy D et al., Rare de novo and transmitted copy number variation in autistic spectrum disorders, Neuron, 2011;70:886–897.

[15] Uvnas Moberg K, Prime DK, Oxytocin effects in mothers and infants during breastfeeding, Infant, 2013;9:201–206.

[16] Volkmar FG, Greenough WT, Rearing complexity affects branching of dendrites in the visual cortex of the rat, Science, 1972;176:1445–1447.

[17] Weaver ICG, Cervoni N, Champagne FA, et al., Epigenetic programming by maternal behaviour, Nature Neuroscience, 2004;7:848–854.

[18] Grewen KM, Davenport RE, Light KC, An investigation of plasma and salivary oxytocin responses in breast and formula feeding mothers of infants, Psychophysiology, 2010;47:285–332.

[19] Insel TR, O'Brien DJ, Leckman JF, Oxytocin, vasopressin and autism, is there a connection, Biological Psychiatry, 1999;45:145–157.

[20] Modahl C, Green L, Fein D, et al., Plasma oxytocin levels in autistic children, Biological Psychiatry, 1998;43:270–277.

[21] Hollander E, Novotney S, Hanratty M, Oxytocin infusion reduces repetitive behaviour in adults with autistic and Asperger disorder, Neuropsychopharmacology, 2003;28:193–198.

[22] Hollander E, Bartz J, Chaplin W, Oxytocin increases the retention of social cognition in autism, Biological Psychiatry, 2007;61:498–503.

[23] Guastella AJ, Einfeld EL, Gray K, Rinehart N, Tonge B, Lambert TJ, Hichie IB, Intra-nasal oxytocin improves emotion recognition for youth with autism spectrum disorder, Biological Psychiatry, 2009;67:692–704.

[24] Green LA, Fein D, Modahl C, Waterhouse C, Morris M, Oxytocin and autistic disorders; alteration in peptide forms, Biological Psychiatry, 2001;50:609–613.

[25] Jacob S, Brune CW, Carter CS, et al., Association of oxytocin receptor gene (OXTR) in Caucasian children and adolescents with autism, Neuroscience Letters, 2007;417:69.

[26] Shafai T, Mustafa M, Hild T, Promotion of exclusive breastfeeding in low-income families by improving the WIC food package for breastfeeding mothers, Breastfeeding Medicine, 2014;9:375–376.

[27] Glaser B, Hessl D, Dyer-Feldman J, et al., Biological and environmental contributions to adaptive behaviour in Fragile X syndrome, American Journal of Medical Genetics, 2003; 117A:21–29.

[28] Tanoue Y, Oda S, Weaning time of children with infantile autism. Journal of Autism and Developmental Disorders, 1989;19:425–434.

[29] Schultz TS, Klonoff-Cohen HS, Wingard DL, et al., Breastfeeding, infant formula supplementation and autistic disorder; the result of a parent survey, International Breastfeeding Journal, 2006;16:1.

[30] Johnson SE, Ball GF, Coirini H, Harbaugh CR, McEwen BS, Insel TR, Time course of estradiol-dependent induction of oxytocin receptor binding in the ventromedial hypothalamic nucleus of the rat, Endocrinology, 1989;125:1414–1419.

[31] Champagne F, Diorio J, Sharma S, Meaney MJ, Naturally occurring variations in maternal behaviour in the rat are associated with differences in estrogen-inducible central oxytocin

receptors, Proceedings of the National Academy of Sciences of the United States of America, 2001;122:12736–12741.

[32] Carter CS, The neuroendocriology of social attachment and love, Psychoneuroendocrinology, 1998;23:779–818.

[33] Carter CS, Altemus M, Integrative functions of lactational hormones in social behaviour and stress management, Annals of the New York Academy of Sciences, 1997;897:164–174.

[34] Uvnas-Moberg K, Oxytocin may mediate the benefits of positive social interaction and emotions, Psychoneuroendocrinology, 1998;23:819–835.

[35] Lucas R, Cutler A, Dysregulated breastfeeding behaviour in children later diagnosed with autism, The Journal of Perinatal Education, 2015;24(3):171–180.

[36] Krol K, Monakhov M, Ebstein R, Grossman T, Genetic variation in CD38 and breastfeeding experience interact to impact infant's attention to social eye cues. www.pnas.org/lookup/suppl/doi:10.1073/pnas.1506352112/-/DCSupplemental.

Section 3

Impact of Autism

Chapter 7

Family Quality of Life in Autism Spectrum Disorders (ASD)

Elena Predescu and Roxana Şipoş

Additional information is available at the end of the chapter

http://dx.doi.org/10.5772/66201

Abstract

In latest years the concept of quality of life (QoL) has been acknowledged as an important outcome in psychiatric pathology fields. Most researchers consider that social indicators and the perception of personal wellbeing also, should be considered when measuring the quality of life. Our purpose was to investigate the QoL of the families of children with autism spectrum disorders (ASD) and to determine whether in this population, the potential mediators (irrational cognitions, negative automatic thoughts, coping strategies) relate significantly with the emotional distress reported. We also aimed to assess the parents' irrational cognitions and negative automatic thoughts as mediators in the relationship between the overall assessment of family QoL and their emotional distress. We found significant correlations between the emotional distress reported by the parents and their automatic negative thoughts, irrational cognitions, and different coping strategies. The relationship between the overall assessment of family QoLand the parents' emotional distress was partially explained by their negative automatic thoughts and irrational cognitions. In this view, the specialised services should include also interventions for the parents of children with developmental disorders (ASD, ADHD) in order to improve their overall assessment of family QoL.

Keywords: family quality of life, autism spectrum disorders, emotion regulation, coping mechanisms

1. Introduction

Quality of life (QoL) is a measure of individual well-being, which includes multiple areas of functioning and is increasingly recognized as a necessary construct in developmental disorder studies. The QoL concept is not new. Happiness and well-being have been discussed by Plato and Aristotle in their writings. QoL has been defined in various ways, from "general conditions for happiness" [2] to "positive life experiences" [3]. Most researchers consider that social indicators, but also the perception of personal well-being should be considered when measuring QoL and that the objective and subjective indicators are two complementary facets that have to be measured separately [1, 4].

QoL is a construct that has been used for a wide range of health problems (drug abuse, mental disorders, oncology, geriatrics, cardiovascular disease, etc.), but lacks a coherent theoretical-derived model or a definition generally accepted [5, 6]. Although there is a general consensus on the main characteristics of the construct [7–9], there are still some issues to be clarified for the development of appropriate QoL measurement instruments: the principles that should guide the measurement process and how should be carried the assessment [10, 11].

The concept of family QoL has been studied systematically only in the recent years. Parents' experience was considered to be a part of the family life and was initially explored as part of the QoL concept. In the late 1990s, there were initiated two large projects on the families' QoL, one at Kansas University and the other led by a team of researchers from Australia, Canada, and Israel. The main rationale for these studies was the tendency of governments and other funding sources to assign to the families the care of children and adults with disabilities. This trend was especially important for the families who had a member with intellectual disability that required constant care and supervision. Even though most families are willing to assume this role, many difficulties arise and affect their quality of life [12, 13].

The concept of family QoL emerged as a viable alternative to the use of multiple measurements, which most often caused difficulties in design studies and results reporting because these measurements, developed individually, are rarely suitable to produce a global profile of family status. Given the increasing interest in health status or economic well-being of families and community, these issues were included in the instruments that measure family QoL. Although some researchers have conceptualized and measured some aspects of the family QoL in terms of services available for the child or the family [14], most of them developed a multidimensional construct, with a number of domains representing different areas of the family life, the sum of their ratings indicating the overall family quality of life. That view was shared by many researchers, each of them describing a framework for the domains of the family quality of life. The International Family Quality of Life Project [13, 15, 16] developed an instrument that organizes family QoL in nine domains. Another research team [17] proposed an instrument with six areas. The third research team [18, 19] conceptualized, developed, and tested an instrument that evaluates five domains: family relationships, parenting style, emotional well-being, physical and material wellbeing, and disability support.

A way to assess families' perceptions and needs is to investigate the areas in which they function. One of the problems that arise from using these questionnaires is the difficulty to convince other family members than mothers to answer to them. However, overall satisfaction with the family quality of life can be high, even if there are problems in some areas. Satisfaction varies significantly in each assessed area of the family life. This variation may be associated with the intensity of child's behavioral problems or family experience. It is also important to note that family members are different in terms of resilience and coping strategies and that they may report high levels in satisfaction, even if they have many difficulties and need support [20]. The concept of family quality of life is a multidimensional construct, involving a variety of physical, economic, and emotional dimensions, which cannot be properly measured by focusing only on the perspective of the mother. In a systematic review on the conceptualization and assessment of the effects on families who have children with disabilities, among the 20 studies evaluated, 14 used assessments focused on family welfare, family adjustment, and functioning. Among these studies, 55% were focused on the maternal perspective, 35% included both parents, and only one study included the siblings of children with disabilities [21].

The use of variables such as stress and depression to study the effect of disability on families has been criticized because these variables do not take an objective view on the families' experience and do not consider the possibility that many families experience positive effects and adapt well to raising a child with disabilities [22].

Stress level was studied in relation to parents' mental health QoL in several studies [23–25]. Lee et al. found stress to be a significant predictor of mental health QoL, after controlling for five demographic variables (e.g., age, education, income, number of children in family, and severity of child with disability). Stress was negatively correlated with all aspects of QoL including physical, psychological, social, and environmental HRQOL [26].

In another study on parents of children with autism spectrum disorders (ASD), Johnson et al. evaluated the relationships between parents' stress, family functioning, and QoL. They found that parents' stress had a negative impact on mental health outcomes [27]. These results are supported by other studies and confirm the negative impact of stress on psychological outcomes among parents of children with ASD (e.g., depression, anxiety, and adjustment) [28, 29].

Smith et al evaluated the depressive symptoms of the mother of children and adolescents with ASD. A third of them had clinically significant depressive symptoms [30]. Wallace et al. suggested that parents' depression is associated with the intensity of child repetitive behaviors and their anxiety with child social communication problems [31]. Family history of depression or shyness had the greatest influence on children socialization scores. Parents of children with autism were more likely to be hospitalized for a mental disorder than those in the control group, and depression and personality disorders were more common in mothers than fathers [32].

Social support, family functioning, and parents' coping mechanisms are factors that mediate the quality of life of parents of children with ASD [33]. High social support is associated with low levels of anxiety, depression, and stress. The high degree of cohesion and adaptability of the family was shown to be protective against the potential negative effects of raising a child with ASD.

Another factors found to be associated with parental QoL are child's symptom severity and behavioral problems [25, 26, 34]. Benson et al. studied the impact of child ASD symptoms severity on parents' depression, the results suggesting that both child symptoms severity and parental stress predicted depression and that the effect of child symptom severity on parental depression was partially mediated by stress [23].

In a study that investigated the QoL of the main caregiver of children with ASD, the results suggested that the most important predictors for caregiver' physical health were the intensity of children behavioral problems and social support and for their mental health, the level of child functional impairment, social support, use of maladaptive coping strategies, and perceived difficulty. The impact on mental health was more important than that on physical health, which was only slightly below the norms for general population [35].

Coping refers to the cognitive and behavioral effort of an individual to adapt to a stressful situation [36]. Studies in autism reported that the frequent use of emotion-oriented coping is associated with parents' low quality of life [37]. In contrast to these findings, Lee et al. found no association between coping strategies and QoL [26].

Family emotional environment, including the expression of different types of emotions, help children to develop emotional competence. A chronically poor emotional expression of parents and high levels of negative emotions have significant implications for children emotion regulation skill development (failure in understanding emotions, poor management of stressful emotional situations, and incorrect social use of emotions). Chronic suppression of emotional experiences is associated with higher subjective distress and on a long term with emotional regulation deficits.

There are some data suggesting that parental capacity to assure their children health and adaptability may be affected by their emotional state and well-being. Parental stress can influence parents' and children's coping resources and affect their ability to perform [38, 39].

A study that investigated the quality of life of 286 children with ASD, compared with the norms for general population and the population with chronic somatic disorders, reported that the children with ASD had lower scores for the psychosocial, emotional, and social functioning, but comparative to the population with chronic somatic disorders for physical and school functioning. QoL did not significantly correlate with the diagnosis of ASD or the intellectual abilities, but was significantly associated with the internalizing/externalizing problems measured by child Behavior checklist (CBCL), with the repetitive behaviors, social responsiveness, and adaptive behaviors. Given the fact that the socialization difficulties that characterize ASD are not specific to chronic somatic disorders, such as asthma or diabetes, it is not surprising that children with ASD had lower scores on the psychosocial functioning domain [39]. Storch et al. found a stronger correlation between the CBCL scores and quality of life for the internalizing problems [40]. This stronger association with the internalizing problems is not necessarily surprising for children with ASD, given that withdrawal is an important clinical feature in ASD and also a significant part of internalization scores measured by CBCL.

Studies on QoL of the caregivers of children with ASD reported different results. Allik et al. found the behavioral problems and not the autism severity as predictors for the mental health of mothers of children with ASD. This study included parents of children with Asperger syndrome and high-functioning autism, which could influence the results related to autism severity, these forms of ASD associating a lower symptoms severity [41].

http://dx.doi.org/10.5772/66201

Stuart and McGrew reported a protective effect for social support and a negative one for the use of maladaptive coping strategies, on the subjective difficulty reported by the parents of children with autism. The problems in family functioning also contributed to the level of difficulties reported [42]. These results are similar to those described by Altiere and von Kluge, who found a more frequent use of the adaptive coping mechanisms and social support for the parents of children with autism who had better family relationships than for those with family problems or separated [43].

For children with autism, it was demonstrated a strong correlation between their behavioral problems, the autism symptoms severity and parental stress. Osborne and Reed reported that the parental stress levels have a negative influence on the child outcomes after receiving different educational interventions. The negative effects were observed in both cognitive and adaptive behavior acquisitions [44]. The reason why high levels of parental stress have a negative impact on child's behavioral problems and are predictive for poor outcomes in therapy has not been elucidated yet. The most plausible explanation is that the parental stress produces changes in the parent's ability to adjust and respond to child's behavioral problems.

The aim of this study was to assess the mediating role of parents' irrational beliefs and automatic negative thoughts in the relationship between the children's emotional/behavioral problems and the parents' emotional distress. Our goal was also to investigate whether in this population (families of the children with ASD or attention deficit hyperactivity disorder (ADHD)), the potential mediators (irrational cognitions, negative automatic thoughts, and coping strategies) relate significantly with the emotional distress reported and to assess the parents irrational cognitions and negative automatic thoughts as mediators in the relationship between the assessment of the overall family quality of life and their emotional distress [1]. Few studies have been reported on this topic, especially, much less in families of the children with ASD or ADHD.

The results from previous studies [45, 46] showed no differences between the two diagnosis categories regarding the parents' levels of emotional distress and the overall assessment of family QoL, so analyses were performed on all studied clinical sample.

2. Method

2.1. Participants

The data were collected from 114 children aged 2–14 years, diagnosed with ASD or ADHD, according to international diagnosis criteria DSM IV-TR and ICD-10 and from their parents (65 children with ASD and 49 children with ADHD).

Children and adolescents included in the study were recruited between January 2011 and November 2011. They were patients in the Child and Adolescent Psychiatry Clinic from Cluj-Napoca, Romania or included in a therapy program in various specialized centers from Romania (ClujNapoca, Sibiu, Oradea, Arad, and Tg. Jiu). Children diagnosed and treated in this clinic come from all parts of the country and are diverse in terms of socioeconomic status.

We included in the study: boys or girls with ages between 2 and 14 years, with diagnosis of autistic spectrum disorder (ASD) or attention deficit hyperactivity disorder (ADHD), according to DSM IV-TR international criteria; sign consent of parents to be included in the study. We excluded from the study: the children with a known medical condition (heart or lung and chronic disorders); children who suffered accidents or had major stress or in the last 6 months, which may significantly affect the family quality of life; the children placed in foster care [1].

2.2. Instruments

Child Behavior Checklist (CBCL) was used to assess the internalizing/externalizing problems. There are two versions of the instrument, depending on the age of the child: the preschool checklist (CBCL/1½-5) and the school-age version (CBCL/6-18). The CBCL is to be filled in by the parent/caretaker who spends the most time with the child and assesses various problems and child functioning over the past 2 months. It has been one of the most widely used standardized measures for evaluating maladaptive behaviors and emotional problems in children and adolescents. CBCL assesses internalizing (i.e., anxious, depressive, and overcontrolled) and externalizing (i.e., aggressive, hyperactive, noncompliant, and under controlled) behaviors, as well as scores on DSM-IV-related scales (emotional problems, anxiety disorders, ADHD, opposition defiant disorder, and pervasive developmental disorders/somatic problems) [47].

To assess parents' emotions and emotional regulation strategies, we used the following instruments: profile of affective distress (PAD)—rating scale with 39 items that assesses subjective dimensions of positive and negative emotions (functional and dysfunctional) [47]; white bear suppression inventory (WBSI)—rating scale with 15 items that assesses the use of suppression as a cognitive and emotional coping strategy; self-efficacy scale (SES)—rating scale with 10 items that assesses the perceived self-efficacy; automatic thoughts questionnaire (ATQ)—rating scale with 30 items that measures the negative automatic thoughts frequency; attitudes and beliefs scale—short form (ABSs)—is a global measure of irrationality into adulthood; it has eight items that assess four types of irrational evaluative beliefs (absolutist claims, catastrophic interpretation, low frustration tolerance and negative overall assessment); cognitive-emotional regulation questionnaire (CERQ)—has 36 items and assesses nine cognitive coping strategies that a person uses when experiencing negative events or situations (self-blame; other-blame; rumination; catastrophizing; putting into perspective; positive refocusing; positive reappraisal; acceptance; refocus on planning) [48, 49].

Family quality of life survey (FQOL) was used to assess the family quality of life, instrument designed to assess the quality of life of the families that have one or more members with intellectual or developmental disability. The family quality of life can be approached from different perspectives.

The FQOL has several sections: first section includes the description of the family members; the following nine assess specific areas of family life (health, financial status, family interactions, support from others, and support from services, values influence, career, leisure activities, and integration in community life). Each of these areas has two sections: Section A

http://dx.doi.org/10.5772/66201

contains questions of a more general nature and Section B contains questions related to six key concepts for the theoretical construction of the instrument: importance, opportunities, initiative, achievement/current status, stability, and satisfaction. The final section is shorter and is designed to collect the overall impressions regarding the family QoL [50].

The demographics and other data of interest were obtained through a questionnaire containing questions about the patient (age, sex, age at diagnosis, school activities, and treatment) and his family (mother and father's age, marital status, education level, and occupation).

2.3. Design

The study is cross-sectional. Parents and children who agreed to participate to the study received additional information and signed the informed consent. Psychiatric and somatic evaluations were performed for the patients who met the study inclusion and exclusion criteria in order to confirm the diagnosis and detect possible comorbidities. Each child was psychologically evaluated in order to determine the developmental level and symptoms severity. After the clinical interview, the parents/caregivers filled in the CBCL for the assessment of child internalizing/externalizing problems, the emotional assessment rating scales (PAD, WBI, SES, ATQ, ABSs, and CERQ) and the family quality of life questionnaire (FQOL) [1]. Data were supplemented with information from the patients' charts and other medical documents. For all the children included in the study, we required and obtained the consent to use medical data, ensuring the privacy and subject's identity protection. The questionnaires were filled in by the mothers for all children included in the study.

2.4. Data analysis

Data were collected into a SPSS database (version 17). Analyses were performed to assess the mediating role of parents' automatic thoughts and irrational beliefs as mediators of the relationship between children's problems (affective, anxiety, behavioral) and parents' emotional distress. The same procedure was used to assess the role of parents' irrational beliefs and automatic thoughts as mediators of the relationship between the global assessment of family QoL and their emotional distress.

The mediation analysis was used following the next steps: first, the mediation criteria were tested according to the following procedure. We tested if the independent variable is a significant predictor of the dependent variable (criterion). In this way, the total effect was identified. Then we tested whether the independent variable is a significant predictor of the mediating variable and if the latter is a significant predictor of the dependent variable. After that, it was tested whether the independent variable predictive value is reduced when it is placed next to the mediating variable in the multiple linear regression equation on the dependent variable. The difference between the total effect and the independent variable predictive value on controlled mediator represents the mediation effect.

Its difference from 0 value was tested using the Sobel test, at a probability of the null hypothesis (mediation effect is null) $p < 0.05$. For the situations where the mediation effect proved to be statistically significant, in the last phase of the analysis, the mediation effect size was calculated. An effect size indicator was used. It represents the proportion of the total effect explained by the mediating variable. This indicator was calculated as: the difference between the total effect and the mediation effect divided by the total effect and multiplied by 100.

2.5. Ethical aspects

The study was conducted in compliance with the international ethical standards set out in the Helsinki Declaration of Human Rights updated. We obtain the approval of the University of Medicine and Pharmacy Cluj-Napoca Ethics Committee to conduct the study. All the parents and children included in the study signed the informed consent and received additional information. Data were used ensuring the privacy and subject's identity protection.

3. Results

3.1. Sample description

One hundred and fourteen subjects were enrolled in the study, with ages ranging between 2 and 14 years ($M = 6.95$ years, SD = 2.67) (see **Table 1**). In terms of gender distribution, the sample included 84 boys (73.7%) and 30 girls (26.3%), with a clear predominance of male subjects. Sixty-five children (57%) were diagnosed with ASD and 49 with ADHD (43%). After psychological evaluations, 54 (47.37%) children had a proper developmental level, 51 (44.74%) had developmental delay in all areas (cognitive, language, independence, communication), and 9 children had language delay (7.89%). Most children were under psychological or pharmacological therapy.

Out of the 114 participants in the study, 32 (28.07%) were from rural and 82 (71.93%) from urban environment. In both diagnosis groups, most parents were married, with secondary education and employed [1].

The results of our previous studies on the comparison of satisfaction for the nine areas of family quality of life (QoL) among families of children with ASD and ADHD highlighted the lack of statistically significant differences between the two categories of diagnosis in all the domains assessed by FQOL. We also found no statistically significant differences between the two diagnosis groups regarding parents' emotional distress, meaning that the diagnostic category does not moderate the intensity and/or direction of the relationship between parental emotional distress and the overall assessment of family QoL, so analyses were performed on the whole clinical sample [45, 46].

3.2. Analysis of parents automatic thoughts and irrational cognitions as mediators in the relationship between children problems (affective, anxiety, behavioral) and parents' emotional distress

Previous analysis on the relationship between the child affective, anxiety, and behavioral problems and the overall assessment of the family QoL revealed no significant relationship for both category of diagnosis, TSA and ADHD.

	ASD (N = 65)	ADHD (N = 49)
Child characteristics		
Age mean (SD)	6.46 (2.17)	7.61 (3.13)
Gender (% male)	58.3	41.7
Developmental level	N (%)	N (%)
Normal	15 (23.07)	39 (79.59)
Developmental delay	44 (67.69)	7 (14.28)
Language delay	6 (9.23)	3 (6.12)
Pharmacological therapy N (%)	43 (66.2)	27 (55.1)
Psychotherapy N (%)	60 (92.3)	24 (48.97)
Family characteristics		
Mothers age mean (SD)	33.21 (5.58)	35.46 (6.37)
Fathers age mean (SD)	36.79 (5.54)	37.78 (6.50)
Marital status N married (%)	55 (84.6)	40 (81.6)
Level of education	N (%)	N (%)
Less than 12th grade	4 (6.2)	8 (16.3)
Bachelor's degree	37 (56.9)	28 (57.1)
Graduate degree	24 (36.9)	13 (26.6)
Employment status		
N employed (%)	58 (89.2)	38 (77.6)

Table 1. Sample demographic description.

The parents included in the study showed high emotional distress mean scores compared with the general population norms (M = 56.21, SD = 19.64). Analyses performed separately for the two diagnosis categories revealed no statistically significant differences (t (112) = −1.08, p > 0.05) on the level of distress reported.

The scores for negative dysfunctional emotions were average to high when compared with the general population norms (M = 25.1, SD = 10.9), 40% of the parents reporting high and very high levels of negative dysfunctional emotions. Analyses performed separately for the two diagnosis categories revealed no statistically significant differences (t (112) = −1.29, p > 0.05), suggesting that for the studied sample, increased levels of negative dysfunctional emotions and emotional distress, may be due to child developmental problems, but they are not specific to diagnosis.

3.2.1. Study on the relationship between the intensity of children affective problems and parents' emotional distress

Analysis of variance (ANOVA) revealed no statistically significant differences between the three groups (non-clinical, sub-clinical, and clinical) for any aspect of parents' emotional distress measured in the study: emotional distress total score (F = 0.40, p > 0.05), negative dysfunctional emotion total score ($F = 0.16$, $p > 0.05$), worry/anxiety dysfunctional emotion score ($F = 0.14$, $p > 0.05$), respectively, sadness/depression dysfunctional emotion score ($F = 0.16$, $p > 0.05$) (see **Table 2**).

3.2.2. Study on the relationship between the intensity of children anxiety problems and parents' emotional distress

Comparative analysis of the parents' emotional distress scores in the three groups (nonclinical, subclinical, and clinical), highlighted a lack of statistically significant differences, as follows: emotional distress total score ($F = 0.37$, $p > 0.05$), negative dysfunctional emotion total score ($F = 0.39$, $p > 0.05$), worry/anxiety dysfunctional emotion score ($F = 0.03$, $p > 0.05$), and sadness/depression dysfunctional emotion score ($F = 1.05$, $p > 0.05$) (see **Table 3**).

3.2.3. Study on the relationship between the intensity of children behavioral problems and parents' emotional distress

Comparative analysis of parents' emotional distress scores in the three groups (nonclinical, subclinical, and clinical) showed a lack of statistically significant differences for the level of emotional distress total score ($F = 0.44$, $p > 0.05$), negative dysfunctional emotion total score

Variable	**Lot**	*N*	**Mean (*M*)**	**Standard deviation (SD)**
Emotional distress total score	Nonclinic	67	55.22	19.86
	Subclinic	25	55.92	18.82
	Clinic	22	59.59	20.41
	Total	114	56.21	19.64
Negative dysfunctional emotion total score	Nonclinic	67	24.80	11.31
	Subclinic	25	24.84	10.66
	Clinic	22	26.31	10.70
	Total	114	25.10	10.98
Worry/anxiety dysfunctional emotion score	Nonclinic	67	11.44	6.54
	Subclinic	25	11.24	4.53
	Clinic	22	12.09	4.17
	Total	114	11.52	5.71
Sadness/depression dysfunctional emotion score	Nonclinic	67	13.35	5.56
	Subclinic	25	13.60	6.55
	Clinic	22	14.22	7.26
	Total	114	13.57	6.09

Table 2. Central tendency and dispersion indicators of parents' emotional distress in relation with the intensity of children affective problems.

http://dx.doi.org/10.5772/66201

Variable	Lot	*N*	Mean (*M*)	Standard deviation (SD)
Emotional distress total score	Nonclinic	58	54.68	17.75
	Subclinic	30	57.30	20.16
	Clinic	26	58.38	23.28
	Total	114	56.21	19.64
Negative dysfunctional emotion total score	Nonclinic	58	24.20	10.33
	Subclinic	30	25.86	10.62
	Clinic	26	26.23	12.90
	Total	114	25.10	10.98
Worry/anxiety dysfunctional emotion score	Nonclinic	58	11.41	6.47
	Subclinic	30	11.76	4.84
	Clinic	26	11.50	4.98
	Total	114	11.52	5.71
Sadness/depression dysfunctional emotion score	Nonclinic	58	12.79	4.78
	Subclinic	30	14.10	6.05
	Clinic	26	14.73	8.35
	Total	114	13.57	6.09

Table 3. Central tendency and dispersion indicators of parents' emotional distress in relation with the intensity of children anxiety problems.

($F = 0.28$, $p > 0.05$), worry/anxiety dysfunctional emotion score ($F = 0.23$, $p > 0.05$), and sadness/depression dysfunctional emotion score ($F = 0.48$, $p > 0.05$) (see **Table 4**) [1].

3.3. Automatic thoughts, irrational beliefs and coping strategies

Assuming that the high levels of parental emotional distress is generated among other factors, by the child developmental disorder, we investigated whether in this population (parents of children diagnosed with ASD or ADHD), the potential mediators (irrational beliefs, negative automatic thoughts, coping strategies) relate statistically significant to the reported emotional distress.

Parents of children included in the study registered high levels of negative automatic thoughts ($M = 30.15$, SD = 10.39) (more than 69.1% of the general population). For the irrational beliefs measured by ABSs, the mean scores were also very high ($M = 11.29$, SD = 3.54). Low to medium levels of self-efficacy were reported ($M = 30.22$, SD = 4.61) (>6.7 of the general population).

Table 5 shows the correlations of parents' automatic thoughts, irrational beliefs, perceived self-efficacy, and suppression coping strategy with their emotional distress scores.

Variable	Lot	*N*	Mean (*M*)	Standard deviation (SD)
Emotional distress total score	Nonclinic	61	55.80	21.05
	Subclinic	22	53.77	16.89
	Clinic	31	58.77	18.86
	Total	114	56.21	19.64
Negative dysfunctional emotion total score	Nonclinic	61	25.04	12.16
	Subclinic	22	23.81	8.53
	Clinic	31	26.12	10.23
	Total	114	25.10	10.98
Worry/anxiety dysfunctional emotion score	Nonclinic	61	11.73	6.90
	Subclinic	22	10.77	3.89
	Clinic	31	11.64	4.07
	Total	114	11.52	5.71
Sadness/depression dysfunctional emotion score	Nonclinic	61	13.31	6.11
	Subclinic	22	13.04	5.07
	Clinic	31	14.48	6.76
	Total	114	13.57	6.09

Table 4. Central tendency and dispersion indicators of parents' emotional distress in relation with the intensity of children behavioral problems.

	Automatic negative thoughts (ATQ)	Irrational beliefs (ABSs)	Self-efficacy (SES)	Suppression coping strategy (WBSI)
Emotional distress total score	0.48**	0.41**	−0.40**	0.38**
Negative dysfunctional emotion total score	0.49**	0.39**	−0.37**	0.36**
Worry/anxiety dysfunctional emotion score	0.37**	0.30**	−0.28**	0.31**
Sadness/depression dysfunctional emotion score	0.53**	0.43**	−0.41**	0.36**

**Correlation significant at $p < 0.01$.

Table 5. The correlation of parents' emotional distress scores with their automatic thoughts, irrational beliefs, perceived self-efficacy and use of suppression coping strategy.

Both automatic negative thoughts and irrational beliefs correlate positively and statistically significant with all emotional distress scores, the intensity varying from medium to high. The relationship is positive, meaning that when the intensity of the negative automatic thoughts increases, the emotional distress increases also. In terms of explanatory value, negative automatic thoughts explain between 13% (R^2 = 0.13 for worry/anxiety dysfunctional emotion score) and 28% (R^2 = 0.28 for sadness/depression dysfunctional emotion score) of the emotional distress variance.

For the irrational beliefs, the relationship is also positive, meaning that when the level of irrationality increases, the emotional distress increases also. The determination coefficients obtained from the square of the correlation coefficients indicate that irrationality explains between 9% ($R^2 = 0.09$ for worry/anxiety dysfunctional emotion scores) and 18% ($R^2 = 0.18$ for sadness/depression dysfunctional emotion score) of the emotional distress variance.

The perceived self-efficacy correlated with all emotional distress scores with values between −0.28 and −0.41. The negative relationship means that, if the self-efficacy reported by parents is higher, the emotional distress will be lower. In terms of explanatory value, the perceived self-efficacy explains between 7.8% ($R^2 = 0.078$ for worry/anxiety dysfunctional emotion score) and 16.8% ($R^2 = 0.168$ for sadness/depression dysfunctional emotion score) of the emotional distress variance.

The suppression coping strategy measured by WBSI correlated with all emotional distress scores with values between $r = 0.31$ and $r = 0.38$, statistically significant at $p < 0.01$. The mean scores ($M = 48.51$, SD = 11.79) did not exceed the critical cut-off ($M > 60$).The use of suppression coping strategy (WBSI) explains between 9 ($R^2 = 0.09$ for worry/anxiety dysfunctional emotion score) and 14% ($R^2 = 0.14$ for the emotional distress total score) of the emotional distress variance.

Regarding the cognitive coping strategies used, the scores reported by the parents showed above average use for catastrophizing ($M = 9.64$, SD = 3.82), average use for self-blame ($M = 9.66$, SD = 3.06), acceptance ($M = 13.51$, SD = 3.49), rumination ($M = 12.24$, SD = 3.52), refocus on planning ($M = 15.9$, SD = 3.25), positive reappraisal ($M = 14.37$, SD = 3.82), putting into perspective ($M = 14.19$, SD = 3.76), and below average for positive refocusing ($M = 10.89$, SD = 3.91) and blame others ($M = 7.05$, SD = 2.90).

As seen in **Table 6**, the reported emotional distress correlated statistically significant with the strategies: self-blame ($r = 0.32$), rumination ($r = 0.20$), positive refocusing ($r = -0.22$), positive reappraisal ($r = -0.23$), catastrophizing ($r = 0.37$), and blame others ($r = 019$). The only coping strategies that correlated with all scores of emotional distress measured were self-blame and catastrophizing strategies. Both registered positive relationships meaning that their frequent use associated with higher emotional distress scores. For the self-blame strategy the intensity was mild. The most intense correlation was obtained for the catastrophizing strategy ($r = 0.37$). The positive refocusing, positive reappraisal, refocus on planning registered negative relationships with different scores of emotional distress, meaning that their frequent use associated with lower emotional distress scores [1].

3.4. The parents' irrational cognitions and negative automatic thoughts as mediators in the relationship between the assessment of the overall family quality of life and their emotional distress

3.4.1. Model 1

This mediation model includes the following variables: overall assessment of family quality of life ($M = 3.57$, SD = 0.65)—predictor variable, emotional distress—criterion variable and irrational cognitions—the mediator variable (**Figure 1**).

CERQ coping strategy	Emotional distress total score	Negative dysfunctional emotion total score	Worry/anxiety dysfunctional emotion score	Sadness/depression dysfunctional emotion score
Self-blame	0.32**	0.32**	0.30**	0.29**
Acceptance	0.07	0.05	0.06	0.03
Rumination	0.20*	0.15	0.13	0.15
Positive refocusing	−0.22*	−0.18*	−0.07	−0.26**
Refocus on planning	−0.10	−0.14	−0.02	−0.23*
Positive reappraisal	−0.23*	−0.25**	−0.13	−0.34**
Putting into perspective	−0.06	−0.09	−0.03	−0.14
Catastrophizing	0.37**	0.38**	0.32**	0.38**
Blame others	0.19*	0.14	0.10	0.15
CERQ coping strategy	Emotional distress total score	Negative dysfunctional emotion total score	Worry/anxiety dysfunctional emotion score	Sadness/depression dysfunctional emotion score

**Correlation significant at $p < 0.01$.
*Correlations significant at $p < 0.05$.

Table 6. Correlation of parents' emotional distress with their coping strategies (CERQ).

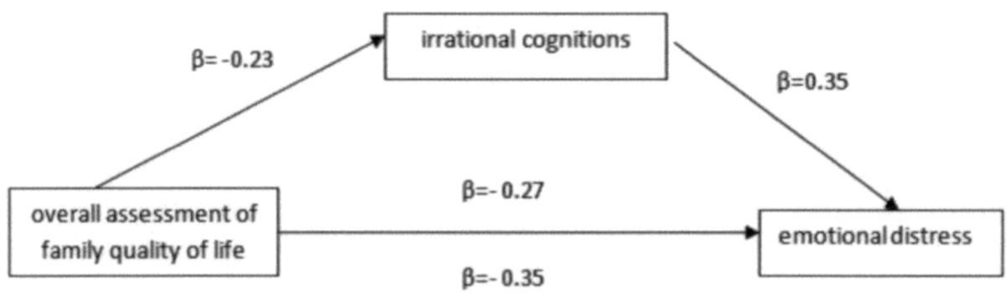

Figure 1. Mediation model 1 diagram.

Mediation model 1 testing included the following steps:

Step 1. Testing the relationship between the overall assessment of family quality of life and parents reported emotional distress. Simple linear regression analysis proved overall assessment of family quality of life to be a significant predictor for the emotional distress ($B = -0.97$, $\beta = -0.35$, SE = 2.27, $p < 0.05$). This represents the total effect of the overall assessment of family quality of life on the parents' emotional distress.

Step 2. Testing the relationship between the overall assessment of family quality of life and parents irrational beliefs. Simple linear regression analysis showed the overall assessment of family quality of life as significant predictor for parents' irrational cognitions ($B = -1.07$, $\beta = -0.23$, SE = 0.42, $p < 0.05$).

Step 3. Testing the simultaneous predictive value of the overall assessment of family quality of life and irrational beliefs on parents' emotional distress. The multiple linear regression analysis showed the predictive value of parents irrational cognitions on their emotional distress, when controlling for the overall assessment of family quality of life ($B = 1.93$, $\beta = 0.35$, SE = 0.47, $p < 0.05$). It showed also a reduction in the predictive value of the overall assessment of family quality of life on the parents emotional distress, when controlling for their irrational cognitions ($B = -6.98$, $\beta = -0.27$, SE = 2.18, $p < 0.05$). The mediation effect (the difference in predictive value), delta $B = -9.07 - (-6.98)$, was tested for statistical significance using the Sobel test. The mediating effect was statistically significant, $Z = -2.16$, $p = 0.03$. Next, the mediation effect size was calculated as follows: the ratio between the mediation effect and the total effect, multiplied by the value $\{[-9.07 - (- 6.98)]/ -9.07\} \times 100$. This indicator shows the proportion of relationship between the overall assessments of family quality and parents' emotional distress explained by irrational cognitions. The mediation size effect was ES = 23%, which expresses a partial mediation effect [1].

3.4.2. Model 2

The second mediation model includes three variables: family quality of life— predictor variable, parents' emotional distress—criterion variable and parents' automatic negative thoughts—the mediator variable (**Figure 2**).

Mediation model 2 testing included, as in the previous case, the following steps:

Step 1. Testing the relationship between the overall assessment of family quality of life and parents reported emotional distress. Simple linear regression analysis showed overall assessment of family quality of life as significant predictor for the emotional distress ($B = -0.97$, $\beta = -0.35$, SE = 2.27, $p < 0.05$).

Step 2. Testing the relationship between the overall assessment of family quality of life and parents automatic negative thoughts. Simple linear regression analysis showed the overall assessment of family quality of life as significant predictor of parents automatic negative thoughts ($B = -4.50$, $\beta = -0.33$, SE = 1.21, $p < 0.05$).

Step 3. Testing the simultaneous predictive value of the overall assessment of family quality of life and automatic negative thoughts on parents' emotional distress. The multiple linear regression analysis showed the predictive value of parents negative automatic thoughts on their emotional distress, when controlling for the overall assessment of family quality of life ($B = 0.78$, $\beta = 0.41$, SE = 0.16, $p < 0.05$). It showed also a reduction of the predictive value

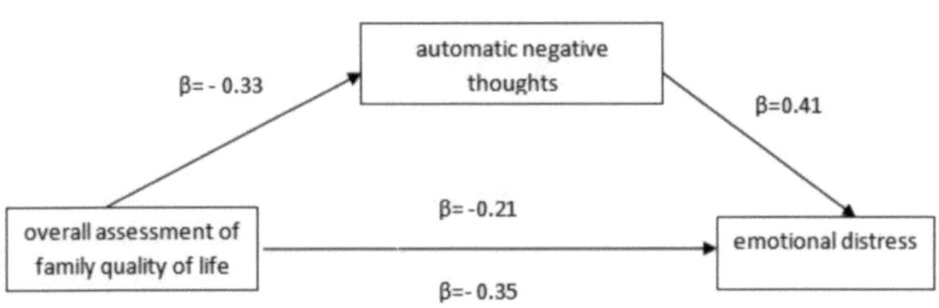

Figure 2. Mediation model 2 diagram.

of the overall assessment of family quality of life on the parents emotional distress, when controlling for their automatic negative thoughts ($B = -5.54$, $\beta = -0.21$, SE = 2.19, $p < 0.05$). The mediation effect, delta $B = -9.07 - (-5.54)$, was tested with the Sobel test. The mediating effect was statistically significant, $Z = -2.95$, $p = 0.003$. ES = effect size was 38.9%, which represents a partial mediator effect. From the total effect of the overall assessment of family quality of life on parents' emotional distress, 38.9% is explained by their automatic negative thoughts [1].

4. Discussion

4.1. Main findings

The impact of an autism spectrum disorder (ASD) diagnosis on families is devastating, particularly because there is no curative pharmacological or psychological treatment.

It has been already proven that having a child with special needs involves child-care-related stress, and less time for parents to fulfill their own needs. Compared to typical children's parents, parents of children with autism have reported higher family difficulties and are at greater risk for developing physical or psychological problems. Lee et al. investigated the main predictors of mental health for the parents of children with high-functioning autism and reported that physical health, financial status, and low stress are the most critical. The study underlined the need for more research on the potential stress of these parents and stated the need for services targeting the parents' mental health, in addition to the therapies addressed to the child problems [26].

Some studies have reported that parents' emotional problems correlated positively with child's behavioral problem severity and low ability to communicate functionally. Also, a strong correlation between child behavioral problems, autism symptom severity and parental stress was demonstrated. Khanna et al. found a correlation between the physical QoL dimension and child's behavioral problems [35]. Tung et al. and McStay et al. reported lower QoL among parents of children with higher levels of externalizing problems [24, 25]. Lower scores on prosocial behaviors and higher scores of hyperactivity and conduct problems indicated lower maternal mental health [51, 52]. Only half of the studies that assessed the impact of child emotional problems on parents QoL indicated a significant correlation between the child's emotional problems and maternal mental health [52, 53].

Although recent studies have suggested that there is a link between the level of parents' emotional distress and the intensity of child internalizing/externalizing problems, the results of this study showed no statistically significant differences between the levels of emotional distress, negative dysfunctional emotions, worry/anxiety dysfunctional emotions, sadness/depression dysfunctional emotions in relation to the intensity of children's affective, anxiety and behavioral problems, measured by CBCL. In this view, we believe that child's developmental disorders may increase parents' emotional distress, but it does not differ significantly depending on the diagnosis or child-associated internalizing/externalizing problems.

Parental stress levels were found to be more pronounced in the parents of children with ASD compared to the parents of children with disabilities or other health problems [54]. Hastings and Johnson reported that increased severity levels of autistic symptoms are associated with higher levels of parental stress [55]. Elevated levels of stress can have a negative impact on parents and can lead to depression, anger, anxiety, and family conflicts [56]. Most studies considered the child with autism the source of stress and the well-being of the other family members as the result, but this relationship is bidirectional, meaning that the family members can influence the children with ASD (e.g., maternal marital stress and depression can influence child behavior) [37]. Another study reported that the most important stressors for the parents of children with ASD are: the permanence of the disorder, lack of acceptance of ASD-associated behaviors by the family members and society and low levels of support available. Among the stressors identified were also included: the financial difficulties due to raising a child with ASD, parents concern about the child's future, behavioral problems and parents' psychological characteristics (perceived self-efficacy, locus of control and coping styles) [57].

Parents of children included in the study showed higher mean scores for emotional distress and average for the negative dysfunctional emotions, compared with the norms for general population. These results can be explained by the impact of raising a child with a developmental disorder, considering that some children did not received any form of psychological intervention to help parents manage the disorder-associated problems. The increased levels of negative dysfunctional emotions and emotional distress may be due to the child developmental problems, but it was not specific to the diagnosis.

Several studies assessed the levels of stress, anxiety, and depression in parents of children with ASD [30, 32]. Stress, coping style, and parental self-efficacy emerged as important factors associated with QoL. The results of a recently published review [58] suggested that parental stress was negatively associated with QoL and also that parents of children with ASD are more likely to experience high levels of stress [59].

Emotional or behavioral problems are probably based on the maladaptive and irrational beliefs about selves, world, and life. The results of an unpublished study showed that people with high levels of distress presented more maladaptive cognitions, irrational beliefs, and dysfunctional attitudes, while having a diminished unconditional acceptance of self, when compared to people with low-distress levels [60].

The frequency of negative automatic thoughts on self is theoretically associated with depression. Parents' mean scores indicated a high level of negative automatic thoughts. For the irrational beliefs measured by ABSs, the mean scores were very high, high level of irrationality being usually associated with emotional distress, anxiety, depression, and various cognitive distortions. Both automatic thoughts and irrational beliefs correlate positively and statistically significant with all measured scores of emotional distress. Self-efficacy represents a person belief that their actions can be/are responsible for the success of a particular activity. Parents reported low to medium levels of self-efficacy. High levels of self-efficacy are positively correlated with unconditional acceptance, optimism, and self-esteem. Studies have shown a negative relation between the levels of anxiety and self-efficacy. It was demonstrated that self-efficacy improved parental well-being [61], but very few studies addressed its impact on parental QoL. Parental self-efficacy in managing their children's problems and dealing with other family problems was found to be an important factor associated with QoL [53, 58].

Coping refers to a person cognitive and behavioral effort to adapt to a stressful situation. Generally, two types of coping strategies are used: problem-oriented (adaptive coping) and emotion-centered (maladaptive coping). Problem-oriented coping strategies address directly the problem causing the stress, while emotion-centered coping involves strategies to reduce the stress created by the problem. Although more studies emphasized the role of coping in parental adjustment, results were conflicting on the specific coping strategies that were associated with QoL due to the variation in the measurements used and in the theoretical conceptualization of coping. Hastings et al. identified four key coping dimensions: active avoidance coping, problem-focused coping, positive coping, and religious/denial coping [62]. Other studies reported that the use of emotion-oriented coping is associated with parents' low quality of life [30, 63]. A chronic and general trend of using suppression as coping strategy may result in increased frequency of the thoughts that the person tries to avoid, and may be a precursor or a maintenance factor to certain psychopathological conditions. Suppression measured by WBSI correlated to all scores of emotional distress. Further research on the relationship between coping dimensions and QoL is necessary to establish which coping styles are helpful when raising a child with ASD. Future studies should aim at distinguishing between ASD and other conditions when examining parental coping and QoL.

The scores reported by the parents on the cognitive coping strategies measured by CERQ showed above average use for catastrophizing, average use for self-blame, acceptance, rumination, refocus on planning, positive reappraisal, putting into perspective, and below average for positive refocusing and blame others. Parents' emotional distress correlated significantly with self-blame, rumination, positive refocusing, catastrophizing, and blame others strategies. For the strategies self-blame, rumination, catastrophizing, and blame others, the positive correlation indicates that their frequent use associated with higher emotional distress levels. The positive refocusing, positive reappraisal, refocus on planning strategies registered negative relationships with different scores of emotional distress, meaning that their frequent use associated with lower emotional distress levels.

The study on parents' irrational beliefs and negative automatic thoughts as mediators of the relationship between the overall assessment of family quality of life and parents' emotional distress showed that of the total effect of the overall assessment of family quality of life on the parents' emotional distress, 38.9% is explained by their negative automatic thoughts and 23% by their irrational cognitions. Therefore, correct identification of parents' irrational cognitions and negative automatic thoughts and their relationship with quality of life (that became the main therapeutic outcome) are essential for adequate family support and therapy efficiency. These results suggest that the development of support services for parents in order to reduce negative automatic thoughts and irrational beliefs could have a beneficial effect on the families' quality of life and level of distress experienced due to raising a child with developmental disorders.

http://dx.doi.org/10.5772/66201

4.2. Study limits

The study is cross-sectional and the results do not allow a causal relationship deduction. Also, the clinical sample size was relatively small. The instruments were filled in by a parent (mother) and the answers reflect its perception on the family quality of life. The parents were asked to answer the questions considering different periods of time (ranging from 2 weeks to the last 2 months) and the reporting accuracy could be reduced. The tested variables were analyzed in relation to the overall assessment of family quality of life. They may have an impact on certain areas or domains included in the family quality of life assessment (e.g., health, financial well-being, etc.), but not change the overall perceived family quality of life. The mediation analyses were also calculated using the overall assessment of family quality of life scores. The psychometric instruments used do not fully identify the emotional regulation mechanisms and some cognitive or noncognitive strategies may be excluded or not considered. Also, emotions and regulation strategies are difficult to separate, but the instruments used were standardized, validated, and proved to be optimal in previous studies. The results will reflect the experience of families of children with ASD and ADHD who receive specialized services in the Child and Adolescent Psychiatry Clinic from Cluj-Napoca and other specialized centers in the country, and that exclude some families with children diagnosed with ASD or ADHD who do not have health insurance, live in rural areas or the financial status does not allow them access to specialized services.

5. Conclusion

There were no statistically significant differences between the levels of emotional distress, negative dysfunctional emotions, worry/anxiety dysfunctional emotions, sadness/depression dysfunctional emotions reported by parents, in relation to the intensity of children's affective, anxiety and behavioral problems. Increased levels of emotional distress may be due to child developmental problems, but it is not specific to the diagnosis. We found significant correlations between the emotional distress reported by the parents and their automatic negative thoughts and irrational cognitions, the relation intensities varying from medium to high [1]. Significant correlations were obtained also for the relationship between parents' emotional distress and the coping strategies: self-blame, rumination, positive refocusing, positive reappraisal, blame others, and catastrophizing. The level of parents' emotional distress proved also to be linked with the use of suppression strategy and self-perceived efficacy. Part of the relationship between the overall assessments of family quality of life with parents' emotional distress was explained by their irrational beliefs and negative automatic thoughts, the mediating effect being partial. In this view, the specialized services should include also interventions for the parents of children with developmental disorders (ASD, ADHD) [1]. Adaptive coping mechanisms, low levels of perceived distress, irrational cognitions, and negative dysfunctional emotions may become relevant outcomes for parents' psychological interventions due to their impact on the assessment of the overall family quality of life.

Future studies should investigate more links between the emotional distress, cognitive strategies used, irrational cognitions, self-efficacy, negative automatic thoughts, and the satisfaction with QoL. These studies should be longitudinal, with large clinical samples and involving different pathologies. Thus, the reported quality of life could be more accurately assessed in the processes of establishing and monitoring the therapeutic outcomes.

Conflict of interests

The authors declare that they have no conflict of interest.

Author details

Elena Predescu* and Roxana Şipoş

*Address all correspondence to: elenepredescu@yahoo.com

Department of Neuroscience, Discipline of Psychiatry and Pediatric Psychiatry, Iuliu Hatieganu University of Medicine and Pharmacy Cluj-Napoca, Romania

References

[1] Sipos. Quality of life, emotion regulation of parents and dimensional diagnosis of children with autism spectrum [dissertation]. http://www.umfcluj.: abstract unpublished doctoral.

[2] Prescott-Allen R. The well-being of nations. Washington, DC: Island Press; 2001.

[3] Campbell A, Converse PE, Rodgers WL. The quality of American life. New York: Russell Sage Foundation; 1976.

[4] Cummins RA. Assessing quality of life. In: Brown RI, editor. Assessing quality of life for people with disabilities: Models, research, and practice. London: Stanley Thornes; 1997. pp. 116–150.

[5] Taillefer MC, Dupuis G, Roberge MA, et al. Health-related quality of life models: Systematic review of the literature. Social Indicators Research. 2003;**64**(2):293–323.

[6] Moon P, Budts W, De Geest S. Critique on the conceptualisation of quality of life: A review and evaluation of different conceptual approaches. International Journal of Nursing Studies. 2006;**43**:891–901.

[7] IASSID World Congress. Quality of life. Journal of Intellectual Disability Research. 2004;**48**(4–5):444–462.

[8] Verdugo MA, Schalock RL, Keith KD, Stancliffe RJ. Quality of life and its measurement: Important principles and guidelines. Journal of Intellectual Disability Research. 2005;**49**(10):707–717.

[9] Inoguchi T, Shin DC. The quality of life in Confucian Asia: From physical welfare to subjective well-being. Social Indicators Research. 2009;**92**(2):183–190.

[10] Cummins RA. Instruments for assessing quality of life. In: Hogg JH, Langa A, editors. Approaches to the assessment of adults with intellectual disabilities: A service providers guide. London: Blackwell; 2004. pp. 130–152.

[11] Cummins RA. Moving from the QOL concept to a theory. Journal of Intellectual Disability Research. 2005;**49**(10):699–706.

[12] Renwick R, Brown I, Raphael D. Quality of life in families that have a son or daughter with a developmental disability. Report to the Ontario ministry of community and social services. Centre for Health Promotion. Toronto: University of Toronto; 1997.

[13] Brown I, Anand S, Fung WLA, Isaacs B, Baum N. Family quality of life: Canadian results from an international study. Journal of Developmental and Physical Disabilities. 2003;**15**(3):207–230.

[14] Hebbeler K, Spiker D, Bailey DB, Scarborough A, Mallik S, Simeonsson R, et al. Early intervention for infants and toddlers with disabilities and their families: Participants, services, and outcomes. Menlo Park: SRI International; 2007.

[15] Brown RI, MacAdam-Crisp J, Wang M, Iarocci G. Family quality of life when there is a child with a developmental disability. Journal of Policy and Practice in Intellectual Disabilities. 2006;**3**:238–245.

[16] Brown TA. Confirmatory factor analysis for applied research. New York: Guildford; 2006.

[17] Aznar AS, Castanon DG. Quality of life from the point of view of Latin American families: A participative research study. Journal of Intellectual Disability Research. 2005;**49**:784–788.

[18] Hoffman L, Marquis JG, Poston DJ, Summers JA, Turnbull AP. Assessing family outcomes: Psychometric evaluation of the family quality of life scale. Journal of Marriage and Family. 2006;**68**:1069–1083.

[19] Summers JA, Poston D, Turnbull AP, Marquis J, Hoffman L, Mannan H, et al. Conceptualizing and measuring family quality of life. Journal of Intellectual Disability Research. 2005;**49**:777–783.

[20] Cummins RA. Living with support in the community: Predictors of satisfaction with life. Mental Retardation and Developmental Disabilities Research Reviews. 2001;**7**:99–104.

[21] Turnbull AP, Summers JA, Lee SH, Kyzar K. Conceptualization and measurement of family outcomes associated with families of individuals with intellectual disabilities. Mental Retardation and Developmental Disabilities Research Reviews. 2007;**13**:346–356.

[22] Hastings RP, Daley D, Burns C, Beck A. Maternal distress and expressed emotion: Crosssectional and longitudinal relationships with behavior problems of children with intellectual disabilities. American Journal on Mental Retardation. 2006;**111**:48–61.

[23] Benson RP. The impact of child symptom severity on depressed mood among parents of children with ASD: The mediating role of stress proliferation. Journal of Autism and Developmental Disorders. 2006;**36**:685–695.

[24] McStay R, Trembath D, Dissanayake C. Stress and family quality of life in parents of children with autism spectrum disorder: Parent gender and the double ABCX model. Journal of Autism and Developmental Disorders. 2014;**44**:3101–3118.

[25] Tung LC, Huang CY, Tseng MH, Yen HC, Tsai YP, Lin YC, et al. Correlates of health-related quality of life and the perception of its importance in caregivers of children with autism. Research in Autism Spectrum Disorders. 2014;**8**:1235–1242.

[26] Lee GK, Lopata C, Volker MA, Thomeer ML, Nida RE, Toomey JA, et al. Health-related quality of life of parents of children with high functioning autism spectrum disorders. Focus on Autism and Other Developmental Disabilities. 2009;**24**:227–239.

[27] Johnson N, Frenn M, Feetham S, Simpson P. Autism spectrum disorder: Parenting stress, family functioning and health-related quality of life. Families, System, & Health. 2011;**29**:232–252.

[28] Ozturk Y, Riccadonna S, Venuti P. Parenting dimensions in mothers and fathers of children with autism spectrum disorders. Research in Autism Spectrum Disorders. 2014;**8**:1295–1306.

[29] Sanders JL, Morgan SB. Family stress and management as perceived by parents of children with autism or Down syndrome: Implications for intervention. Child and Family Behavior Therapy. 1997;**19**:15–32.

[30] Smith LE, Seltzer MM, Tager-flusberg H, Greenberg JS, Carter AS. A comparative analysis of well-being and coping among mothers of toddlers and mothers of adolescents with ASD. Journal of Autism and Developmental Disorders. 2008;**38**:876–889.

[31] Wallace AE, Anderson GM, Dubrow R. Obstetric and parental psychiatric variables as potential predictors of autism severity. Journal of Autism and Development Disorders. 2008;**38**:1542–1554.

[32] Daniels JL, Forssen U, Hultman CM, et al. Parental psychiatric disorders associated with autism spectrum disorders in the offspring. Parental psychiatric disorders associated with autism spectrum disorders in the offspring. Pediatric. 2008;**121**:1357–1362.

[33] Leavy RL. Social support and psychological disorder: A review. Journal of Community Psychology. 1983;**11**:3–21.

[34] Reed P, Osborne L. Diagnostic practice and its impacts on parental health and child behavior problems in autism spectrum disorders. Archives of Disease in Childhood. 2012;**97**:927–931.

[35] Khanna R, Madhavan SS, Smith JM, Patrick HJ, Tworek C, Becker-Cottrill B. Assessment of health-related quality of life among primary caregivers of children with autism spectrum disorders. Journal of Autism and Developmental Disorders. 2011;**41**:1214–1227.

[36] Folkman S, Lazarus RS. An analysis of coping in a middle-aged community sample. Journal of Health and Social Behavior. 1980;**21**:219–239.

[37] Hastings RP, Kovshoff H, Ward NJ, degli Espinosa F, Brown T, Remington B. Systems analysis of stress and positive perceptions in mothers and fathers of pre-school children with autism. Journal of Autism and Developmental Disorders. 2005;**35**:635–644.

[38] Friedman RJ, Chase-Lansdale PL. Chronic adversities. In: M. Rutter, E. Taylor, editors. Child and adolescent psychiatry. 4th Ed. London: Blackwell Publishing; 2002. pp. 261–276.

[39] Kuhlthau K, Orlich F, Hall AT, Sikora D, Kovacs AE, Delahaye J, Clemons ET. Health-related quality of life in children with autism spectrum disorders: Results from the autism treatment network. Journal of Autism and Development Disorder. 2010;**40**:721–729.

[40] Storch EA, Merlo LJ, Lack C, Milsom VA, Geffken GR, Goodman WK, et al. Quality of life in youth with tourette's syndrome and chronic tic disorder. Journal of Clinical Child and Adolescent Psychology: The Official Journal for the Society of Clinical Child and Adolescent Psychology, American Psychological Association, Division 53. 2007;**36**(2):217–227.

[41] Allik H, Larsson JO, Smedje H. Health-related quality of life in parents of school-age children with Asperger syndrome or high-functioning autism. Health and Quality of Life Outcomes. 2006;**4**:1.

[42] Stuart M, McGrew JH. Caregiver burden after receiving a diagnosis of autism spectrum disorder year. Research in Autism Spectrum Disorder. 2009;**3**:86–97.

[43] Altiere MJ, von Kluge S. Family functioning and coping behaviors in parents of children with autism. Journal of Child and Family Studies. 2009;**18**:83–92.

[44] Osborne LA, Reed P. The relationship between parenting stress and behavior problems of children with autistic spectrum disorders. Exceptional Children. 2009;**76**(1):54–73.

[45] Sipos R, Predescu E, Muresan G, Iftene F. The evaluation of family quality of life of children with autism spectrum disorder and attention deficit hyperactive disorder. Applied Medical Informatics. 2012;**30**:1–8.

[46] Predescu E, Şipoş R. Cognitive coping strategies, emotional distress and quality of life in mothers of children with ASD and ADHD—A comparative study in a Romanian population sample. Open Journal of Psychiatry. 2013;**3**:11–17.

[47] Achenbach TM, Rescorla LA. Manual for ASEBA school-age forms and profiles. Burlington: University of Vermont, Research Center for Children, Youth, and Families; 2000.

[48] Garnefski N, Kraaij V, Spinhoven P. Negative life events, cognitive emotion regulation and emotional problems. Personality and Individual Differences. 2001;**30**:1311–1327. DOI: 10.1016/S0191-8869(00)00113-6

[49] Garnefski N, van den Kommer T, Kraaij V, Teerds J, Legerstee J, Onstein E. The relationship between cognitive emotion regulation strategies and emotional problems. European Journal of Personality. 2002;**16**:403–420. DOI: 10.1002/per.458

[50] Isaacs BJ, Brown I, Brown RI, Baum N, Myerscough T, Neikrug S, Roth D, Shearer J, Wang M. The international family quality of life project: Goals and description of a survey tool. Journal of Policy and Practice in Intellectual Disabilities. 2007;**4**:177–185. DOI: 10.1111/j.1741-1130.2007.00116.x

[51] Hsiao YJ. Pathways to mental health-related quality of life for parents of children with autism spectrum disorder: roles of parental stress, children's performance, medical support, and neighbour support. Research in Autism Spectrum Disorders. 2016;**23**:122–130.

[52] Totsika V, Hastings RP, Emerson E, Berridge DM, Lancaster GA. Behavior problems at 5 years of age and maternal mental health in autism and intellectual disability. Journal of Abnormal Child Psychology. 2011;**39**(8):1137–1147.

[53] Bourke-Taylor H, Pallant J, Law M, Howie L. Predicting mental health status of mothers of school-aged children with developmental disabilities: The relative contribution of child, maternal and environmental factors. Developmental Medicine and Child Neurology. 2012;**54**:23.

[54] Blacher J, McIntyre LL. Syndrome specificity and behavioural disorders in young adults with intellectual disability: Cultural differences in family impact. Journal of Intellectual and Developmental Disabilities. 2006;**50**:184–198.

[55] Hastings RP, Johnson E. Stress in UK families conducting intensive home-based behavioral intervention for their young child with autism. Journal of Autism and Developmental Disorders. 2001;**31**:327–336.

[56] Bromley J, Hare D, Davison K, Emerson E. Mothers supporting children with autistic spectrum disorders: Social support, mental health status and satisfaction with services. Autism. 2004;**8**:409–423.

[57] Meadan H, Halle JW, Ebata AT. Families with children who have autism spectrum disorders: Stress and support. Exceptional Children. 2010;**77**(1):7–36.

[58] Vasilopoulou E, Nisbet J. The quality of life of parents of children with autism spectrum disorder: A systematic review. Research in Autism Spectrum Disorders. 2016;**23**:36–49.

[59] Hoffman CD, Sweeney DP, Hodge D, Lopez-Wagner MC, Looney L. Parenting stress and closeness mothers of typically developing children and mothers of children with autism. Focus on Autism and Other Developmental Disabilities. 2009;**24**(3):178–187.

[60] Opriş D, Macavei B. The profile of emotional distress. Cluj-Napoca: Romanian Psychological Testing Services; 2007.

[61] Jones TL, Prinz R.J. Potential roles of parental self-efficacy in parent and child adjustment: A review. Clinical Psychology Review. 2005;**25**(3):341–363.

[62] Hastings RP, Kovshoff H, Brown T, Ward NJ, degli Espinosa F, et al. Coping strategies in mothers and fathers of preschool and school-age children with autism. Autism. 2005;**9**(4):377–391.

[63] van der Veek S, Kraaij V, Garnefski N. Cognitive coping strategies and stress in parents of children with down syndrome: A prospective study. Intellectual and Developmental Disabilities. 2009;**47**:295–306. DOI: 10.1352/1934-9556-47.4.295

Section 4

Neurobiology, Genetics and Autism

Chapter 8

The Genetic and Epigenetic Basis Involved in the Pathophysiology of ASD: Therapeutic Implications

Maria Carmen Carrascosa-Romero and
Carlos De Cabo-De La Vega

Additional information is available at the end of the chapter

http://dx.doi.org/10.5772/66854

Abstract

The prevalence of autism has increased in an exponential way in the past few years. Many monogenetic mutations as well as copy number variants and single nucleotide polymorphisms have been associated with autism spectrum disorders (ASD), a large proportion of which occur in genes associated with synaptogenesis and synaptic function. However, the increase in appearance of genetic alterations does not explain the etiology of an elevated number of ASD cases. Recent research is now focusing on the role of environmental/epigenetic factors, which by themselves and/or in combination with classical genetic factors, may be the root cause of a large number of ASDs. In this chapter we review the current literature regarding the epigenetic changes involved in ASD, including their possible mechanisms of action such as oxidative stress, altered fatty acid metabolism, mitochondrial dysfunction, DNA methylation and histone methylation (via the one-carbon metabolism cycle), histone variants, and ATP-dependent chromatin remodeling. We discuss possible new biochemical markers related to autism as well as new lines of research for therapeutic targets.

Keywords: ASD, autism, children, betaine, choline, genetics, epigenetics, fatty acid, lipid, one-carbon metabolism cycle, PUFAs, peroxidation, methylation, mitochondrial dysfunction, oxidative stress, phospholipases, research

1. Introduction

Autism spectrum disorder (ASD) etiopathogenesis occurs result of a complex, engaging multiple environmental factors and epigenetic modifications, interacting with the genetic basis of the developmental processes. Although the ADS-risk genes are numerous, and many of them have a dual function involved in different neural networks, they seem to converge in a limited number of molecular pathways. It has been proposed that genes implicated in "monogenic" variants of syndromic and nonsyndromic ASD converge on molecular pathways and mechanisms related to synaptic dysfunction also known as "developmental synaptopathy." The interplay between mutations in different genes can produce "idiopathic" autism, but the exposure to environmental modifiers as well as epigenetic factors may add up to a varying expression of autistic features, allowing to define autism as "synaptic and chromatin-remodeling disorders."

Congenital epigenetic diseases are a newly delineated group of multiple congenital anomalies, intellectual disabilities, and ASD syndromes resulting from "Classical imprinting disorders" and "Mendelian disorders of the epigenetic machinery." The advances in the identification of the DNA-methylation level of specific genes, histones modifications (highlighted dysregulation of histone methylation as a major contributing factor), histone variants, and ATP-dependent chromatin remodeling complexes throw light about the epigenetic effects of nongenetic biological risk factors and environmental factors in ASD.

Currently, new biochemical markers have been implicated in the etiology of autism, such as increased oxidative stress and lipid peroxidation, phospholipase release of fatty acid, and the formation of toxic metabolites, mitochondrial dysfunction, or alteration of DNA-methylation. In addition, other relevant epigenetic mechanisms such as impaired methylation via the "one-carbon metabolism cycle" including the folate metabolism, the methionine-homocysteine remethylation cycle (involving choline and betaine), and the transsulfuration pathway also help to complete the difficult puzzle of autism.

Therefore, epigenetic mechanisms constitute new lines of research and may open the door for new targets in the treatment of autism. The epigenetic changes are potentially reversible, and, therefore, a thorough understanding of these modifications may identify new therapeutic targets for the disease. So finally several questions arise: Is autism also an acquired and therefore preventable, treatable, and potentially curable epigenetic disease? Could alteration in diet and fat supplementation result in neuronal repair and reverse the deficit in autism? How could this knowledge be applied to clinical practice?

In this chapter, we conducted an updated review of the role of genetic and epigenetic changes involved in the pathophysiology of ASD including their possible mechanisms of action. We also included the latest lines, perspectives, and future directions of therapeutic approaches.

2. The etiopathogenesis of ASD

The autism, a debilitating neurological handicap in children, is a highly heterogeneous set of disorders with wide variations in symptom severity, intellectual level, and functional disability. Classically in DSM IV-TR [1] "*Pervasive developmental disorders*" (PDD) encompass a heterogeneous group of children characterized by severe and pervasive impairment in several areas of development: (1) reciprocal social interaction skills, (2) communication skills, and (3) the presence of stereotyped behavior, interests, and activities. The qualitative impairments that define these conditions are distinctly deviant relative to the individual's developmental level or mental age. The specific disorders included five subtypes in this section: autistic disorder (AD), Rett's disorder (RD), childhood disintegrative disorder (CDD), Asperger's disorder, and pervasive developmental disorder not otherwise specified (PDD-NOS). These disorders are usually evident in the first years of life and are often associated with some degree of *"intellectual disability."*

At present, a new edition of the DSM ("Diagnostic and Statistical Manual of Mental Disorders," from the American Psychiatric Association) has been published: DSM-5® [2]. In the new DSM-5 there is a single category of ASD (autism spectrum disorder) instead of five subtypes, and has deleted the term "pervasive developmental disorders." Scientific evidence and clinical practice show that a single spectrum better reflects the symptom presentation, time course, and response to treatment. ASDs is a new DSM-5® name that reflects a scientific consensus of four previously separate five subtypes disorders, and are actually a single condition. The three domains of DSM IV are combined into two core domains: (a) Deficits in social communication and social interaction. The rationale is that deficits in communication and social behaviors are inseparable. Social communication domain will be created by merger of key symptoms from the DSM-IV social and communication domains. This de-emphasizes language skills not employed in the context of social communication. (b) The second major criterion remains restricted repetitive behaviors, interests, and activities (RRBs).

In multiple communities of the United States (CDC surveillance data, 2010) [3], the overall prevalence of ASD was 14.7 per 1000 (1 in 68) children aged 8 years. Overall ASD prevalence estimates varied among sites from at least 5.7 to 21.9 per 1000 children aged 8 years. Consistent with previous reports, findings were marked by significant variations in ASD prevalence by geographic area, sex, race/ethnicity, and level of intellectual ability. The extent to which this variation might be attributable to diagnostic practices, underrecognition of ASD symptoms in some racial/ethnic groups, socioeconomic disparities in access to services, and regional differences in clinical or school-based practices that might influence the findings in this report is unclear.

The importance of accurately identifying individuals with autism has never been greater, particularly given the growing prevalence [4], considerable family and societal costs [5], and recognized importance of early diagnosis and intervention. The ASD frequency has been increasing for decades, with an astonishing 556% reported increase in pediatric prevalence between 1991 and 1997 (a prevalence higher than that of spina bifida, cancer, or Down syndrome). Even though researchers cannot agree on whether the trend is a result of increased awareness, improved detection and changing diagnostic criteria with expanding definition and reduced stringency of diagnostic criteria, rather than to new environmental influences and other factors of unknown nature [6, 7]. The classification systems used strongly affect prevalence studies, and is important to consider the changes that have occurred at this level when analyzing the possible causes of the increase in previously known as *pervasive developmental disorders* [8]. But this increased ASD prevalence cannot be attributed entirely to "nonetiological factors" such as changes in reporting practices, diagnostic ascertainment, and "diagnostic substitution" (i.e., ID diagnoses decreased at the same time ASD diagnoses increased) [9–11].

Because people with autism can have very different features and symptoms with very high degree of phenotypic heterogeneity, autism is a multifactorial condition and is thought of as a spectrum disorder [12, 13]. Autism is one of the most complex heritable disorders, and a paradigmatic complex genetic disorder, with convincing evidence for genetic factors and little or no support for the influence of the environment factors [14]. However, it is essential that the ASD not be reflected alone in overly restrictive genetic approaches if we want to better understand its pathogenesis. Today, different studies support that the etiopathogenesis of ADS involves an interaction between both susceptible genetic loci and a wide range of environmental risk factors on the developmental trajectory. So the pathogenesis of ASD is considered an authentic "puzzle," for a multifactorial threshold model underlying ASD with all types of genetic variation (SNV/indel/CNV in coding and noncoding DNA, germline, somatic, epigenetic) and environmental factors (the most significant: toxic, immune dysregulation, and nutritional status) involved in clinical, neuropsychological, and neurobiological perspectives [13, 15–18].

Since there are no definitive biological markers of autism, for a majority of cases, diagnosis depends on a range of behavioral signs. But advances in system biology are becoming strategic for carrying out knowledge on the ASD etiology and for early diagnosis. The most relevant metabolic pathways and discriminant metabolites in ASD belong among other, amino acid metabolism, antioxidant status, mitochondrial metabolism, nicotinic acid metabolism, and altered fatty acid metabolic pathways. So, for the study of this "autism epidemic" it is of great interest to identify risk factors (genetic and nongenetic) as well as metabolic routes that can contribute to ASD; but not separately if not collectively and simultaneously through common pathways, allowing to insert the pieces of the ASD puzzle together. That is, from the approach to the different disciplines: genomics, epigenomics, metabolomics, and environmental metabolomics.

3. Genetic in ASD

Children with dysmorphic features, congenital anomalies, intellectual disability, or family members with developmental disorders are those most likely to benefit from extensive medical testing and genetic consultation. Increased diagnosis of ASD associated with genetic abnormalities has allowed its new specification in the DSM5: "associated with known medical or genetic condition." However, for children with "nonsyndromic or idiopathic" autism the studies of genetic risk factors have been less conclusive

3.1. ASD associated with "known medical or genetic condition"

It is known that several monogenic disorders (Mendelian disorders) are associated with autism. The most common of these single-gene defects, including CGG trinucleotide repeats within the FMR1 gene as the cause of Fragile X syndrome, mutations in the *MECP2* gene in Rett syndrome and related disorders, tuberous sclerosis, and PTEN mutation account for but a small minority of cases (for up to 5% of ASDs) [19]. Less often and among other genetic diseases consistently associated with autism include: rare genetic developmental disorder

http://dx.doi.org/10.5772/66854

(*inter alia* examples the Cohen syndrome caused by a mutation in the vacuolar protein sorting 13B (*VPS13B*) gene on locus 8q22-8q23, or the Smith-Lemli-Opitz syndrome caused by mutations in the *DHCR7* gene on locus 11q13.4 leading to deficiency of the enzyme 3 beta-hydroxysterol-delta 7-reductase); and metabolic diseases like phenylketonuria, adenylosuccinate lyase deficiency, or mucopolysaccharidosis III (Sanfilippo syndrome). (For more comprehensive listing see [20].)

There are also many anecdotal reports of autism with visible chromosomopathies [21, 22], and Down syndrome have been found with high rates of ASD of up to 42% [23]; and well-known microdeletion syndromes like 22q11 deletion syndrome divided into distinct syndromes (e.g., DiGeorge syndrome, velocardiofacial syndrome, and cardiofacial syndrome) in which more than 40% meet the criteria for either ASD, ADHD, or both [24]; as well as Angelman syndrome, or Smith-Magenis syndrome, are well known autism. Although the latter mentioned can be produced by different genetic mechanisms, Angelman syndrome is caused by deletion of the 15q11.2-q13 critical region (60–75%), paternal uniparental disomy (2–5%), imprinting defect (2–5%), and mutation in the *UBE3A* gene (10%); and Smith-Magenis syndrome is caused either by a 17p11.2 deletion encompassing the retinoic acid-induced 1 (RAI1) gene (90%) or a mutation of the gene (10%) [25].

Currently, these diagnosable medical conditions, cytogenetic abnormalities, and single-gene defects together account for <10% of cases of ASD. The latest advances made in genetics and technology, mainly the widespread use of molecular techniques by chromosomal microarray studies have increased the diagnostic cost-effectiveness of conventional techniques (karyotype, subtelomeric analyses, etc.) from 3–5% to 30–40% in patients with developmental delay/intellectual disability (DD/ID) or ASD, describing numerous genetic alterations. Overall, identified genetic causes of autism can be classified as single-gene disorders (5%), cytogenetically visible chromosomal abnormalities (5%), and copy number variants (CNV) (10–20%) [26].

Chromosomal microarray analysis (CMA) is increasingly utilized for genetic testing of individuals with unexplained DD/ID, multiple congenital anomalies (MCA), and has become increasingly important in the assessment of patients' ASD. CMA was initially restricted to ASD patients with specific additional phenotypic characteristics or comorbidities (DD/ID or MCA); at present, it has been established as the general recommendation and consensus statement that CMA should be offered as a first-tier diagnostic test in the assessment of patients with ASD in place of G-banded karyotyping [27]. Since CMA is higher (8.9%) than conventional karyotyping (1.6%) and other genetic analyses (3.8%) they are changing the frequency of the causes of ASD [28].

CNV is the most prevalent type of structural variation in the human genome [29] and they have been described as having strong association of "*de novo*" CNV with autism [30]. So, at least 8% of sporadic ASD cases carried a *de novo* CNV and they are clarifying the etiology for many cases of autism previously considered idiopathic [31, 32]. The *de novo* nature of these CNVs, together with their absence in the general population, suggests they represent a class of highly deleterious and highly penetrant mutations. Smaller microdeletions or microduplications may occur within this highly dynamic with frequent rearrangements using alternative low-copy repeats (LCRs), also known as segmental duplications (SDs), as recombination substrates during nonallelic homologous recombination (NAHR).

The presence of these sequences in LCRs concentrated on "hotspots," in recurring break points, it confers great instability, with frequent deletions, duplications, and the formation of small chromosome markers, since these repeated sequences can lead to incorrect meiotic recombination by NAHR and can be interchromosomal (between homologous chromosomes) or intrachromosomal (in the same chromosome); and every day are described new loci for recurrent NAHR-mediated CNV [33]. Specially "recurrent microdeletions" in ASD include: 22q13 deletion or Phelan-McDermid syndrome, 15q13.2-q13.3 (BP4–BP5) deletion, 16p11.2 deletion syndrome, 17q12 deletion. And "recurrent microduplications" like: duplication of 15q11-q13 or Dup15q syndrome in Prader Willi/Angelman region; duplication 7q11.23 in Williams's syndrome region; duplication of 22q11.2 in DiGeorge syndrome region (for review see [34]). Some of the genes contained within the *de novo* CNVs we identified are good candidates for autism [35]. Although specific "rare *de novo*" CNVs are individually infrequent, but combined they account for a significant fraction of patients with autism and their study could contribute to a better understanding of the phenotypic manifestations in ASD [36, 37].

We want to highlight as Phelan-McDermid syndrome (22q13.3 deletion syndrome) with a disruption of the *SHANK3* gene, it is believed to be underdiagnosed due to lack of specific clinical features, and because until recently it has inadequate genetic testing [38]. So when ASD is associated with intellectual disability, *SHANK3* mutations or deletions have been found in up to 2.3% of cases of ASD individuals [39].

The region 15q11 contains a number of LCRs (regions of repetitive DNA which are susceptible to rearrangements) known as breakpoint (bp) bp1, bp2, bp3, bp4, and bp5; and is especially linked to autism. The 15q11.2 BP1-BP2 microdeletion is emerging as a recognized new syndrome, its appearance ranging from 0.57 to 1.27% of patients sent for microarray analysis. Its expression can be variable: patients may present with developmental and language delay, neurobehavioral disturbances, and ASD in 27% of patients. The BP1-BP2 region include four genes (*TUBGCP5*, *CYFIP1*, *NIPA1*, and *NIPA2*) which are not subject to imprinting (a differential expression depending on maternal or paternal origin gene) and therefore with expression biallelicis [40]. Larger deletions involving BP3 (BP1-BP3 and BP2-BP3) cause either Prader-Willi or Angelman syndrome (PWS/AS) depending on which parent the deleted chromosome is inherited from (paternal or maternal, respectively). And also worth noting is duplications of the chromosome 15q11-q13.1 region (Dup15q syndrome) typically of maternal origin, which are associated with an estimated 1–3% of all autism cases, making this CNV one of the most frequent chromosome abnormalities associated with ASD. The region including ubiquitin protein ligase E3A (*UBE3A*)—the gene disrupted in Angelman syndrome—is involved in neural function and may play important roles in the neurobehavioral phenotypes associated with Dup15q syndrome. Genome-wide analyses suggest that common neuronal pathways may be disrupted in both the AS and Dup15q syndromes [31].

3.2. Genetic factors in ASD "nonsyndromic or idiopathic"

The concordance remarkably from 60 to 92% in monozygotic twins and from 0 to 10% in dizygotic pairs suggests a strong genetic component [41, 42]. Nevertheless, the recurrence rate of ADS in siblings of affected children is approximately 2% [43], which is 16 times higher than in the general population but much lower than in single-gene diseases, so the underlying genetic determinants are still largely unknown [41]. Recent advances in genetic screening (as next-generation sequencing, NGS, and whole-exome sequencing, WES) and systems biology approaches have extended our knowledge of the genetic etiology of ASD, and may lead to the discovery of underlying genetic factors for ASD, and may thereby identify novel therapeutic targets for this disorder [35].

3.2.1. Linkage and candidate gene association studies

During the past decade, research about the genetic variations that underlie susceptibility to ASD has been focusing on linkage and candidate gene studies. Even though genetics is considered to play a significant role in ASD, until recently solely 16–17% of autistics are carriers of a known genetic variant. A large number of linkage studies have been conducted and have identified possible susceptibility loci on multiple chromosomes. Although there is no full agreement among different studies, certain regions, such as those on chromosomes 2q, 3, 7q, 11, 16, 17q, and 19, have been involved in multiple occasions (for review see [44]), but only few common alterations were recognized as candidate genes in association studies including support from meta-analysis [45, 46]. So, only a few loci show recurrent mutations (particularly the 7q22-q37 and the 11p12-p13 locus) [47, 48], and these "recurrent mutations" account for only about 1–2% of patients [49]. The studies have identified several ASD candidates including genes encoding neuroligins [50], neurexins [47], or *SHANK3* [51].

This is now changing, linkage data with WES data has achieved great success for identifying many Mendelian disease genes [52–55] and the number of such studies is increasing gradually (for review see [35]). Studies carried out in twins, in which one sibling had a diagnosis of autism and the other was not affected, bioinformatics and gene ontological analyses implicate genes which are involved in nervous system development, inflammation, and cytoskeletal organization, in addition to genes which may be relevant to gastrointestinal or other physiological symptoms often associated with autism; and these processes may be modulated by cholesterol/steroid metabolism, especially at the level of androgenic hormones (higher levels of testosterone in the autistic sibling) [56].

3.2.2. Genome-wide association studies (GWAS)

The genetic architecture of ASD comprises a diversity of rare single nucleotide variants (SNVs), copy number variations (CNVs), chromosomal abnormalities, and common polymorphic variations [57–59]. Genome-wide association study (GWAS) is an examination of a genome-wide set of genetics variants in different individuals to see if any variant is associated with a trait. Advances in genomic technology, including GWAS of single nucleotide polymorphisms (SNPs), and CNV studies, allow the detection of *de novo* or inherited mutations in the coding regions and new candidate genes for ASD. Principally, CNVs implicate many ASD-associated genes like *CHD2, HDAC4, GDI1 SETD5, MIR137, HDAC9, SHANK2, SYNGAP1, DLGAP2*, and the *X-linked DDX53-PTCHD1* locus [60, 61]. But this only represents a selected sample of examples of the numerous studies in this field; inasmuch as these CNVs are widely distributed across the genome, at more than 100 different loci. The statistical distribution of influences across the genome suggests that hundreds of different human genes can mutate to influence autism risk [53]. Also, there is recent interest in rare highly penetrant SNV analogous to these traditional genetic models that may influence risk for "idiopathic autism." SNVs most commonly identified in ASD cohort including among others: *NRXN1, SHANK3, CTNNA3, CHD8, SCN1A* and *2A, ADNP, PTEN, DYRK1A*, and *SYNGAP1* [52, 53, 55, 62, 63]. Genes affected by *de novo* CNVs and/or loss-of-function SNVs converged on networks related to neuronal signaling and development, synapse function, and chromatin regulation [61].

Up to now, estimates suggest that CNVs and SNVs acting in dominant, recessive, or X-linked models might account for a small proportion of ASD (as many as 15% of cases), and common SNP can account for nearly half the variation in autism. Several GWASs [61, 64–66] have been performed to decipher the genetic etiology of autism that is attributable to common variants (i.e., SNPs) with only a few variants having shown significant associations and replicated in an independent population or in endophenotypes. Based on results from individual SNPs and their *en masse* effect on risk, as inferred from the allele score results, it is reasonable to conclude that common variants affect the risk for ASD but their individual effects are modest.

3.2.3. Molecular pathways ASD: "developmental synaptopathies"

As it has been mentioned previously, recent advancements in NGS and WES have enabled the discovery of an overwhelming number of *de novo* mutations (from 500 to 1000 genes) distributed along all chromosomes that confer a risk for ASD demonstrating a heterogeneous genetic landscape [35]. For an up-to-date database of ASD-associated genes, the reader is referred to the SFARI Gene database (Simons Foundation Autism Research Initiative; https://gene.sfari.org/). As of June 2016, there were 826 genes and 2163 CNV loci in this database. This resource reviews the evidence for each gene implicated in autism susceptibility and assigns a score, from "Category 1" ("high confidence," with 16 listed: *ADNP, ANK2, ARID1B, ASH1L, ASXL3, CHD8, DYRK1A, GRIN2B, POGZ, PTEN, SCN2A, SETD5, SHANK3, SUV420H1, SYNGAP1*, and *TBR1* genes), to "Category 6" ("not supported"). Genes associated with syndromic ASD are categorized separately ("Category S," including 78 genes, among the best known are: *FMR1* cause Fragile X syndrome, *MECP2* cause Rett syndrome, *SHANK3* is part of a multigenic region that is deleted in Phelan-McDermid syndrome, *UBE3A* present in common 15q11-13 duplications syndrome or deletion in Angelman syndrome, *RERE* in 1p36 deletion syndrome, *PTEN* in Cowden syndrome, etc.).

Fortunately, although the ADS-risk genes are numerous, and many of them have a dual function involved in different neural networks, they seem to converge in a limited number of molecular pathways [67], allowing the study from single gene to a pathway perspective [68]. So, it has been proposed that, rather than as a result of dysfunction of specific genes, ASD

http://dx.doi.org/10.5772/66854

result in dysfunction of specific genetic pathways [69]. The identified several potential genetic pathways to ASD including wnt signaling during development, synaptic function, chromatin remodeling, mRNA translation, and metabolism seem to converge in common functional pathways affecting neuronal and synaptic homeostasis [70]. Just like that, 88% of high-risk genes for autism influence neural induction and early maturation of the neuroblast. In addition, 80% of these same genes influence later stages of differentiation, including neurite and synapse development [71].

Rare mutations-ASD include mutations in synaptic proteins such as ProSAPs/SHANKS proteins (with a crucial role in the assembly of the postsynaptic density during synaptogenesis, in synaptic plasticity and in the regulation of dendritic spine morphology) [72–74]; synaptic vesicle-associated proteins (*SYN2* gene) [75]; and neuroligins/neurexins (synaptic cell adhesion molecules) for excitatory glutamatergic and inhibitory GABAergic synapses [neurexins (NRXN) (trigger postsynaptic differentiation), and neuroligins (NLGN) (trigger presynaptic differentiation)] [76] and play a pivotal role in synaptic function, especially at GABAergic synapses [77]. It has been shown that many genes associated with ASDs are involved in the neuroligin-neurexin interaction at the glutamate synapse: *NLGN3*, and *NLGN4* on the X chromosome [50, 78, 79], NRXN1 on chromosome 2p16 [80], CNTNAP2 on chromosome 7q35 [81], and *SHANK3* on chromosome 22q13 [51, 82]. Autism-associated *NLGN3* mutations commonly disrupt tonic endocannabinoid signaling, providing evidence that alterations in the endocannabinoid pathway may contribute to autism pathophysiology [83]. Besides the neurotrophic factors as well as the neurotransmitter systems are thought to be good candidates for ASD [84]. Thereby, elevated platelet serotonin (5-HT) in 20–25% of ASD cases points to the 5-HT transporter (*5-HTT*; *SERT*) as a strong candidate gene, and also allelic heterogeneity at serotonin transporter locus (*SLC6A4*) may be connected with susceptibility to autism [85]. Also, it has been implicated in the catecholaminergic pathways (allelic variants in the dopamine decarboxylase (DDC) gene) [86].

It has been proposed that genes involved in "monogenic" forms of syndromic and nonsyndromic ASD converge on common molecular pathways and mechanisms of synaptic dysfunction ("developmental synaptopathies"): control synaptic protein synthesis and degradation with postsynaptic scaffold architecture and neurotransmitter receptors; and that are involved in synaptic development, plasticity, and signaling [87]. Many studies have suggested that neurites and synapses associated gene products, in fact, may be involved in the early stages of neural differentiation normally recognized, resulting in defects of migration and other indications of disturbance to premigratory cell fate determination [88–90].

However, it is yet unclear whether the same genes may performance through rare, highly penetrant mutations and common genetic risk factors. Additionally, although many approaches have attempted to identify "molecular pathways" implicated in ASDs to unify disparate genes, these data have not converged to provide conclusive and well-replicated evidence. How these mutations lead to ASD phenotypes is poorly understood (for review see [91, 92]). Hence, most cases still remain unknown, but potentially, including additional less penetrant rare variants or complex mechanisms, such as gene-gene interaction or gene-environment interaction. In this way, one might conclude that interactions between multiple genes cause "idiopathic" autism, but that "epigenetic dysregulation" and exposure to environmental modifiers might contribute to variable expression of autism-related traits [93] and to significant proportion of ASD cases [94–96].

4. Epigenetic and chromatin structure

Definition: Epigenetics is an important aspect of research in current biology, defined as the study of mitotically and meiotically heritable changes in gene function that are not dependent on DNA sequence [97]. So "an epigenetic trait is a stably heritable phenotype resulting from changes in a chromosome without alterations in the DNA sequence." Epigenetics shows that gene expression undergoes changes more complex than modifications in the DNA sequence; it includes the influence of the environment on the gametes prior to conception. Berger et al. [98] proposed three categories of signals that culminate in the establishment of a stably heritable epigenetic state:

- A signal that we propose to call the "Epigenator," which emanates from the environment and triggers an intracellular pathway.
- An "Epigenetic Initiator" signal, which responds to the Epigenator and is necessary to define the precise location of the epigenetic chromatin environment. The Initiator could be a DNA-binding protein, a noncoding RNA, or any other entity that can define the coordinates of the chromatin structure to be assembled.
- An "Epigenetic Maintainer" signal, which sustains the chromatin environment in the first and subsequent generations.

The molecular basis of epigenetic processes: is complex and this signal involves many different mechanisms, including major epigenetic silencing pathways: DNA methylation, modifications (like methylation and acetylation) of histones (H), positioning of histone variants, and gene regulation by small noncoding RNAs [99].

The study of chromatin structure has taken an important impetus in recent years and has transcended to the point to understand various diseases in humans including ASD. Chromatin is the structure in which the DNA is organized and packed into the nucleus of the eukaryotic cell. The main components of chromatin are DNA and histone proteins; both units are the target of epigenetic modifications. The primary unit is the nucleosome, formed for a segment of DNA (approximately 200 base pairs) wound in sequence around eight histone protein cores (H2A, H2B, H3, and H4), and linker subunit H1 that connects the nucleosomes. A region of chromatin is in a more or less favorable to gene expression depending on the type of sequences that form and also epigenetic modifications at that level state. The regulation mechanism of transcriptional activity is mainly mediated by DNA methylation and chromatin remodeling.

DNA methylation: Methylation of DNA and mainly 5-methylcytosine methylation is a major mechanism of epigenetic gene silencing, essential for cell division and normal development, and plays an important role of key processes including inactivation of the X-chromosome, genomic imprinting, gene silencing, and repression of repetitive elements. DNA methylation may affect the transcription of genes in two ways:

- Directly impede the binding of transcriptional proteins to the gene.
- Methylated DNA may be bound by proteins known as methyl-CpG-binding domain proteins (MBDs) which later recruit additional proteins to the locus, such as histone deacetylases (HDAC) and other chromatin remodeling proteins that can modify histones, thereby forming heterochromatin.

Chromatin remodeling: Modulate chromatin structure and function can involve covalent modification of histones (acetylation, methylation, or ubiquitination of lysine; methylation of arginine; and phosphorylation of serine), the incorporation of histone variants, and noncovalent ATP-dependent chromatin remodeling complexes. One of the most significant epigenetic processes is to strengthen or weaken the interactions between DNA and histones ("histone code" as epigenetic histone chemical modifications in nucleosomes). The regulation of each histone modification requires specific enzymes that add or remove the methyl or acetyl group. The histone modifications affect interactions between nucleosomes and therefore the degree of chromatin condensation, so a region will behave as euchromatin, lightly packed, and accessible to active transcription; or in reverse when the interaction is strong, the histones are attached firmly to the DNA chromatin (heterochromatin), this means in a closed or dormant state, and it is tightly packed and inaccessible to polymerases and therefore not transcribed [100].

In the transition from the closed conformation to a more open chromatin, the interactions between histones and DNA must be dissolved. This process requires epigenetic "writer" as transferases that add specific small molecules such as the methyl and acetyl groups to DNA, or proteins to alter its pack aging proteins—the histones—such as histone acetyltransferases (HATs), histone methyltransferases (HMTs), protein arginine methyltransferases (PRMTs), and kinases lay down epigenetic marks on amino acid residues on histone tails. This modification (e.g., by adding an acetyl group) blocks the ability of the histone to bind DNA and thus making the chromatin more open and is associated with active gene expression. In contrast, epigenetic "eraser" proteins, such as histone deacetylases (HDACs), lysine demethylases (KDMs), and phosphatases catalyse, remove the epigenetic marks from the histones restoring the interaction between the histone and DNA, leaving the DNA once again in a closed conformation tends to be present in transcriptionally silent regions. The epigenetic "readers" (such as proteins containing bromodomains, chromodomains, and Tudor domains) are transcriptional regulators proteins that do not alter the histone but rather detect the acetyl group within the histones.

Proteins that contain reader domains can be usually classified into four groups: chromatin architectural proteins (induce chromatin compaction), chromatin remodeling enzymes (prompt a more open chromatin architecture driven by the energy of ATP hydrolysis), chromatin modifiers, and adaptor proteins that recruit other machinery involved in gene expression. Enzymes which "write" or "erase" epigenetic marks may also contain such reader domains, leading to the coordination of "read-write" or "read-erase" epigenetic processes [101]. The proper gene expression requires the attainment of a balance between the activities of the two opposing systems (writers and erasers) and subsequently the placement of their respective marks, which ensures that the appropriate composition of chromatin is present at particular gene promoters. Opposite histone systems are susceptible to be dynamic, allowing the cell to quickly respond to changes in environmental signals by altering gene expression at specific loci. Epigenetic machinery is highly redundant, perhaps reflecting the critical importance of maintaining this balance in many different cell types

5. Epigenetic changes involved in ASD

As we mentioned previously, the rates of ADS diagnosis have dramatically increased in the past three decades to constitute "autism epidemic" and have been well documented in public health surveillance studies [102]. New advances in genetic studies (*Linkage and candidate gene association studies and GWAS*) identifying multifarious loci associated with ASD, especially mutations in genes encoding synapse-associated proteins (Shank/ProSAP proteins, synaptic vesicle-associated proteins, synaptic cell adhesion molecules, neurotransmitter…); however so far, genetic analyses have mainly been on the ~1.5% of the genome encoding genes. Although genetic contributions to autism etiology are well accepted, genetics alone does not explain the underlying cause in a substantial proportion of cases. So, the rising prevalence and inconsistent finding from genetic studies suggest a role for interactions between susceptibility genes and relevance of environmental factors and other potential contributors. Now there is convincing evidence that gene interactions with the environment are important in the etiology of ASD. However, the mechanisms by which environmental factors interact with genetic susceptibilities to confer individual risk for ASD remain significant knowledge emptiness in the field. It has been suggested that environmental factors linked to epigenetic mechanisms as DNA methylation and/or histone modifications; they may be involved in ASD by changes into the function of the genome.

A number of rare Mendelian disorders, such as Rett syndrome (by mutation in *MECP2*, locus Xq28), Cornelia de Lange syndrome-2 (by mutations of the *SMC1A* gene locus Xp11.2 encodes a subunit of the cohesin complex, essential for sister chromatid cohesion during mitosis, with broad roles in chromosome condensation, and DNA repair), and Coffin-Siris syndrome (chromatin remodeling complex gene *ARID1B* which encodes an epigenetic modifier of chromatin structure) have pointed to the importance of DNA methylation and chromatin remodeling factors, mainly histones in human brain development. At present the identification of other ATP-dependent chromatin remodelers (e.g., *CHD8*) and transcription factors (e.g., *ADNP, ASH1L, FOXG1*), which are also typically involved in regulation of gene expression but without alterations in the DNA sequence, have aroused the interest toward the epigenetics of autism and how environmental factors may be playing a key role in transcriptional regulatory influences [94–96, 103, 104].

Recent advances in genomic technologies allow a position to initiate large-scale studies of human disease-associated epigenetic variation, specifically variation in DNA methylation, and highlight the contribution of noncoding variants to the etiology of ASD. Epigenetic state in ASD, mainly epigenetic mark of DNA CpG methylation, can be used as biomarker of disease risk, diagnosis, prognosis, and response to treatments; but also, clues to the causal factors and mechanisms of the disorder [105]. So, aberrant methylation profiles in 1.1% of

ASD cases have been reported [13]. A significant overrepresentation of genes with functions in chromatin regulation and early developmental expression was found in ASD probands but not in unaffected siblings [106]. Also, oxidative protein/DNA damage and DNA hypomethylation (epigenetic alteration) were found in autistic children but not paired siblings or controls [107]. So, nowadays attention has turned to environmental factors but also with epigenetic changes as potential etiological agents predisposing to autism susceptibility. New genetics analyses have displayed a multitude of novel candidate ASD-genes in networks that involve epigenetic change, encoding nuclear factors implicated in chromatin remodeling, histone demethylation, histone variants, and the recognition of DNA methylation [13, 108]. This approach is described as an "epigenome-wide association study" (EWAS) and takes its cue from the association of genetic variability with phenotypes in GWAS. However until today and in contradistinction to GWAS, EWAS are scarce related to ASD (for review see [109]).

Just like that functionally, ASD-risk genes often converge in key molecular pathways early in development, which modulate synaptic transmission but also chromatin remodeling and transcriptional regulation, allowing to define autism as "synaptic and chromatin-remodeling disorders" [110]. All of the above can be added to state that epigenetic changes are potentially reversible, and, therefore, a thorough understanding of these modifications may identify new therapeutic targets for the disease. So finally the question arises: Is autism also an acquired and therefore preventable, treatable, and potentially curable epigenetic disease?

Epigenetic studies besides being keys to the causal factors, also clues to the biomarkers and physiological mechanisms predisposing or resulting from the onset of ASD, and may have an important role in the therapeutic implications. So this chapter will focus on developing the main aspects related to epigenetics of autism, according to the following scheme:

- Congenital epigenetic diseases in ASD:
  - Imprinted-x liability. Sex differences.
  - Classical imprinting disorders.
  - Mendelian ASD disorders of the epigenetic machinery:
    - Mendelian ASD disorders in DNA methylation machinery.
    - Mendelian ASD disorders in the histone machinery.
    - Mendelian ASD disorders in other chromatin remodelers and transcription factors.
- Acquired epigenetics disorders in ASD.

6. Congenital epigenetic diseases in ASD

Congenital epigenetic diseases are a newly delineated group of multiple congenital anomalies, intellectual disabilities, and ASD syndromes resulting from:

- **Classic epigenetic processes:** X chromosome inactivation and genomic imprinting are classic epigenetic processes that cause disease when not appropriately regulated. "Classical imprinting disorders" or epigenetic alterations at specific loci result mainly from disruptions occurring in *cis* (acting in cis).
- **"Mendelian disorders of the epigenetic machinery"** or mutations in genes encoding components of the DNA methylation machinery and histone modifications machinery, which implicate *trans*-acting factors (acting in trans), and are thus expected to have widespread downstream epigenetic consequences (for review see [111–113]).

6.1. The imprinted-X liability: sex differences

X chromosome inactivation (XCI) evolved to solve the problem of gene dosage compensation between XY males and XX females by random inactivation of one of the two female X chromosomes in placental mammals. X inactivation is controlled by a single X-linked cis-acting locus called the X inactivation center (Xic), which contains the noncoding RNA encoding X-inactive specific transcript (Xist) locus. However, there are regions on the XCI that sustain active transcription and "escape" inactivation by looping out of the chromosomal territory covered by Xist.

The male predominance universally observed in ASD (male:female ratio approximately 4:1) is one of the best known, and at the same time, one of the least understood characteristics of these disorders. The mechanisms underlying this male preponderance have been associated with genetic, epigenetic, hormonal (e.g., early exposure to androgenic hormones), and environmental factors (e.g., prenatal stress, early maternal immune activation) [114]. It has been proposed that the pronounced sex ratio of ASD could be related to genetic loci expressed on the noninactivated X chromosome modulate the phenotypic expression of autosomal loci conferring risk for ASD [115]. Females have detectably lower global levels of DNA methylation, and increasing the number of X chromosomes further reduces the methylation on autosomes [116]. The mechanism of female protective effect is unknown, yet genome scans have not revealed any predisposing loci on the sex chromosomes [117]. It has been hypothesized as "the imprinted-X liability threshold model," so imprinted X-linked gene(s) that is ASD protective in nature and raises the threshold for phenotypic expression is expressed only in the X-chromosome inherited from the father. It is normally silenced when transmitted maternally, so because only females have a paternal X-chromosome, the threshold for phenotypic expression is higher in them than in males [118]. Evidence for the existence of the genetic locus was found in a study of females with Turner's syndrome (X-monosomy), in which females had either a single paternal or maternal X-chromosome [119].

The studies of sex differences in normal human brain development at the genomic level are lacking; a recent large transcriptomic study shows that male-biased genes are enriched for pathways repeatedly implicated in autism like the processes of extracellular matrix formation/glycoproteins, immune response, chromatin, and cell cytoskeleton [120]. X chromosome inactivation status in female human induced pluripotent stem cells (hiPSCs) and their differentiation into neurons have shown complexities. A small number of recent papers have begun to explore cellular phenotypes of autism observed in hiPSC-derived neurons [121–123].

However, at present there are major gaps and inconsistencies in the existing literature regarding XCI status during the derivation and maintenance of hiPSCs (for review see [124, 125]).

Moreover, not all genes on the inactive X chromosome are inactivated, and the genes that "escape" X inactivation in females are revealing some interesting ideas on chromatin and brain transcriptional sex differences in understanding the female protective effect in autism [126]. An example is X-chromosome-linked ichthyosis caused by mutation or deletion of the *STS* gene associated with a deficiency of the enzyme steroid sulphatase, located in the distal part of the short arm of the X chromosome (Xp22.3-pter) and the importance of the region in the higher incidence of neurological disorders among males like attention deficit hyperactivity disorder, autism, and X-linked mental retardation [127]. Other gene that escapes X chromosome inactivation is *KDM5C locus* Xp11.22, encoding O-linked-*N*-acetylglucosamine (*O-GlcNAc*) transferase (*OGT*) that regulates chromatin remodeling factors (histone demethylase of H3K4, implicated in gene repression), is expressed lower in males than females and further reduced by prenatal stress [128].

6.2. Classical imprinting disorders

As X chromosome inactivation, gene-imprinting process is a selective differential gene expression regulated by epigenetic mechanisms that are different, but in this case, determined by the parental origin of the alleles. Human-imprinting disorders are a group of eight rare but probably underdiagnosed congenital disorders of growth, development, and metabolism, and represent a curious defiance of normal Mendelian genetics. They are caused by similar molecular changes affecting regulation, dosage, or the genomic sequence of imprinted genes, associated with disturbance of parent of origin-specific DNA methylation across the genome. Humans inherit two alleles from mother and father, both are functional for the majority of the genes, but sometimes one is turned off or "stamped" and does not show in offspring, that the gene is imprinted. The term imprinting refers to the differential expression of alleles (the repressed allele is methylated, while the active allele is unmethylated) for a particular gene depending on the parental origin of the allele. Each allele contains a distinct set of epigenetic modifications or marks, which influence chromatin structure and regulate gene expression at particular imprinted loci [129].

At present there are more than 200 genes subject to imprinting in humans, 97 demonstrated and 107 predicted, generally grouped into different chromosomal regions. For an up-to-date database of imprinted genes, the reader is referred to the Geneimprint database (Geneimprint database; http://www.geneimprint.com). Nevertheless, it remains to be identified the overall role of human imprinted genes and their regulatory elements implicated in the puzzle of ASD. The regulation of the differential expression of genes at imprinted loci is quite complex and involves DNA methylation, characteristic epigenetic signatures of associated covalent posttranslational modifications of histone tails, noncoding RNAs, and *trans*acting factors, all of which play a key role in the process [130]. Epigenetic imbalances in the effects of imprinted genes has been associated with different abnormalities in development: Psychotic spectrum conditions (schizophrenia, bipolar disorder, major depression, PWS, Klinefelter syndrome) have been mediated in part by alterations of imprinted genes with maternal expression or other genes favoring maternal interests. By contrast, ASD (like Kanner autism, Asperger syndrome, Turner syndrome, AS, and Beckwith-Wiedemann syndrome), commonly engender increased relative effects from paternally expressed imprinted genes, or reduced effects from genes favoring maternal interests [131].

Imprinting disorders may result by different genetic mechanisms: deletion of the critical region, paternal/maternal uniparental disomy (UPD), imprinting center defect, and mutation in the imprinting gene (for review see [132]). For most chromosomes, no obvious phenotypic effect from UPD has been observed. However, UPD of certain chromosomes affecting imprinted region leads to clinically recognizable syndromes (e.g., UPD affecting the chromosome 14q32.2 imprinted region is one that causes a distinct disorder: Temple syndrome (or maternal UPD) and Kagami-Ogata syndrome (or paternal UPD), although different, are two sides of the same coin [133–135]).

The association of so-called "classical imprinting diseases" and autism is well known. For example, **imprinted gene locus on 15q11 region**, results from the loss of function or overexpression of at least 1 imprinted gene [136]. Prader-Willi syndrome (PWS) is caused by a lack of the paternal contribution of genes, and Angelman syndrome (AS) is caused by a lack of maternal *UBE3A* expression resulting from disrupted imprinting via a variety of genetic and epigenetic mechanisms occurring in cis [137]. Duplication of 15q11-q13: As we mentioned previously, microduplication of the 15q11-q13 segment is the most consistently known chromosomal abnormality reported in ASD (1–3% of all autism cases), which occurred on the maternally derived chromosome. It represents a contiguous gene duplication syndrome, and reveals epigenetic alterations in gene expression. The segment contains a cluster of three GABA (A) receptor subunit (GABR) genes (imprinted key genes) essential for normal neurodevelopment [138]. Genome-wide analyses suggest that common neuronal pathways can be disrupted in both the Angelman and Dup15q syndromes. mRNA-Seq experiments show that there is substantial overlap of differentially expressed genes between 15q11-q13.1 deletion and duplication neurons. UBE3A transcripts can be pharmacologically rescued to normal levels in induced pluripotent stem cell (iPSC)-derived neurons with 15q11-q13.1 duplication [139].

Another **imprinted region 11p15** contains two separate imprinting domains: the *IGF2/H19* locus [imprinting control region 1 (ICR1)] and the *CDKN1C/KCNQOT1* locus (ICR2). When either locus is disrupted, tipping the balance toward increased expression of paternal genes, the Beckwith-Wiedemann syndrome (BWS) overgrowth disorder occurs. This dosage imbalance occurs primarily via epigenetic mechanisms acting in *cis*, most commonly loss of methylation at ICR2, gain of methylation at ICR1, or paternal uniparental disomy (UPD) of the entire 11p15 region [140]. In BWS 6.8% of patients had been diagnosed of ASD, and occurred in children with UPD and ICR2 defects [141]. By contrast, Russell-Silver syndrome (RSS) with growth failure can result from paternal hypomethylation at ICR1, a gene dosage imbalance that leads to increased maternal gene expression with no paternal contribution [142].

We highlighted as BWS and AS occur with an increased incidence in the offspring of infertile couples conceived following assisted reproductive technologies, which involve a multitude of environmental disruptions that could potentially impact malleable epigenetic marks [143].

However, earlier investigations on possible links between artificial reproductive technologies and autism have shown inconsistent findings [144, 145]. More recent epidemiological studies involving larger populations display that IVF is not associated with ASD [146]; but the risk for autism is associated with a small increased risk of intellectual disability, and was significantly higher following intracytoplasmic spermatozoid injection (ICSI) using surgically extracted sperm and fresh embryos compared to *in vitro* fertilization (IVF) without ICSI [147].

6.3. Mendelian ASD disorders of the "epigenetic machinery"

Mendelian disorders of the epigenetic machinery are a newly delineated group of multiple congenital anomaly, intellectual disability, and autism syndromes arising from mutations in genes encoding components of the chromatin remodeling epigenetic pathways.

6.3.1. Mendelian ASD disorders in DNA methylation machinery

- **Rett syndrome (RTT)** is an X-linked dominant (Xq28) and severe neurological disorder caused by mutations in the gene that encode a single polypeptide MeCP2 (methyl-CpG-binding protein 2), a chromatin-associated protein [148] that contains both a methyl-CpG binding domain (MBD) and transcriptional repression domain (TRD) associated with the regulation of gene expression by activating or repressing transcription, or by functioning at a posttranscriptional level. *MeCP2* is capable of binding specifically to methylated DNA and form a complex with histone deacetylase (HDAC/Sin3A complex). MeCP2-mediated transcriptional repression may involve two distinct mechanisms one being dependent on chromatin modification by histone deacetylation and the other being chromatin independent (block transcription factors directly) [149–151]. In RTT patients' lymphocytes compared with controls have been shown to be increased in the density of histone H3, and decreased levels of trimethylation of lysine 4 on histone H3 (H3K4me3), a modification associated with transcriptional activation [152]. *MeCP2* results in the alteration of the chromatin state by suppressing a number of target genes associated with synaptic function and disrupted synaptic plasticity mechanisms (e.g., *BDNF, DLX5, ID, CRH, IGFBP3, CDKL1, PCDHB1*, and *PCDH7, LIN7A*) in neurons and other types of brain cells [153, 154]. Thereby controlling excitatory synaptic strength by regulating the number of glutamatergic synapse number [155].
- **Fragile X syndrome** (FXS, OMIM #300624) is the most common known genetic cause of inherited intellectual disability. Despite early controversy, it is now accepted that a substantial proportion (50–75%) of children with FXS meets diagnostic criteria for ASD [156]. FXS is associated with a fragile site at Xq27.3, results from a repeat expansion mutation near the *FMR1* (X-linked gene fragile X mental retardation 1) gene promoter. Full mutations larger than 200 CGG repeats in the 5'UTR (5' untranslated region) of the *FMR1* are able to trigger FMR1 subsequent heterochromatinization by DNA methylation of the promoter region [157, 158], accompanied by additional epigenetic histone modifications (as DNA hypermethylation coupled with histone H3 and H4 tail deacetylation, and trimethylation at critical residues H3K9 and H3K27) that result in a block of transcription in FMR1 and absence of the fragile X mental retardation protein (FMRP), involved in multiple

aspects of mRNA metabolism in the brain. Future studies could investigate a therapeutic approach to FXS based on the pharmacological reactivation of the *FMR1* expression [159].

- **MBD5** (methyl-CpG-binding domain 5) is an important factor in methylation patterning and epigenetic regulation and key on the autistic spectrum. Although it was known that the loss of one copy of this gene is the major causative factor in 2q23.1 microdeletion syndrome and point mutations are associated with autism and intellectual disability [160, 161], the duplication of this gene also causes disorders similar to those described in cases with abnormal loss of gene function development [162].

- **Methylation level of specific genes in nonsyndromic ASD:** The postmortem brain tissues from ASD patients show increased DNA methylation within the genes of: oxytocin receptor (*OXTR*) [163], RORA [164], Engrailed-2 (*EN2*) homeobox gene [165], Reelin (*RELN*) [166], and *BCL2 gene* [167].

○ **Oxytocin receptor (OXTR)** is a G-protein coupled receptor for the peptide hormone and neurotransmitter oxytocin that activates the frontal cortex. OXTR is known to be involved in modeling human social behavior (social memory and recognition, anxiety, sexual and aggressive behaviors, and maternal-offspring bonding), and a potential role of the "prosocial" hormone in autism [168]. The involvement of this gene was suggested by its deletion in an autistic patient. The subsequent analysis of a group of unrelated autistic subjects did not show an OXTR deletion, but rather hypermethylation of the gene promoter, with a reduced mRNA expression [163]. These findings address two major points of the current debate on the etiology and pathogenesis of autism: the role of the oxytocin-vasopressin pathway and the possible social processes under epigenetic control. Several studies have begun to explore the so-called OXT deficit hypothesis of ASD, but they have yielded conflicting results. Dysregulated OXT biology is not uniquely associated with ASD social phenotypes as widely theorized, but instead variation in OXT biology contributes to important individual differences in human social functioning, including the severe social impairments, which characterize ASD [169].

○ **RORA** (retinoic acid-related orphan receptor alpha) is a proposed risk factor for autism because it is reduced in the brain and lymphoblastoid cell lines of multiple cohorts of individuals with ASD, and oppositely regulated by male and female hormones. *RORA* and several of its transcriptional targets might contribute to the sex bias in autism by differentially regulating target genes, including CYP19A1 (aromatase) in certain regions of the brain of both mice and humans; in a sex-dependent manner that can also lead to elevated testosterone levels. An important sex-dependent difference has been found in the level of RORA protein in brain tissues of males and females. Specifically, females without autism have a slightly higher level of *RORA* in the frontal cortex of the brain than males without autism, while the levels of the protein are comparably lower in the brain of both males and females with autism. RORA-deficient males may experience greater dysregulation of genes relevant to ASD in certain brain regions during development [164].

○ **Engrailed-2 (EN2) homeobox gene:** contributes to neurodevelopmental disorders, especially ASD. En2 knockout mice (En2-/-) display subtle cerebellar neuropathological changes and reduced levels of tyrosine hydroxylase, noradrenaline, and serotonin in the hippocampus and cerebral cortex similar to those ones which have been observed in the ASD brain [170]. The disruption of hindbrain patterning genes can alter monoamine system development and thereby produce forebrain defects that are relevant to human neurodevelopmental disorders [171].

- **Others:** In addition, significant correlations were also identified between the severity of the autistic phenotype and differential DNA methylation at several multiple loci implicated in the pathogenesis of ASDs. Genes that control synaptic molecules are subjected to a specific epigenetic control mechanism, for example, DNA methylation regulates the tissue-specific expression of SHANK3 gene [172]. Other prominent genes regulated by epigenetic mechanisms include *AFF2, APC, ARHGAP15, AUTS2, JMJD1C, GABRB3, KCNJ10 MAP2, MBD4, NLGN3, NRXN1, PIK3C3, SNRPN, SLC6A4, THAP10, TSNAX,* and *UBE3A* [173].

6.3.2. Mendelian ASD disorders in the histone machinery

- **Histone modifications** include acetylation, methylation, ubiquitylation, phosphorylation, sumoylation, ribosylation, and citrullination. Histone lysine acetylation and histone lysine methylation are the most highly studied of these modifications. But histone demethylases are now emerging as important players in developmental processes and have been linked to human diseases such as neurological disorders and cancer.

- **Histone acetylation**

Brain-derived neurotrophic factor (BDNF) is a protein encoded by the BDNF gene localized to 11p13, whose transcription is controlled by eight different promoters and activity is strongly stimulated by calcium. BDNF is a prosurvival factor induced by cortical neurons that centrally mediates growth, differentiation, and survival of neurons, and essential to promote synaptic plasticity that underlies learning and persistence of long-term memory storage [174]. BDNF binds at least two receptors on the surface of cells: TrkB and LNGFR. It may also modulate the activity of various neurotransmitter receptors, like in serotonergic neurons. Histone modulation of BDNF particularly increased H3 acetylation at the BDNF gene in the medial prefrontal cortex (mPFC), and may be one of the molecular mechanisms that mediated the cognitive dysfunction [175]. Accumulating evidence suggests that BDNF may be implicated in the developmental outcomes of children with ASD. Three recent meta-analysis show as children with ASD have increased peripheral blood levels of BDNF, strengthening the clinical evidence of an abnormal neurotrophic factor profile in this population. Peripheral BDNF levels are a potential biomarker of ASD [176–178].

Proteins involved in the "readout" of lysine acetylation marks, referred to as **BET bromodomain proteins** (including BRD2, BRD3, BRD4, and BRDT), have been shown to be key regulators of chromatin dynamics and disease, and BET inhibitors are currently being studied in several clinical trials. Pharmacological suppression of BET proteins in the brain of young mice, by the novel, highly specific, brain-permeable inhibitor I-BET858 leads to selective suppression of neuronal gene expression followed by the development of an autism-like syndrome.

So, environmental factors controlling BET proteins or their target genes may contribute to the epigenetic mechanism of ASD [179].

- **Histone methylation**

Recent large-scale exome sequencing studies highlighted dysregulation of histone methylation as a major contributing factor of ASD [180, 108]. Methylation of lysine 4 of histone H3 (H3K4me) is one such modification, which is associated with gene activation. Two families of proteins serve as primary regulators of H3K4me: histone lysine methyltransferases (KMTs) are the "writers," which place the methyl marks onto histones; and histone lysine demethylases (KDMs) are the "erasers," which remove them. The mutations in histone lysine methyltransferase KMT2D are a major cause of Kabuki syndrome. Dysregulation of histone methyltransferases and histone deacetylases (HDACs) associated with low activity of methyl CpG binding protein-2 at cytosine-guanine sites in genes may reduce the capacity for condensing chromatin and silencing genes in the frontal cortex, a site characterized by decreased cortical interconnectivity in autistic subjects (for review of mechanisms for altering DNA-histone interactions see [181]).

To date, several genes were found mutated in autism encode histone methylation enzymes such as:

- Methyltransferase complex genes: *KMT2A, KMT2C, KMT2D, KMT2F* encodes H3K4 methyltransferase [182]. *EHMT1, EHTM2,* and *WIZ* encode H3K9 methyltransferase [183]. Histone methyltransferase Ash1L mediates activity-dependent repression of neurexin-1α [184].
- Histone demethylases: *KDM5C* encodes an H3K4-specific eraser enzyme that directly catalyzes the demethylation of mono-, di-, and tri-methylated H3K4, implicated in gene repression; and *JMJD1C,* a demethylase for histone H3K9 implicated in hormone-dependent transcriptional activation.

- **Histone variants: Macrohistones** (mH) are unusual histone variants found exclusively in vertebrate chromatin.

- The histone H2A subunit has a variant -macroH2A1.1 encoded by the autosomal gene H2AFY. The macroH2A1.1 is generally associated with repressed chromatin, such as the inactive X chromosome [185] and could explain the 4:1 male:female gender distortion present in autism. But because it also contains binding sites for cellular metabolites in through the macrodomain, macroH2A1.1 may have a more dynamic role in the modulation of gene expression in response to environmental signals [186]. Although macroH2A1.1 was identified as an autism candidate gene by a GWAS, no association was found [187].
- A related family member encoding gene, *MACROD2* (*macro domain containing* 2) on chromosome 20p12 was also found on a separate chromosome in ASD GWAS [65, 188], so MACROD2 gene is a strong positional candidate risk factor for autistic-like traits in the general population. The macrodomain of MacroD2 binds a cellular metabolite that emerges from histone deacetylation reactions linking both histone variant and histone modification events. There is also evidence that suggests that *MACROD2* could act to regulate the

expression of the phospholipase D2 (PLD2) gene [65]. Phospholipase proteins could play an important role in risk for ASD. The protein derived from PLD2 has been shown to regulate axonal growth [189] and metabotropic receptor signaling [190].

6.3.3. Mendelian ASD disorders in others chromatin remodelers and transcription factors

- **ATP-dependent chromatin remodeling complexes:**

As we have detailed above, the importance of histones (particularly HAT and HDAC complexes) and chromatin structure in the regulation of eukaryotic gene transcription has become much more widely accepted over the past few years. Today it is known as a specific type of chromatin remodeling machine involved in transcription regulation and can use the energy of ATP hydrolysis to alter interactions between histones and DNA within the nucleosome. Changing chromatin states is an active process that requires appropriate external signal, as well as energy in the form of ATP. The engines that carry out the active process are called "ATP-dependent chromatin remodeling complexes"; they utilize the energy from ATP hydrolysis, and are key players in the reorganization and regulation of chromatin accessibility and nucleosome positioning on the eukaryotic DNA, regulating gene expression; and particularly modulates transient extracellular signals to influence neural lineage commitment [191]. These complexes contain an ATPase subunit that belongs to the SNF2 superfamily of proteins. Based on the identity of the sequence homology of their conserved ATPase domains, SNF2 proteins have been into three main groups, the SWI2/SNF2 group, imitation SWI (ISWI) group, and a third class that contain a SNF2-like protein family ATPase and also show deacetylase activity. The diverse subunits together provide a multitude of functions, from early embryogenesis through cell differentiation to organogenesis (for review see [192–194]).

Several components of the ATP-dependent SWI/SNF complex also known as the BAF complex, one of the best characterized ATP-dependent chromatin remodeling complexes, are encoded by genes in which rare autism mutations have been observed, including *ARID1A* and *ARID1B* in Coffin-Siris syndrome, *ATRX* in X-linked alpha-thalassemia/mental retardation syndrome, and *SMARCC1* (*BAF 155*) and *SMARCC2* (*BAF170*) genes [195]. A neuron-specific protein ATPase subunit BAF53b defines a neuronal chromatin-remodeling complex that is necessary for long-term memory and synaptic plasticity in mice [196].

Forms of Coffin-Siris syndrome (CSS) have been shown to be caused by mutations in each of five genes encoding subunits of the SWI/SNF complex. These include CSS1 caused by heterozygous mutation in the *ARID1B* gene (614556) on chromosome 6q25; CSS2 (614607), caused by mutation in the *ARID1A* gene (603024); CSS3 (614608), caused by mutation in the *SMARCB1* gene (601607); CSS4 (614609), caused by mutation in the *SMARCA4* gene (603254); and CSS5 (616938), caused by mutation in the *SMARCE1* gene (603111) [197].

In addition, several exome sequencing studies in autism have identified rare mutations in genes encoding the ATP-dependent chromatin helicases CHD8 (CHD8-chromodomain helicase binding protein 8) [198]. CHD8 is a chromatin remodeling ATPase of the SNF2-like protein family and an important regulator of beta-catenin and Wnt signaling pathways in neuronal development, and is typically involved in the regulation of gene expression (e.g., CHD8 insufficiency results in altered expression of 1715 genes, including both protein-coding and noncoding RNAs) [199]. Another novel ATPase of SNF2-like protein family termed ARIP4 interacts with androgen receptors and modulates androgen-dependent transcription [200].

- **Transcription factors:**

Transcription factor (TF) is a protein that binds to specific DNA sequences, just like that controlling the rate of transcription of DNA to mRNA. A defining feature of TF is that they include one or more DNA-binding domains, which attach to specific sequences of DNA adjacent to the genes that they regulate [201]. At present there are numerous transcriptional changes associated with autism, so *MECP2* gene is also a transcription factor.

- **ADNP:** ASD caused by a mutation in ADNP, a transcription factor involved in the SWI/SNF. ADNP is known to be mutated in at least 0.17% of ASD cases, making it one of the most frequent ASD genes known to date [202].

- **FOXG1:** Overexpression of the transcription factor FOXG1 is responsible for the overproduction of GABAergic neurons. Altered expression of gene network modules and FOXG1 are positively correlated with ASD symptom severity, and likely a shift toward GABAergic neuron fate caused by FOXG1 is a developmental precursor of ASD [104].

- **PITX1** (paired-like homeodomain transcription factor 1) is a key regulator of hormones within the pituitary-hypothalamic axis (as ACTH, cortisol, and betaendorphin) and may be implicated in the etiology of autism [187]. The ACTH-cortisol system, which also plays an important role in stress-related responses, is impaired in autistic individuals in whom lower cortisol levels and higher ACTH levels have been reported.

7. Acquired epigenetics disorders in ASD

Compared with the magnitude of genetic studies in ASD, nongenetic biological risk factors were studied to a lesser extent. Even though in the last decade, the number of publications that address epidemiological factors and autism has grown tremendously. Although there are numerous risk factors (prenatal, perinatal, and postnatal risk factors) that have been linked to autism [203–206], in some cases their involvement has been or is still considered controversial, and as a possible hypothesis, postulates that improvements in obstetric and neonatal management have resulted in an increased frequency of survivors with preexisting brain damage, which has subsequently led to autism [203]. For each infant, an environmental challenge during a critical window of development can have particularly serious consequences, causing the abnormal functioning of the CNS, perhaps autism.

Among the most significant environmental factors linked to epigenetic mechanisms in autism include the following (for review see [95, 110]).

7.1. Toxic exposures teratogens and medications

The particular vulnerability of the developing nervous system for low-level exposure to chemicals is well established. Some degree of developmental neurotoxicity was found for a large number of industrial chemicals and environmental pollutants. However, for only few of these (lead, arsenic, organic mercury, and polychlorinated biphenyls, PCBs), human moderate evidence has emerged for a potential role of environmental pollutants in neurodevelopmental adversity and may, thus, be involved in contributing to neurodevelopmental disorders like autism, ADHD, ID, or cerebral palsy (for review see: [207–209]). However, the mechanisms by which environmental factors produce neurotoxicity during early development are not well stated. Heritable genetic vulnerabilities in ASD may amplify adverse effects triggered by environmental chemicals exposures if genetic and environmental factors converge to dysregulate the same signaling systems at critical times of development.

Among the several major signaling pathways linked to altered neuronal connectivity in the developing brain, as a convergent molecular mechanisms target of gene and environment chemicals interactions, they have been involved in dysfunctional signaling via cytokine dysregulation [210], Ca(2+)-dependent mechanisms, extracellular signal-regulated kinases (ERK)/phosphatidylinositol-3-kinases (PI3K), and neuroligin-neurexin-SHANK (for review see [211]). As well as, exposure to environmental chemicals (using PCBs, lead, and bisphenol A, BPA, as examples) may contribute to adverse neurodevelopmental outcomes of relevance to ASD via effects on DNA methylation in the developing brain (for review see [212]). *In utero* exposure to environmental pollutants increases autism-like behavioral phenotypes in adult animals and induces epigenetic changes, so exposure to heavy metals resulted in multiple behavioral abnormalities that persisted into adulthood. Valproic acid and manganese induced changes in perseverative/impulsive behavior and social dominance behavior, arsenic caused changes only in perseverative/impulsive behavior, and lead induced abnormalities in social interaction in comparison to the control animals. The Chd7 gene, essential for neural crest cell migration and patterning, was found to be hypomethylated in each experimental animal [213].

- **Heavy metals** like lead and mercury are widespread environmental toxins. Developmental exposure to these compounds is associated with lower IQ, endocrine disruptions, and behavioral disturbances. They also have immunotoxic properties. These features have made them possible, though controversial, candidates in ASD. There are conflicting reports regarding lead in autism. A few studies have documented higher serum lead levels [214] often associated with pica [215], although more recent studies show no difference between autism and control populations [216, 217]. Association between mercury levels and autism is also somewhat contradictory [218]. Ethyl mercury is a component in the vaccine preservative thimerosal, which has received attention in recent years. It has neurotoxic capacities, while *in vitro* studies suggest toxic potential for thimerosal (can alter calcium signaling and cytokine production), a large number of independent epidemiological studies show no link to autism [219, 220].

- **Bisphenol A (BPA)**, an epoxy resin, is an endocrine-disrupting chemical (xenoestrogen), employed to make certain polycarbonate plastic products as food containers and baby bottle, and it is the major estrogenic compound that leaches into nearby water and food supplies. BPA has been detected in 95% of human urine samples, which indicates that environmental exposure is widespread [221]. Exposure to BPA during development may affect brain organization and behavior, perhaps as a consequence of its actions as a steroid hormone agonist/antagonist and/or as an epigenetic modifier that alters DNA methylation. Fetal and prenatal BPA exposure was suggested to perturb the serotonergic system in rat and mice models. Epigenetic mechanisms are suggested by a mouse study that demonstrated that BPA prenatal exposure had long lasting, transgenerational effects on social recognition [222]. BPA affects the mRNA levels (lower transcript levels) of several genes encoded for estrogen receptors, oxytocin, and vasopressin, recognized as important neuropeptides modulators of various social behaviors. BPA is not metabolized well in children with ASD. The most recent FDA updates (Administration January 2010) points to "some concern about the potential effects of Bisphenol A on the brain, behavior, and prostate gland in fetuses, infants, and young children." In France, BPA was banned in baby bottles in 2010, and in any food or beverage packaging since January 2015 [223].

- **Other environmental pollutants and toxic products** have also been controversial in its possible relationship with neurodevelopment and ASD. There was weak evidence of an association between nickel exposure during pregnancy and ASD [224]. Also, gestational exposure to inorganic arsenic (an important natural pollutant of water) affected the expression of cysteine/glutamate transporters in the cortex and hippocampus and induced a negative modulation of glutamate receptor N-methyl-D-aspartate (NMDAR) subunits NR2A in the hippocampus. Behavioral tasks showed significant spatial memory impairment in males while the effect was marginal in females [225]. Developmental neurotoxicity and autism risk a positive association with pesticides (organochlorines, organophosphates, pyrethroids) [226, 227]; halogenated aromatic hydrocarbons [PCBs and polybrominated diphenyl ethers (PBDEs)] [210, 228].

- **Exposure to drugs:** Prenatal exposure to valproic acid, ethanol, thalidomide, and misoprostol has been shown to be associated with an increased incidence of autism. These drugs are able to modulate the expression of many genes involved in processes such as proliferation, apoptosis, neuronal differentiation and migration, synaptogenesis, and synaptic activity [229]. Exposure to selective serotonin reuptake inhibitors (SSRI) in depressed pregnant women might be involved in the etiology of autism, as well as the prenatal valproic acid (VPA) exposure, which is also thought to interfere with serotonin levels [230], by disruption of early serotonergic neuronal development [231] or via the reduction of *PTEN* level [232].

Children exposed to valproate *in utero* were seven times more likely to develop autism than those not exposed to antiepileptic drugs. Qin et al. [233] have shown that VPA exposure sequentially activates Wnt signaling and mTOR signaling in rats. Suppression of the Wnt signaling pathway relieves autistic-like behaviors partially by deactivating the mTor-signaling pathway in VPA-exposed rats.

As we have previously redesigned previous research has not been able to prove that administrations of the measles-mumps-rubella vaccine were connected with the autism upsurge [6], but it has been suggested that acetaminophen systematically administered during vaccination, may mediate oxidative stress and neurotoxicity in autism [234], and exposure during pregnancy enhances the probability of appearance of ADHD-like behaviors [235].

http://dx.doi.org/10.5772/66854

These are data from an ecological analysis, not considered optimal as evidence of causality. Nonetheless, there is accumulating clinical and experimental evidence connecting acetaminophen metabolism to biochemical routes known to be relevant for autism and related developmental disorders. Taking into account both ecological and mechanistic evidence, the role of acetaminophen in autism should be formally studied [236]. In rat liver, acetaminophen overdose has been implicated in Id2 (a pleiotropic protein whose function depends on its expression levels) down-regulation vía histone-H3 hypoacetylation [237].

7.2. Immune dysregulation or inflammation

The immune system and the nervous system interact widely. Therefore, it is not surprising that immune dysfunction is often observed in neurological disorders. There is accumulating evidence for immune dysregulation playing a role in the pathogenesis of ASD. Early-life infections can skew fetal development, leading to aberrant neural and immune activity. Several infections [238, 239] including measles, cytomegalovirus, and rubella during pre- and perinatal periods have been associated with autism [240–244]. A large-scale epidemiological study showed that infection-related hospitalizations during pregnancy significantly increased the risk of ASD [245], and also worth noting is prenatal inflammation, particularly prenatal urinary tract infection [204]. A multidirectional interaction between immune system activation in the mother during pregnancy and epigenetic regulation in the brain of the fetus may cooperate to produce an autistic phenotype. This interaction includes immune factor-induced changes in epigenetic signatures in the brain, dysregulation of epigenetic modifications specifically in genomic regions that encode immune functions, and aberrant epigenetic regulation of microglia (for review see [246]).

Numerous immune system abnormalities including T and B cell lineages of adaptive immune responses have been described in individuals with autism, for example:

FOXP3 (Forkhead box P3) is a marker of (+) regulatory T cells [T (Reg)] which are potent mediators of dominant self-tolerance in the periphery. A subset of CD4+ T cells is primed in early life, to recognize common environmental antigens and inhibit later inappropriate immune responses. The expression of the *FOXP3* locus is intimately linked to its chromatin structure [di- and trimethylation of lysine 4 of histone H3 (H3K4me2 and -3)]. Interestingly, T (Reg) fate determination is an epigenetic event of *FOXP3* promoter demethylation induced by repeated Ca+2-mediated signal transduction and prevented by the mTOR pathway [247, 248]. Abnormalities in the ratio of Th1/Th2/Th17 cells and T (Reg) cell-related transcription factor signaling in ASD is characterized by a systemic deficit of *FOXP3*$^+$ (TReg) and increased RORγt$^+$, T-bet$^+$, GATA-3$^+$, and production by CD4$^+$ T cells [249].

Also immune aberrations, with increased levels of plasma cytokines, have been reported in ASD especially in those autistic children with a regressive form of the disease [250]; and mothers of children with ASD exhibit altered cytokine profiles and autoantibodies indicative of systemic immune activation [210]. There are many reports of cytokine imbalances in autism, including IL-1B, IL-6, IL-4, IFN-γ, and TGF-B. Cytokines act mainly as mediators of immune activity, but they also have meaningful interactions with the nervous system. They take part in normal neural development and function, and improper activity can have a variety of neurological implications. These imbalances could have a pathogenic role, or they may be markers of underlying genetic and environmental influences (for review see [210]). Histone modifications play critical roles in the regulation of the innate immune response; for example, histone lysine methyltransferase Ezh1 promotes TLR-triggered inflammatory cytokine production by suppressing Toll-interacting protein [251], and histone H3 phosphorylation by IκB kinases-α is critical for cytokine-induced gene expression [252].

Even though infections and inflammation have profound effects on epigenetic modifications and trigger susceptibility to diseases as ASD, however, very little is known about the epigenetic pathways involved in the modulation of inflammatory and anti-inflammatory genes (for review see [246, 253]).

A novel unifying hypothesis of the etiopathogenesis of ASD for fitting the pieces of the puzzle together (collectively and simultaneously), suggest that ASD are disorders of the immune system that occur in a very early phase of embryonic development. In a background of genetic predisposition and environmental predisposition (like vitamin D deficiency), an infection (notably a viral infection) or food allergy could trigger a deranged immune response which, in turn, results in damage to specific areas of the CNS [254].

mTOR pathway: Postnatal pathogenic exposures and/or Immunological disturbances in autistic individuals have been reported and a role for food allergy has been suggested in ASD. Single gene mutations in mammalian target of rapamycin (mTOR) signaling pathway are associated with the development of ASD and enhanced mTOR signaling plays a central role in directing immune responses toward allergy as well [255, 256]. Multiple ASD syndromes are caused by mutations in genes that act to inhibit mTOR kinase, including Tsc1/Tsc2, NF1, and Pten [257]. In mouse models of ASD mTOR dysregulation causes spine-pruning defects in Tsc-deficient mouse [258]. Increased dendritic spine density with reduced developmental spine pruning in layer V pyramidal neurons are observed in postmortem ASD temporal lobe, and these spine deficits correlate with hyperactivated mTOR and impaired autophagy [259]. Synaptic mTOR integrates signaling from various ASD synaptic and regulatory proteins, including SHANK3, FMRP, and the glutamate receptors mGluR1/5 [257, 260]. It has been proposed that mTOR pathway plays a central role in directing immune responses toward allergy (e.g., cow's milk allergy, or valproic acid exposure) as well, and may be a pivotal link between the immune disturbances and behavioral deficits observed in ASD [233, 261, 262]. Inhibition of mTORC1 activity by rapamycin improved the behavioral and immunological deficits of cow's milk allergic mice [256]. And also, sulindac (nonsteroidal anti-inflammatory drugs) by suppression of the Wnt signaling pathway relieves autistic-like behaviors partially by deactivating the mTOR-signaling pathway in valproic acid-exposed rats [233].

7.3. Nutritional status

There is consensus that children with autism are nutritionally vulnerable because they have selective or picky eating patterns, food neophobia, limited food repertoire, and abnormal sensory processing ("neurosensorial aversion" can affect both the taste and the texture) that predisposes them to food avoidance and restricted food intake in many children with ASD

http://dx.doi.org/10.5772/66854

[263]. "Insistence on sameness" and compulsive repetitive behaviors reinforce rigid dietary preferences and lead to a limited food repertoire [264].

Although inadequate micronutrient but adequate macronutrient intakes are increasingly reported, there are inconsistent results about the extent and type of nutrient deficiencies (for review see [265]). Micronutrient as essential amino acids, minerals, and vitamins are indispensable for human health, primarily due to their critical function as enzymatic cofactors for numerous reactions in the body, such as the production of neurotransmitters and fatty acid metabolism.

A growing body of literature suggests that certain modifiable risk factors such as maternal metabolic syndrome and nutritional risk factors as certain vitamins, like vitamin D, and folic acid either *in utero* or early life, may be associated with increased risk of autism [266]. Several studies with biomarkers of the nutritional and metabolic status of children with autism have demonstrated statistically significant differences in their nutritional and metabolic status, including biomarkers indicative of vitamin insufficiency, decreased glutathione and increased oxidative stress, reduced capacity for energy transport, sulfation and detoxification, and also impaired methylation [267–269]. Nutrition also influences programming of an offspring's epigenome, so nutritional factors, particularly folate, B vitamins (B2, B6, and B12), and choline, have been studied in ASD, and a likely pathway of this action is the one-carbon metabolism cycle, including the folate metabolism, the methionine-homocysteine remethylation cycle (involving choline and betaine), and the transsulfuration pathway.

7.3.1. Amino acids

The essential amino acids tryptophan and serotonin are precursors of neurotransmitters. It has been seen that plasma-free tryptophan and blood serotonin level are significantly higher in autistic children than in normal control subjects. These results suggest that autistic children have some defects in tryptophan-serotonin metabolism in the brain [270]. And disorders of serotonin metabolism are associated with disturbances of platelet catecholamines, and also with elevated immunoglobulins and enhanced cellular immunity reactions [271].

Multivariate statistical analysis in children with autism from their unaffected siblings and age-matched controls, indicated urinary patterns of the free amino acids glutamate and taurine were significantly different between groups with the autistic children showing higher levels of urinary taurine and a lower level of urinary glutamate, indicating perturbation in sulfur and amino acid metabolism in these children [272]. The metabolomic analyses showed variations in essential amino acid metabolism pathways in children with ASD, related to lowered dietary protein intake or to abnormal catabolism, but their role in the etiology and therapeutic use are contradictory [273]. For body fluid levels of neuroactive amino acids, including glutamate, glutamine, taurine, gamma-aminobutyric acid (GABA), glycine, tryptophan, D-serine, and others, in ASD the results reported in the literature are generally inconclusive (for review see [274]).

7.3.2. Minerals

- **Iron** is critical for early neurodevelopmental processes. Low serum iron occurs more frequently in children with autism compared with children with typical development. The prevalence of iron deficiency and anemia in subjects with autism is reported between 24 and 32% and 8 and 16%, respectively. Because iron deficiency, with or without anemia, results in impaired cognition and developmental defects, iron deficiency in children with autism could further compromise their communication and behavioral impairments [265]. Thus, ferritin levels should be measured in subjects with autism as a part of routine investigation [275]. Studies consistently show link between maternal supplemental iron and ASD. Maternal intake of supplemental iron (from 3 months before pregnancy through the end of pregnancy and during breastfeeding) was associated with reduced ASD, especially during breastfeeding. Low iron intake significantly interacted with advanced maternal age and metabolic conditions [276].

- **Other minerals:** Yasuda et al. [277] examined scalp hair concentrations of 26 trace elements for 1967 children with autistic disorders and found deficient in zinc (29.7%), magnesium (17.6%), and calcium (5.8%); and 2.0% or less in other essential metals. The incidence rate of mineral deficiency was highly observed in infants aged 0–3 years old. By contrast, individuals were found suffering from high burden of aluminum (17.2%), cadmium (8.5%), and lead (4.8%), and 2.8% or less from mercury and arsenic burden. Findings by other authors also include deficient in: calcium [269, 278], magnesium [269, 279], iodine [269], chromium [269], and selenium [279]. These findings suggest that infantile zinc and magnesium deficiency and/or toxic metal burdens may epigenetically play principal roles as environmental factors in autistic disorders. Also compared with controls and/or reference ranges of healthy children, children with autism have lower concentrations of lithium [269]. Low concentrations of lithium are particularly interesting because its deficiency has been linked to a wide range of psychiatric disorders including autism. The low concentrations of lithium can be translated into decreased activity of enzymes involved in growth factor signaling pathways and regulation of neurotransmitter, and suggest that low-level lithium supplementation may be beneficial for mood stabilization in this group [280].

7.3.3. Vitamins

Children with autism had many statistically significant differences in their nutritional and others vitamin insufficiency, such as low levels of vitamin D, vitamin B6, biotin, vitamin A, and vitamin C, and also trend toward lower levels of vitamin B5 and vitamin E, and total carotenoids, although could not objectify constant data for different populations [269, 281].

- **Dietary vitamin D** could regulate epigenetic machinery. Epidemiologic evidence supporting the role of vitamin D deficiency either during pregnancy [282, 283] or early childhood may be an environmental trigger for ASD in individuals who are genetically predisposed (for review see [254, 284, 285]). Vitamin D and its receptor (VDR) also known as calcitriol receptor NR1I1 (nuclear receptor subfamily 1, group I, member 1) belongs to the family of trans-acting transcriptional regulatory factors, and are involved principally through two main areas: (1) in the brain homeostasis and mineral metabolism the receptor regulates a variety of other metabolic pathways and several genes controlling anti-inflammatory actions, immune response, and neurodevelopment (cellular proliferation, differentiation, and apoptosis); mainly vitamin D might play a role in the regulation of the production of

http://dx.doi.org/10.5772/66854

autoantibodies not only through modulation of T-helper cell function, but also through induction of CD4(+)CD25(high) regulatory T cells. Vitamin D might also protect the mitochondria, and upregulate glutathione, which scavenges oxidative by-products and chelates (captures and excretes) heavy metals. (2) In gene regulation the calcitriol receptor play ball with some chromatin modification enzymes (i.e., histone acetyltransferases and histone deacetylases), taking a role in complex epigenetic events [285, 286].

Recent studies in ASD children have shown that fifty-seven 40–57% of the patients had vitamin D deficiency (serum 25-OHD levels10–30 ng/mL), and 30–48% had vitamin D insufficiency (serum 25-OHD levels <10 ng/m); also in patients with severe autism the mean 25-OHD levels were significantly lower than those in patients with mild/moderate autism. Increased levels of serum anti-MAG autoantibodies were found in 70% of autistic patients; and this deficiency may contribute to the induction of the production of serum anti-MAG autoantibodies in these children [287]. Additionally, vitamin D supplementation may have beneficial effects in ASD subject [288].

- **Vitamin B complex**

○ **Folic acid and folate** (anionic form) also known as vitamin B9, is a water-soluble vitamin, listed in vitamin B complex, necessary for the formation of structural proteins and hemoglobin and are essential for basic cellular processes including DNA replication as well as DNA, RNA, and protein methylation. Folic acid is essential for the proper development of the central nervous system, and their deficiency during pregnancy has been associated with a wide range of disorders. Randomized controlled trials have found that periconceptional folic acid supplementation reduces the risk of neural tube birth defects up to 70%. So, in several countries, public health policies recommend periconceptional supplementation with folic acid (400 μg/d) to decrease the risk of neural tube defects [289]. But also findings from a large multicenter case-control study, CHildhood Autism Risks from Genetics and Environment (CHARGE), suggest that periconceptional folic acid may reduce ASD risk in those with inefficient folate metabolism [290].

The vitamin folate regulates the metabolic pathway catalyzed by the methylenetetrahydrofolate reductase (MTHFR), encoded by the MTHFR gene (locus 1p36.3), it is the rate-limiting enzyme in the methyl cycle and a key source of the "one-carbon group," it acts as methyl donor (for homocysteine remethylation to methionine), which critically influences in epigenetic mechanisms to methylate DNA (for review see [291]). But the genomic regions in the offspring that may be sensitive to folate exposure during *in utero* development have not been characterized. Genome-wide DNA methylation profiling identifies a folate-sensitive region of differential methylation upstream of ZFP57-imprinting regulator in humans [292]. The underlying mechanisms of action also includeregulation of two microRNAs—let-7 and miR-34—by methylation [293].

The time period at which periconceptional folic acid was added to the diet of women of childbearing age coincides with the seeming onset of a steady increase in the prevalence of autism. Some studies have reported that periconceptional folic acid supplementation, depending on timing and dose, could be associated with a higher incidence of autism. But nevertheless, a recent meta-analysis shows that the few and contradictory studies present inconsistent conclusions, and epidemiological associations are not reproduced in most of the other types of studies [294]. On the other hand, a well-controlled epidemiological study including a sample of 85,176 children disconfirms this claim and reports a lower incidence of ASD in children whose mothers received prenatal folic acid supplementation around the time of conception (0.10%) compared with those unexposed to folic acid (0.21%) [295]. However, these findings have not been verified in other studies [296]. This could be attributed to periconceptional folic acid, which may reduce ASD risk in those with inefficient folate metabolism (for mothers and children with MTHFR variant genotypes, like MTHFR C677T polymorphism) [290, 297]. Besides, folate receptor autoantibodies (FRAs) that interfere with folate transport across the blood-brain barrier may be important in ASD (a high prevalence to 75.3%) and that FRA-positive children with ASD may benefit from leucovorin (folinic acid) treatment [298]. Also, some studies have reported lower folate levels in patients with ASD [299, 300] and high levels of homocysteine [299, 301]. Folic acid supplementation may have a certain role in the treatment of children with autism, and this treatment also improved the concentrations of folic acid, homocysteine, and normalized glutathione redox metabolism [302]; but the effects of folate-enhancing interventions on the clinical symptoms have yet to be confirmed [294].

- **B-Group vitamins B2, B6 and B12:**
  Studies in autistic children report decreased concentrations likely below the reference range of vitamin B-12 and folate by dietary deficits [300]. Vitamin B6 and B12 (or cobalamin) acts as coenzymes in the metabolism, with a close metabolic interrelation in the methylation of homocysteine to obtain methionine (Met). The name "one-carbon metabolism" involving folic acid, vitamins B2, B6, and B12, and folate metabolism does not only generate methyl groups, thus determining epigenetic processes, modifications of the genome and carcinogenesis, it also provides the compounds involved in the DNA synthesis and repair processes, especially the synthesis of purines and pyrimidines [303]. Nutritional supplementation with vitamin methyl-B12, folinic acid, and trimethylglycine might be beneficial on glutathione redox status in children with autism [304].

  Elevated and unusually broad vitamin B-6 (pyridoxine) concentrations have been reported in children with autism which may be due to low activity of pyridoxal kinase that converts pyridoxal and pyridoxine into the active form pyridoxal 5-phosphate (P5P), which is the active cofactor for several enzymatic reactions, including the formation of many key neurotransmitters [305]. This explains the benefits of high-dose vitamin B-6 supplementation in individuals with autism with low P5P [269, 306].

- **Biotin** or vitamin B7 (and also H or $B_{8)}$ is a water-soluble vitamin involved in the metabolism of carbohydrates, fats, amino acids, and purine. Decreased concentrations below the reference range of biotin have been reported in nutritional status of children with autism [269]. Also, it is evident for treatable inborn errors of metabolism patients with ASD. So detailed metabolic revealed biomarkers (urine 3-hydroxyisovaleric acid and serum beta hydroxybutyrate) in 7% of patients for whom biotin supplementation resulted in mild to significant clinical improvement in autistic features [307].

http://dx.doi.org/10.5772/66854

7.3.4. Vitamin-like substances: choline

Other nutrients whose effects are similar to those of vitamins including choline and is among the most prominent associated with ASD. Choline is an essential nutrient soluble in water usually grouped with B vitamins. Choline is an endogenous compound that is synthesized by all cells of mammals, as an intermediary in the major route of transformation of the hill in phosphatidylcholine, an essential phospholipid of the neuronal membrane in the CNS and is essential for proper brain maturation, including astroglia. Choline is a major source of methyl groups needed for methylation of DNA and histones [308]. There is growing evidence that this nutrient also modulates epigenetic regulation of gene expression in both neuronal and endothelial progenitor cells, thereby modifying brain development [309].

Choline is the precursor for betaine and methyl groups derived from betaine, which are used for S-adenosylmethionine (SAM)-dependent methylation reactions including the synthesis of membrane phosphatidylcholine. In this way, choline indirectly serves as a precursor for the synthesis of membrane phospholipids that are essential for normal membrane fluidity, signal transduction, membrane transport, and integrity for synaptic efficiency. Choline is needed by fetal progenitor cells (proliferate, migrate, differentiate, and undergo apoptosis at specific times during fetal development) for membrane synthesis and for methylation (redox-dependent methylation regulates neuronal mRNA). Choline is also a precursor for the synthesis of acetylcholine (ACh), an important neurotransmitter in both the central and autonomic nervous systems [310, 311].

Inadequate choline and betaine can negatively affect folate-dependent "one-carbon metabolism" and in turn downstream methylation and antioxidant capacity (**Figure 1**.) The metabolism of folate, vitamin B12, vitamin B6, choline, and methionine are interrelated and disturbances in one of these metabolic pathways are associated with compensatory changes in the others. So, when humans and animals are fed a diet deficient in choline, it increases the need for dietary folate [312, 313]. Alternatively, if they are fed a diet deficient in folate, dietary choline requirements increase as choline becomes the primary methyl group donor [314–316].

Choline is found primarily in foods that contain fat and cholesterol, and intake of such foods has decreased in recent years. Estrogen induces the gene for enzyme that catalyzes the biosynthesis of the choline-containing phospholipid phosphatidylcholine. Nevertheless, many women have a SNP that blocks the induction of endogenous biosynthesis, which makes longer requirement of choline in the diet. When these women consume diets low in choline, it is likely to be in insufficient supply of this nutrient for the fetus, and may disrupt the progenitor cell proliferation, migration, differentiation, and apoptosis [309].

Low plasma SAM levels and DNA hypomethylation have been shown to be present in children with autism [107]. Choline deficiency has been also shown in animal models to contribute to global and gene-specific DNA hypomethylation and epigenetic abnormalities [317]. There are inconsistent findings on the amounts of free/total choline in autistic individuals. Free choline levels were similar in the autistic and control groups, but total choline was 17% higher in the autistic group ($p < 0.0001$) [269]. Hamlin et al.'s [318] study of 288 children with autism found that 69–93% had less than adequate choline intake, and 18–30% had betaine intake of

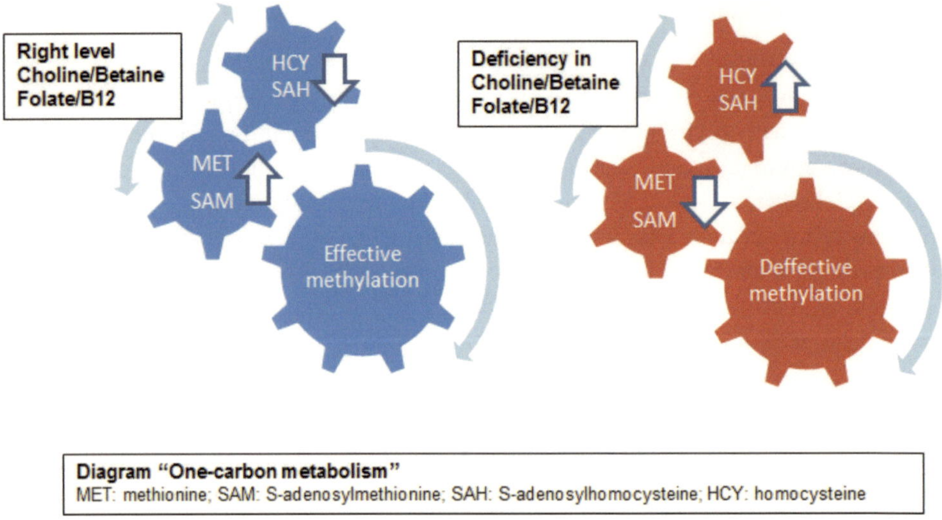

Figure 1. "One-carbon metabolism" implication in epigenetics.

<3.5 mg/Kg. Lower choline and betaine intakes were also correlated with lower plasma choline and betaine concentrations among children with ASD. This suggests that the choline-betaine-homocysteine pathway for Met synthesis may be compromised in children with ASDs.

In a rat model of diet-induced fetal-neonatal iron deficiency, the choline supplementation reduced the effects of iron deficiency, including those on gene networks associated with autism [319]. And also prenatal choline supplementation mitigates the adverse effects of prenatal alcohol exposure on development in rats [320]. A pilot study suggests that an additional evaluation of choline supplementation as an intervention for memory functioning in children with fetal alcohol spectrum disorders is warranted [321]. We have observed improvement after administration of citicoline in a patient with autism and X-chromosome-linked ichthyosis caused by deletion Xp22.3-pte; thanks to the role this nootropic plays in the biosynthesis of structural phospholipids involved in the formation and repair of the neuronal membrane, and a possible contribution of the gene *PNPLA4*, which codes for calcium-independent phospholipase A2 beta, involved in lipoprotein metabolism [127]. Future research should consider whether these metabolic imbalances could be corrected with dietary counseling or supplement interventions.

7.3.5. Fatty acids (FAs)

The inability of the human body to synthesize acid, known as essential fatty acids (EFAs), implies that they must be obtained through diet or supplementation. The EFAs are all omega-3 and -6 methylene-interrupted fatty acids. Polyunsaturated fatty acids (PUFA) are a family of lipids including some subgroups identified by the position of the last double bond in their structure. PUFA omega-3 fatty acids (n-3 or ω-3) include alpha linolenic acid (ALA), eicosapentaenoic acid [EPA, 20:5 (3)], and docosahexaenoic acid [DHA, 22:2 (3)], while PUFA ω-6 include linoleic acid [LA, 18:2 (6)] and arachidonic acid [AA, 20:4 (6)].

The CNS is rich in PUFAs, and in particular AA and DHA are essentials for brain development and play a key role in the maturation and signaling of the brain network. Clinical and animal studies illustrate the importance of long-chain polyunsaturated fatty acids (LCPUFAs) in neural development and neurodegeneration and FAs metabolic pathways may affect proper functioning of the CNS [322]. However, whether or not the levels of these PUFAs are altered in individuals with autism remains debatable.

In female mice maternal ω-3 PUFA deficiency during pregnancy and lactation imprints long-term changes of brain development neurogenesis and apoptosis in adult offspring, associated with DNA methylation of brain-derived neurotrophic factor transcripts [323]. Children with ASD had lower dietary consumption of foodstuff containing DHA, as well as lower serum levels of DHA than controls [324]. In an analysis of the FAs composition of red blood cell (RBC) membrane phospholipids showed that the percentage of total PUFA was lower in autistic patients than in controls; and levels of AA and DHA were particularly decreased ($p < 0.001$) [325]. Reported abnormalities associated with the synthesis of lipid bilayer in ASD as a result of FAs insufficient dietary supplementation or genetic defects can contribute to the symptomatology of autism and individual variety (for review see [326]). A growing body of evidence suggests that individuals who have ASD may have low levels of these PUFAs, particularly DHA and the AA:DHA ratio. Studies also reported significantly higher plasma in the ratios: EPA:AA; linoleic acid:AA; a-linolenic acid:DHA; and ω-3 to ω-6 FA ratios [327–329]. In ASD genetic abnormalities have been reported in the enzymes involved in phospholipid metabolism; e.g., functional abnormalities of the solute carrier 27A (SLC27A) gene family encoding fatty acid transport proteins (FATPs) [330]. But there appears to be no evidence of altered phospholipid-related signal transduction in autism [331].

On the other hand, deficits associated with the release of AA from the membrane phospholipids and its subsequent metabolism to bioactive prostaglandins via phospholipase A (2)-cyclooxygenase biosynthetic pathway have been shown. So, plasma levels of the proinflammatory AA metabolite prostaglandin E2 (PGE2) [325, 331, 332] and leukotrienes (two important lipid mediators) as well as isoprostanes (as marker of oxidative stress) recorded significantly elevated levels in autistics participants compared to controls [333]. The COX/PGE2 pathway and plasma transferrin (an iron mediator related to eicosanoid signaling) play an important role in synaptic plasticity and may be included in pathophysiology ASD [333]. In addition, Wong et al. [334] found that PGE2 activated the canonical Wnt signaling pathway and Wnt-dependent migration and proliferation in neuroectodermal stem cells. In Wnt-induced cells the level of β-catenin protein was increased and the expression levels of Wnt-target genes (Ctnnb1, Ptgs2, Ccnd1, Mmp9) was significantly upregulated in response to PGE2 treatment. This confirms that PGE2 activated the canonical Wnt signaling pathway. Furthermore, the upregulated genes have been previously associated with ASD.

There is strong mechanistic evidence to suggest that vitamin D and n-3 LCPUFAs, specifically DHA, have the potential to significantly improve the symptoms of ASD [335]. But the efficacy of Omega-3 FA supplementation in terms of ASD-symptom management is controversial, so many authors show that DHA supplementation does not improve the core symptoms of autism [336, 337]. A Cochrane review did not find any evidence of effects of omega-3 FA in ASD [338]; by contrast, a recent study by Mazahery et al. [339] have shown that either vitamin D, DHA, or both are effective; the trial would reveal a noninvasive approach to managing ASD symptoms.

7.4. Gastrointestinal dysbiosis

Gut bacteria are an important component of the microbiota ecosystem in the human gut. The intestinal flora is composed of more than 1014 bacteria spread over more than 400 species, of which between 30 and 40 are dominant. The profile of an individual's microbiota is continually influenced by a variety of factors, including but not limited to genetics, age, sex, diet, and lifestyle. Although the microbial profile of each person is different, the relative abundance and distribution of bacterial species is similar among healthy individuals. All these bacteria, in continuous competition, produce a huge variety of enzymatic reactions that necessarily interact with the metabolism and physiology of the host (nutritional functions, immunological, toxicological, etc.), in situations of health or disease in the intestine. Activity microbial biochemistry acts collectively like an organ, intervening in the improvement of nutrient bioavailability and degradation of compounds from the nondigestible diet, the supply of new nutrients, and the elimination of harmful and antinutritional compounds. However, they can also be potentially harmful due to the change of their composition when the gut ecosystem undergoes abnormal changes in the light of the use of antibiotics, illness, stress, aging, bad dietary habits, and lifestyle. Perturbations in gut microbiome composition have an emerging role in health and disease including brain function (development of emotional behavior, stress- and pain-modulation systems, and brain neurotransmitter systems); but also may be environmental contributors in neurodevelopmental disorders including ASD. The ability of the intestinal microbiota to communicate bidirectionally with the brain, known as the "gut-brain axis," in modulating human health by multiple mechanisms, including endocrine and neurocrine pathways, is at the forefront of current research [340, 341]. There is still debate as to whether or not these changes are core to the pathophysiology or merely epiphenomenal [342].

An inconsiderable number of patients with ASD have a history (fetal, neonatal, and infant) of previous antibiotic exposure or hospitalization and GI symptoms; it is important to think about the importance of perturbations in gut microbiome during the first postnatal years of life in modulation of brain development, cognitive functions, and behavior [343]. In the first year of life, decreasing maternal immune protection and child immune system immaturity create an immune vulnerability to disease infection, especially if it is treated with antibiotics, and could facilitate gastrointestinal disorders and dysbiosis. This condition causes a vicious circle between the deterioration of the immune system and increase dysbiosis leading to leaky gut and neurochemical compounds and/or neurotoxic xenobiotics production and absorption. This alteration affects communication "gut-brain axis" that connects the intestine to the CNS through the immune system [344].

The complex carbohydrates (oligo- and polysaccharides) provided by diet are the group of fermentable substrates most abundant. Members gut flora has developed a complex system

http://dx.doi.org/10.5772/66854

of glycohydrolases that allow them to use, thus favoring survival, while generating metabolic energy for enterocytes. Main products of fermentation (enteric bacterial metabolites) are enteric short-chain fatty acids (SCFA) mainly propionic (PPA), butyric acid (BA), and acetic acid, which constitute between 83 and 95% of the total SCFAs. SCFAs represent a group of compounds derived from the host microbiome that are plausibly linked to ASDs. Intraventricular administration of PPA and SCFAs in rats induces abnormal motor movements, repetitive interests, cognitive deficits, perseveration, and impaired social interactions. The brain tissue of PPA-treated rats shows a number of ASD-linked neurochemical changes, including innate neuroinflammation, increased oxidative stress, glutathione depletion, and altered phospholipid/acylcarnitine profiles. These directly or indirectly contribute to acquire mitochondrial dysfunction via impairment in carnitine-dependent pathways; common antibiotics may impair carnitine-dependent processes by altering gut flora favoring PPA-producing bacteria and by directly inhibiting carnitine transport across the gut [345]. GI microbiota and their fermentation products are of potential use as biomarkers for early identification of the etiology and/or symptoms of ASD [346]. Therefore, a significant number of autistic children with chronic digestive disease (most with ileo-colonic lymphoid nodular hyperplasia and inflammation of the colorectum, small bowel and/or stomach) had low serum levels of myeloperoxidase (MPO). However, there was no significant relationship between these levels and severity of GI disease, including the presence of antineutrophil cytoplasmic antibodies (ANCA) [347]. Also, slow intestinal transit contributes to elevate urinary p-cresol level in autistic children [348]. But metabolomics studies in ASD are far to be definitive and univocal [349].

By establishing the hypothesis the role that enteric SCFA, particularly PPA, produced from ASD-associated gastrointestinal bacteria, may be a potential environmental trigger in some forms of ASD. Propionic acid has bioactive effects on (1) neurotransmitter systems, (2) intracellular acidification and calcium release, (3) fatty acid metabolism, (4) gap junction gating, (5) immune function, and (6) alteration of gene expression [350]. SCFA acts as gut-related environmental signals and are capable of altering host gene expression (including CREB-dependent catecholaminergic neurotransmission), partly due to their histone deacetylase inhibitor activity and induced broad alterations in gene expression including neurotransmitter systems (monoaminergic pathways) neuronal cell adhesion molecules, inflammation, oxidative stress, lipid metabolism, and mitochondrial function, all of which have been implicated in ASD [351].

This modulation of the intestinal microbiota is currently a growing area of investigation and it just might be the key to treatment [352]. Studies have also suggested that the intestinal microbiota may be modulated with the use of prebiotics, probiotics, symbiotics, postbiotics, antibiotics, and fecal microbiota transplants and activated charcoal, as an opportunity for therapy in microbiota-associated diseases as ASD [353]. The literature contains information about autism being improved after treatment with common antibiotics (amoxicillin) [354]. Also, ceftriaxone, a beta-lactam antibiotic, increases the expression of the glutamate transporter 1 which decreases extracellular glutamate levels. It is hypothesized that modulating astrocyte glutamate transporter expression by ceftriaxone or cefixime might improve some symptoms of ASD [355].

7.5. Mental stress

Stressor exposure during early life has the potential to increase an individual's susceptibility to a number of neuropsychiatric conditions as anxiety disorders. In the gene-environment interactions underlying ASD, also are implicate early prenatal stress as being especially detrimental to boys with a vulnerable genotype. So, stressful events during pregnancy significantly predicted autistic traits in the offspring in males only [356].

The mechanisms underlying in the nature of this vulnerability have not yet been established. Potentially, etiologic mechanisms of the early postnatal stress including genes involved in the regulation of hypothalamic-pituitary-adrenal axis could be involved. Therefore, in autistic individuals a lower cortisol and higher ACTH levels is described [357, 358]. In experimental animals early life stress increases stress vulnerability through BDNF (brain-derived neurotrophic factor) gene epigenetic changes with decreased levels of acetylated histone H3 and H4 [359]. Recent human epidemiological and animal studies indicate that stressful experiences *in utero* or during early life may increase the risk of neurological and psychiatric disorders, arguably via altered epigenetic regulation and transgenerational epigenetic inheritance (for review see [360]).

7.6. Others prenatal and perinatal environmental factors

7.6.1. Prenatal risk factors

Among the risk factors described for children with ASD those related to the gestational period should be noted. The pregnancy-related risk factors that have been associated with ASD account for few cases, but show the importance of susceptibility of developing brain for certain noxas. As previously mentioned the importance of teratogens toxic, nutritional factors, and immune system, among other factors, has been implicated as prenatal environmental risk. Among these risk factors it should be noted among other things:

- **Maternal chronic disease,** like maternal diabetes, prepregnancy obesity, and pre-eclampsia, is modifiable environmental factor in ASD pathophysiology. Similarly, studies on maternal autoimmune disorders during pregnancy have reported different associated disorders (psoriasis with ASD; thyroid antibodies with ADHD) [361]. Group B streptococcus (GBS) is the most frequent commensal bacterium colonizing or infecting pregnant women. SGB is present in the lower genital tract of 15–30% of healthy pregnant women. In experimental animals, first time gestational exposure to GBS, autistic-like behavior has been reported predominantly affecting male. So, GBS-induced maternal immune activation plays a role in offspring perinatal brain damage (white matter injury) and subsequent neurodisabilities such as autism [362, 363].
- **Maternal smoking during pregnancy:** Growing evidence links prenatal exposure to maternal smoking with disruption of DNA methylation (DNAm) profile in the blood of newborns. An EWAS was conducted using linear regression of methylation values against *in utero* smoke exposure; this study confirms differential methylation in *MYO1G*, *CNTNAP2*, and *FRMD4A* [364]. The association between maternal smoking during pregnancy and ASD risk in offspring has been investigated in several studies, but the evidence

is not conclusive. A recent meta-analysis (including 15 observational studies with 17,890 ASD cases and 1,810,258 participants) indicates that maternal smoking during pregnancy is not associated with ASD risk in offspring [365].

- **Advancing paternal and grandpaternal age and risk of autism:** the father's age is not a factor gene (with genetic implications), which has been associated with ASD, especially in sporadic cases. In men, with age increase *de novo* mutations in their germ cells and there is a greater chance that the children carry a harmful mutation that could increase susceptibility to these disorders [366, 367]. Further, it identifies an association between advanced age (50 or older) males' grandparents when they had their children and diagnosis of autism in the grandsons [368].

7.6.2. Perinatal and neonatal risk factors

Numerous risk factors perinatal and neonatal have been studied in relation to autism, and although there is insufficient evidence to implicate any factor perinatal or neonatal in the etiology of autism, however, there is some evidence to suggest that exposure to a broad class of conditions reflecting general commitments for perinatal and neonatal health may increase the risk [369], with special mention to prematurity [370, 205]. The prevalence (in the range 3.65–12.9%) of ASD among preterm births is 10–12 times more than in the general population [371, 372]. The ASD diagnosis was associated with shorter gestation times and longer hospital stays [373]. Preterm children with very low birth weight (VLBW; 1000–1500 g) or extremely low birth weight (ELBW; under 1000 g) are at increased risk for ASD [374–376]. A number of hypotheses have been put forward to explain these high rates of ASD: prenatal and neonatal complications like sensory impairment associated with prematurity, white matter abnormalities, and cerebellar impairment which occurred more commonly among preterm infants [372, 377, 378]; as well as altered androgen exposure observed in premature infants [379]. Also, gene-environment interactions and prematurity may combine to increase the risk for poor neurodevelopmental outcomes [380]. Thus, fetal membranes from spontaneous preterm birth demonstrate differences in *OXTR* methylation and regulation and expression, but not in *SHANK3*, *BCL2*, and *RORA*, which suggest that epigenetic alteration of OXTR in fetal membrane may likely be indicating an *in utero* programming of this gene and serve as a surrogate in a subset of spontaneous preterm birth [381].

Other risk factors involved in the neonatal period include: higher incidence of hyperbilirubinemia [205, 382], birth defect, a birth weight small for gestational age, acute fetal distress, difficult labor and respiratory infection [204], delayed birth cry and birth asphyxia [205], or low Apgar scores [203]. Factors associated with autism risk in a meta-analysis of 40 studies in 2007 [369] were abnormal presentation, umbilical-cord complications, fetal distress, birth injury or trauma, multiple birth, maternal hemorrhage, summer birth, low birth weight, small for gestational age, congenital malformation, low 5-minute Apgar score, feeding difficulties, meconium aspiration, neonatal anemia, ABO or Rh incompatibility, and hyperbilirubinemia. But the authors conclude that there is insufficient evidence to implicate any one perinatal or neonatal factor in autism etiology, although there is some evidence to suggest that exposure to a broad class of conditions reflecting general compromises to perinatal and neonatal health may increase the risk.

8. Conclusion

Although the knowledge about risk factors for ASD increases day by day, the biological basis of ASD remains largely elusive. Up to now, a large percentage of publications have implicated physiological and metabolic abnormalities (examining peripheral biomarkers such as blood and urine) in ASD and other psychiatric disorders. In particular, "four major areas" have been seen to be involved: immune dysregulation or inflammation, oxidative stress, mitochondrial dysfunction, and environmental toxicant exposures. More recent studies have also reported these physiological abnormalities in brain tissue derived from individuals diagnosed with ASD, suggesting that ASD has a clear biological basis with features more related to known "medical disorders" than "psychiatric disorders."

Genes implicated in ASD alter ratios of excitatory to inhibitory signaling in the CNS (with increased ratio of excitation/inhibition in key neocortical systems) affecting molecular pathways and mechanisms related to synaptic dysfunction, in a process known as "developmental synaptopathy." The interplay between mutations in different genes can produce "idiopathic" autism, but the exposure to environmental modifiers as well as the epigenetic factors may add up to a varying expression of autistic features, allowing to include autism among the "synaptic and chromatin-remodeling disorders." In the last years, the role of nutritional and metabolic status in ASD has also gained importance, particularly the "one-carbon metabolism cycle," including the folate metabolism, the methionine-homocysteine remethylation cycle (involving choline and betaine), and fatty acid metabolism, as well as alterations in gut microbiome composition of children with autism. Furthermore, research in these physiological areas may lead to breakthroughs, in general, as well as subset-specific processes, that could contribute to elucidate the development of ASD. Epigenetic studies besides being useful to discover causal factors, they may also help to unravel the physiological mechanisms predisposing or resulting from the onset of ASD. Therefore, it is also important to follow the epigenetic approach to investigate the possible impairment of metabolic systems in ASD as well as in the search for promising metabolic biomarkers and therapeutic targets.

Nomenclature/Abbreviations

AD	autistic disorder
ADHD	attention=deficit/hyperactivity disorder
AS	Angelman syndrome
ASD	autism spectrum disorder
BA	butyric acid
BDNF	brain=derived neurotrophic factor
BPA	bisphenol A
BWS	Beckwithâ€"Wiedemann syndrome
CDD	childhood disintegrative disorder

http://dx.doi.org/10.5772/66854

CDC	Centers for Disease Control and Prevention
CSS	Coffin=Siris syndrome
CMA	chromosomal microarray analysis
CNS	central nervous system.
CNV	copy number variants
DD	developmental delay
DSM	Diagnostic and Statistical Manual of Mental Disorders
EFAs	essential fatty acids
EWAS	epigenome=wide association study
FAs	fatty acids
FXS	Fragile X syndrome
GWAS	genome=wide association study
H	histone
HATs	histone acetyltransferases
HDACs	histone deacetylases
hiPSCs	human induced pluripotent stem cells
HMTs	histone methyltransferases
ICR	imprinting control region
ICSI	intra=cytoplasmic spermatozoid injection
ID	intellectual disability
IVF	in vitro fertilization
KDMs	histone lysine demethylases
KMTs	histone lysine methyltransferases
LCPUFAs	long=chain polyunsaturated fatty acids
LCRs	low=copy repeats
MBDs	methyl=CpG=binding domain proteins
MCA	multiple congenital anomalies
mPFC	medial prefrontal cortex
NAHR	nonallelic homologous recombination
NDD	neurodevelopmental disorders
NLGN	neuroligins
NGS	next=generation sequencing
NRXN	neurexins
OXTR	oxytocin receptor
PBDEs	polybrominated diphenyl ethers

PCBs	polychlorinated biphenyls
PDD	pervasive developmental disorders
PDD=NOS	pervasive developmental disorder not otherwise specified
PPA	propionic acid
PRMTs	protein arginine methyltransferases
PUFA	polyunsaturated fatty acids
PWS	Prader=Willi syndrome
RORA	retinoic acid=related orphan receptor alpha
SCFA	short chain fatty acids
SDs	segmental duplications
SNP	single nucleotide polymorphisms
SNV	single nucleotide variants
SWI/SNF	SWItch/Sucrose nonfermentable
RSS	Russell=Silver syndrome
RTT	Rett syndrome
TF	transcription factor
T(Reg)	regulatory T cells
TRD	transcriptional repression domain
WES	whole=exome sequencing
Xic	X inactivation center
XCI	X chromosome inactivation

Author details

Maria Carmen Carrascosa-Romero[1] and Carlos De Cabo-De La Vega[2*]

*Address all correspondence to: carlosd@sescam.jccm.es

1 Department of Neuropediatrics; Albacete General Hospital, Spain

2 Neuropsychopharmacology Unit, Albacete General Hospital, Spain

References

[1] American Psychiatric Association. Diagnostic and Statistical Manual of Mental Disorders. Fourth Edition. Washington, DC: American Psychiatric Association; 2000. Text Revision 5

[2] American Psychiatric Association. The Diagnostic and Statistical Manual of Mental Disorders, Fifth Edition: DSM 5. American Psychiatric Association; 2013. BookpointUS

[3] Autism and Developmental Disabilities Monitoring Network Surveillance Year 2010 Principal Investigators. Prevalence of Autism Spectrum Disorders Among Children Aged 8 years – Autism and Developmental Disabilities Monitoring Network, 11 Sites, United States, 2010. Centers for Disease Control and Prevention. MMWR Surveill Summ. 2014;63(SS02):1–21.

[4] Fombonne E. Epidemiology of pervasive developmental disorders. Pediatr. Res. Jun. 2009;65(6):591–598.

[5] Ganz ML. The lifetime distribution of incremental societal costs of autism. Arch. Pediatr. Adolesc. Med. 2007;161:343–349.

[6] Muhle R, Trentacoste SV, Rapin I. The genetics of autism. Pediatrics. 2004;113(5):e472-86.

[7] Neggers YH. Increasing prevalence, changes in diagnostic criteria, and nutritional risk factors for autism spectrum disorders. ISRN Nutr. 2014;13;2014.

[8] Baird G, Simonoff E, Pickles A, Chandler S, Loucas T, Meldrum D, et al. Prevalence of disorders of the autism spectrum in a population cohort of children in South Thames: the special needs and autism proyect. Lancet. 2006;368:179–181.

[9] Coo H, Ouellette-Kuntz H, Lloyd JE, Kasmara L, Holden JJ, Lewis ME. Trends in autism prevalence: diagnostic substitution revisite. J Autism Dev Disord. 2008;38(6):1036–1046.

[10] Rice CE, Rosanoff M, Dawson G, Durkin MS, Croen LA, Singer A, Yeargin-Allsopp M. Evaluating changes in the prevalence of the autism spectrum disorders (ASDs). Public Health Rev. 2013;34:1–22

[11] Hansen SN, Schendel DE, Parner ET. Explaining the increase in the prevalence of autism spectrum disorders: the proportion attributable to changes in reporting practices. JAMA Pediatr. 2015;169:56–62

[12] Durkin SA Maenner MJ, Newschaffer CJ, Lee LC, Cunniff CM, Daniels JL, et al. Advanced parental age and risk of autism spectrum disorder. Am J Epidemiol. 2008;168(11):1268–1276.

[13] Yuen RK, Merico D, Cao H, Pellecchia G, Alipanahi B, Thiruvahindrapuram B, et al. Genome-wide characteristics of de novo mutations in autism. NPJ Genom Med. 2016;3:160271–1602710.

[14] Veenstra-Vanderweele J, Christian SL, Cook EH Jr. Autism as a paradigmatic complex genetic disorder. Annu Rev Genomics Hum Genet. 2004;5:379–405.

[15] Bailey A, Phillips W, Rutter M. Autism: towards an integration of clinical, genetic, neuropsychological, and neurobiological perspectives. J Child Psychol Psychiatry. 1996;37:89–126.

[16] Bourgeron T. From the genetic architecture to synaptic plasticity in autism spectrum disorder. Nat Rev Neurosci. 2015;16:551–563.

[17] Devlin B, Scherer SW. Genetic architecture in autism spectrum disorder. Curr Opin Genet Dev. 2012;22:229–237.

[18] He X, Sanders SJ, Liu L, De Rubeis S, Lim ET, Sutcliffe JS, et al. Integrated model of de novo and inherited genetic variants yields greater power to identify risk genes. PLoS Genet. 2013;9:e1003671

[19] Carter MT, Scherer SW. Autism spectrum disorder in the genetics clinic: a review. Clin Genet. 2013;83:399–407.

[20] Casanova EL, Sharp JL, Chakraborty H, Sumi NS, Casanova MF. Genes with high penetrance for syndromic and non-syndromic autism typically function within the nucleus and regulate gene expression. Mol Autism. 2016;7:18. doi: 10.1186/s13229-016-0082-z. eCollection 2016.

[21] Gillberg C. Chromosomal disorders and autism. J Autism Dev Disord. 1998;28:415–425

[22] Lauritsen M, Mors O, Mortensen PB, Ewald H. Infantile autism and associated autosomal chromosome abnormalities: a registerbased study and a literature survey. J Child Psychol Psychiatry. 1999;40:335–345.

[23] Oxelgren UW, Myrelid Å, Annerén G, Ekstam B, Göransson C, Holmbom A, Isaksson A, Åberg M, Gustafsson J, Fernell E. Prevalence of autism and attention-deficit-hyperactivity disorder in Down syndrome: a population-based study. Dev Med Child Neurol. 2016; doi: 10.1111/dmcn.13217. [Epub ahead of print] PubMed PMID: 27503703.

[24] Niklasson L, Rasmussen P, Oskarsdóttir S, Gillberg C. Autism, ADHD, mental retardation and behavior problems in 100 individuals with 22q11 deletion syndrome. Res Dev Disabil. 2009;30:763–773.

[25] Cohen D, Pichard N, Tordjman S, Baumann C, Burglen L, Excoffier E, et al. Specific genetic disorders and autism: clinical contribution towards their identification. J Autism Dev Disord. 2005;35:103–116.

[26] Miles JH. Autism spectrum disorders – a genetics review. Genet Med. 2011;13:278–294.

[27] Miller DT, Adam MP, Aradhya S, Biesecker LG, Brothman AR, Carter NP, et al. Consensus statement: chromosomal microarray is a first-tier clinical diagnostic test for individuals with developmental disabilities or congenital anomalies. Am J Hum Genet. 2010;86(5):749–764.

[28] Sys M, Van den Bogaert A, Roosens B, Lampo A, Jansen A, Wouters S, et al. Can clinical lcharacteristics be criteria to perform chromosomal microarray-analysis in children and adolescents with autism spectrum disorders? Minerva Pediatr. 2016; [Epub ahead of print] PubMed PMID: 27607483.

[29] Sebat J, Lakshmi B, Troge J, Alexander J, Young J, Lundin P, et al. Large-scale copy number polymorphism in the human genome. Science. 2004;305:525–528.

[30] Sebat J, Lakshmi B, Malhotra D, Troge J, Lese-Martin C, Walsh T, et al. Strong association of de novo copy number mutations with autism. Science. 2007;20;316(5823):445–459.

[31] Germain ND, Chen PF, Plocik AM, Glatt-Deeley H, Brown J, Fink JJ, et al. Gene expression analysis of human induced pluripotent stem cell-derived neurons carrying copy number variants of chromosome 15q11-q13.1. Mol Autism. 2014;5:44. doi: 10.1186/2040-2392-5-44. eCollection 2014

[32] Levy D, Ronemus M, Yamrom B, Lee YH, Leotta A, Kendall J, et al. Rare de novo and transmitted copy-number variation in autistic spectrum disorders. Neuron. 2011;70:886–897

[33] Sanders SJ, Ercan-Sencicek AG, Hus V, Luo R, Murtha MT, Moreno-De-Luca D, et al. Multiple recurrent de novo CNVs, including duplications of the 7q11.23 Williams syndrome region, are strongly associated with autism. Neuron. 2011;70:863–885.

[34] Dittwald P, Gambin T, Szafranski P, Li J, Amato S, Divon MY, et al. NAHR-mediated copy-number variants in a clinical population: mechanistic insights into both genomic disorders and Mendelizing traits. Genome Res. 2013;23(9):1395–1409.

[35] Sener EF, Canatan H, Ozkul Y. Recent advances in autism spectrum disorders: applications of whole exome sequencing technology. Psychiatry Investig. 2016;13(3):255–264.

[36] Merikangas AK, Segurado R, Heron EA, Anney RJ, Paterson AD, Cook EH, et al. The phenotypic manifestations of rare genic CNVs in autism spectrum disorder. Mol Psychiatry. 2015;20(11):1366-1372.

[37] Carrascosa-Romero MC, Suela J, Pardal-Fernández JM, Bermejo-Sánchez E, Vidal-Company A, MacDonald, et al. A 2.84 Mb deletion at 21q22.11 in a patient clinically diagnosed with Marden-Walker syndrome. Am J Med Genet A. 2013;161A(9):2281–2290.

[38] Oberman LM, Boccuto L, Cascio L, Sarasua S, Kaufmann WE. Autism spectrum disorder in Phelan-McDermid syndrome: initial characterization and genotype-phenotype correlations. Orphanet J Rare Dis. 2015;10:105. doi: 10.1186/s13023-015-0323-9

[39] Boccuto L, Lauri M, Sarasua SM, Skinner CD, Buccella D, Dwivedi A, et al. Prevalence of SHANK3 variants in patients with different subtypes of autism spectrum disorders. Eur J Hum Genet. 2013;21(3):310–316.

[40] Cox DM, Butler MG. The 15q11.2 BP1-BP2 microdeletion syndrome: a review. Int J Mol Sci. 2015;16(2):4068–4082.

[41] Bailey A, Le Couteur A, Gottesman I, Bolton P, Simonoff E, Yuzda E, Rutter M. Autism as a strongly genetic disorder: evidence from a British twin study. Psychol Med. 1995;25:63–77.

[42] Tick B, Bolton P, Happe' F, Rutter M, Rijsdijk F. Heritability of autism spectrum disorders: a meta-analysis of twin studies. J Child Psychol Psychiatry. 2016;57(5):585–595.

[43] Ozonoff S, Young GS, Carter A, Messinger D, Yirmiya N, Zwaigenbaum L, et al. Recurrence risk for autism spectrum disorders: a baby siblings research consortium study. Pediatrics. 2011;128:e488-e495.

[44] Freitag CM. The genetics of autistic disorders and its clinical relevance: a review of the literature. Mol Psychiatry. 2007;12:2–22.

[45] Levy SE, Mandell DS, Schultz RT. Autism. Lancet. 2009;374:1627–1628.

[46] Holt R, Barnby G, Maestrini E, Bacchelli E, Brocklebank D, Sousa I, et al. Linkage and candidate gene studies of autism spectrum disorders in European populations. Eur J Hum Genet. 2010;18(9):1013–1019.

[47] Autism Genome Project Consortium, Szatmari P, Paterson AD, Zwaigenbaum L, Roberts W, Brian J, Liu XQ, et al. Mapping autism risk loci using genetic linkage and chromosomal rearrangements. Nat Genet. 2007;39:319–328.

[48] Trikalinos TA, Karvouni A, Zintzaras E, Ylisaukko-oja T, Peltonen L, Jarvela I, et al. A heterogeneity-based genome search meta-analysis for autism-spectrum disorders. Mol Psychiatry 2006;11:29–36.

[49] Abrahams B S, Geschwind DH. Advances in autism genetics: on the threshold of a new neurobiology. Nat. Rev. Genet. 2008;9:341–355.

[50] Jamain S, Quach H, Betancur C, Råstam M, Colineaux C, Gillberg IC, Soderstrom H, et al. Mutations of the X-linked genes encoding neuroligins NLGN3 and NLGN4 are associated with autism. Nat Genet. 2003;34:27–29.

[51] Durand CM, Betancur C, Boeckers TM, Bockmann J, Chaste P, Fauchereau F, et al. Mutations in the gene encoding the synaptic scaffolding protein SHANK3 are associated with autism spectrum disorders. Nat Genet. Nat Genet. 2007;39(1):25–27.

[52] O'Roak BJ, Deriziotis P, Lee C, Vives L, Schwartz JJ, Girirajan S, et al. Exome sequencing in sporadic autism spectrum disorders identifies severe de novo mutations. Nat Genet 2011;43:585–589.

[53] Sanders SJ, Murtha MT, Gupta AR, Murdoch JD, Raubeson MJ, Willsey AJ, et al. De novo mutations revealed by whole exome sequencing are strongly associated with autism. Nature 2012;485:237–241.

[54] O'Roak BJ, Vives L, Girirajan S, Karakoc E, Krumm N, Coe BP, et al. Sporadic autism exomes reveal a highly interconnected protein network Of de novo mutations. Nature. 2012;485:246–250.

[55] Neale BM, Kou Y, Liu L, Ma'ayan A, Samocha KE, Sabo A, et al. Patterns and rates of exonic de novo mutations in autism spectrum disorders. Nature. 2012;485:242–245.

[56] Hu VW, Nguyen A, Kim KS, Steinberg ME, Sarachana T, Scully MA, Soldin SJ, Luu T, Lee NH. Gene expression profiling of lymphoblasts from autistic and nonaffected sib pairs: altered pathways in neuronal development and steroid biosynthesis. PLoS One. 2009;4(6):e5775. doi: 10.1371/journal.pone.0005775

[57] Bourgeron T. From the genetic architecture to synaptic plasticity in autism spectrum disorder. Nat Rev Neurosci. 2015;16:551–563.

[58] De Rubeis S, Buxbaum JD. Genetics and genomics of autism spectrum disorder: embracing complexity. Hum Mol Genet. 2015;24:R24–R31.

[59] Gaugler T, Klei L, Sanders SJ, Bodea CA, Goldberg AP, Lee AB, et al. Most genetic risk for autism resides with common variation. Nat Genet. 2014;46:881–885.

[60] Pinto D, Pagnamenta AT, Klei L, Anney R, Merico D. Functional Impact of Global Rare Copy Number Variation in Autism Spectrum Disorder. Nature. 2010;466(7304):368–372.

[61] Pinto D, Delaby E, Merico D, Barbosa M, Merikangas A, Klei L, et al. Convergence of genes and cellular pathways dysregulated in autism spectrum disorders. Am J Hum Genet. 2014;94(5):677–694.

[62] Iossifov I, Ronemus M, Levy D, Wang Z, Hakker I, Rosenbaum J, De novo gene disruptions in children on the autistic spectrum. Neuron. 2012;74:285–299.

[63] Lim ET, Raychaudhuri S, Sanders SJ, Stevens C, Sabo A, MacArthur DG. Rare complete knockouts in humans: population distribution and significant role in autism spectrum disorders. Neuron. 2013;77:235–242.

[64] Carayol J, Schellenberg GD, Dombroski B, Amiet C, Génin B, Fontaine K, et al. A scoring strategy combining statistics and functional genomics supports a possible role for common polygenic variation in autism. Front Genet. 2014;5:33. doi: 10.3389/fgene.2014.00033. eCollection 2014.

[65] Anney R, Klei L, Pinto D, Regan R, Conroy J, Magalhaes TR et al. A genome-wide scan for common alleles affecting risk for autism. Hum Mol Genet. 2010;19(20):4072–4082.

[66] Anney R, Klei L, Pinto D, Almeida J, Bacchelli E, Baird G, et al. Individual common variants exert weak effects on the risk for autism spectrum disorderspi. Hum Mol Genet. 2012;21(21):4781–4792.

[67] Sala C, Verpelli C (editors). Neuronal and Synaptic Dysfunction in Autism Spectrum Disorder and Intellectual Disability. First Edition. 2016; Elsevier Science & Technology Books- Academis Press, London, San Diego, Cambridge, Oxford. 379 pages. ISBN: 9780128001097.

[68] An JY, Claudianos C. Genetic heterogeneity in autism: From single gene to a pathway perspective. Neurosci Biobehav Rev. 2016;68:442–453.

[69] Hoischen A, Krumm N, Eichler EE. Prioritization of neurodevelopmental disease genes by discovery of new mutations. Nat Neurosci. 2014;17:764–772.

[70] Huguet G, Ey E, Bourgeron T. The genetic landscapes of autism spectrum disorders. Annu Rev Genomics Hum Genet. 2013;14:191–213.

[71] Casanova EL, Casanova MF. Genetics studies indicate that neural induction and early neuronal maturation are disturbed in autism. Front Cell Neurosci. 2014;8:397. doi: 10.3389/fncel. 2014.00397. eCollection 2014

[72] Boeckers TM, Bockmann J, Kreutz MR, Gundelfinger ED. ProSAP/Shank proteins - a family of higher order organizing molecules of the postsynaptic density with an emerging role in human neurological disease. J Neurochem. 2002;81(5):903–910.

[73] Sala C, Vicidomini C, Bigi I, Mossa A, Verpelli C. Shank synaptic scaffold proteins: Keys to understanding the pathogenesis of autism and other synaptic disorders. J. Neurochem. 2015;135:849–858.

[74] Leblond CS, Nava C, Polge A, Gauthier J, Huguet G, Lumbroso S, et al. Meta-analysis of SHANK mutations in autism spectrum disorders: a gradient of severity in cognitive impairments. PLoS Genet. 2014;10:e1004580

[75] Corradi A, Fadda M, Piton A, Patry L, Marte A, Rossi P, et al. SYN2 is an autism predisposing gene: loss-of-function mutations alter synaptic vesicle cycling and axon outgrowth. Hum Mol Genet. 2014;23:90–103.

[76] Graf ER, Zhang X, Jin SX, Linhoff MW, Craig AM. Neurexins induce differentiation of GABA and glutamate postsynaptic specializations via neuroligins. Cell. 2004;119:1013–1026.

[77] Südhof TC. Neuroligins and neurexins link synaptic function to cognitive disease. Nature. 2008;455:903–911.

[78] Talebizadeh Z, Lam DY, Theodoro MF, Bittel DC, Lushington GH, Butler MG Novel splice isoforms for NLGN3 and NLGN4 with possible implications in autism. J Med Genet. 2006;43(5):e21.

[79] Hill-Yardin EL, Argyropoulos A, Hosie S, Rind G, Anderson P, Hannan J, et al. Reduced susceptibility to induced seizures in the Neuroligin-3(R451C) mouse model of autism. Neurosci. 2015;589:57–61.

[80] Szatmari P, Paterson AD, et al. Autism Genome Project Consortium (AGPC). Mapping autism risk loci using genetic linkage and chromosomal rearrangements. Nat Genet. 2007;39:319–328.

[81] Alarco'n M, Abrahams BS, Stone JL Duvall JA, Perederiy JV, Bomar JM, et al. Linkage, association, and gene-expression analyses identify CNTNAP2 as an autism-susceptibility gene. Am J Hum Genet. 2008;82:150–159.

[82] Durand CM, Perroy J, Loll F, Perrais D, Fagni L, Bourgeron T, Montcouquiol M, Sans N. SHANK3 mutations identified in autism lead to modification of dendritic spine morphology via an actin-dependent mechanism. Mol Psychiatry. 2012;17(1):71–84.

[83] Földy C, Malenka RC, Südhof TC. Autism-associated neuroligin-3 mutations commonly disrupt tonic endocannabinoid signaling. Neuron. 2013;78:498–509.

[84] Hamilton PJ, Campbell NG, Sharma S, Erreger K, Herborg Hansen F, Saunders C, NIH ARRA Autism Sequencing Consortium, et al. De novo mutation in the dopamine transporter gene associates dopamine dysfunction with autism spectrum disorder. Mol. Psychiatry. 2013; 18:1315–1323.

[85] Sutcliffe JS, Delahanty RJ, Prasad HC, McCauley JL, Han Q, Jiang L, et al. Allelic heterogeneity at the serotonin transporter locus (SLC6A4) confers susceptibility to autism and rigid-compulsive behaviors. Am J Hum Genet. 2005;77(2):265–279.

[86] Toma C, Hervás A, Balmaña N, Salgado M, Maristany M, Vilella E, et al. Neurotransmitter systems and neurotrophic factors in autism: association study of 37 genes suggests involvement of DDC. World J Biol Psychiatry. 2013;14(7):516–527.

[87] Ebrahimi-Fakhari D, Sahin M. Autism and the synapse: emerging mechanisms and mechanism-based therapies. Curr Opin Neurol. 2015;28(2):91–102.

[88] Peñagarikano O, Abrahams BS, Herman EI, Winden KD, Gdalyahu A, Dong H, et al. Absence of CNTNAP2 leads to epilepsy, neuronal migration abnormalities, and core autism-related deficits. Cell. 2011;147:235–246.

[89] Shi L, Chang X, Zhang P, Coba MP, Lu W, Wang, K. The functional genetic link of NLGN4X knockdown and neurodevelopment in neural stem cells. Hum. Mol. Genet. 2013;22:3749–3760.

[90] Zeng L, Zhang P, Shi L, Yamamoto V, Lu W, Wang K. Functional impacts of NRXN1 knockdown on neurodevelopment in stem cell models. PLoS One. 2013;8:e59685. doi: 10.1371/journal.pone. 0059685

[91] Won H, Mah W, Kim E. Autism spectrum disorder causes, mechanisms, and treatments: focus on neuronal synapses. Front Mol Neurosci. 2013;6:19. doi: 10.3389/fnmol.2013.00019. eCollection 2013

[92] Chang J, Gilman SR, Chiang AH, Sanders SJ, Vitkup D. Genotype to phenotype relationships in autism spectrum disorders. Nat Neurosci. 2015;18(2):191–198.

[93] Stein JL, Parikshak NN, Geschwind DH. Rare inherited variation in autism: beginning to see the forest and a few trees. Neuron. 2013;77:209–211.

[94] Siniscalco D, Cirillo A, Bradstreet JJ, Antonucci N. Epigenetic findings in autism: new perspectives for therapy. Int J Environ Res Public Health. 2013;10:4261–4273.

[95] Tordjman S, Somogyi E, Coulon N, Kermarrec S, Cohen D, Bronsard G, et al. Gene×Environment interactions in autism spectrum disorders: role of epigenetic mechanisms. Front Psychiatry. 2014;5:53

[96] Schanen NC. Epigenetics of autism spectrum disorders. Hum Mol Genet. 2006; 15:R138–R150.

[97] Feinberg AP. Phenotypic plasticity and the epigenetics of human disease. Nature. 2007;447:433–440.

[98] Berger SL, Kouzarides T, Shiekhattar R, Shilatifard A. An operational definition of epigenetics. Genes Dev. 2009;23(7):781–783.

[99] Moore DS. The Developing Genome. An Introduction to Behavioral Epigenetics, First Edition, 2015. Oxford University Press, New York. 320 Pages. ISBN: 9780199922345.

[100] Zentner GE, Henikoff S. Regulation of nucleosome dynamics by histone modifications. Nat Struct Mol Biol. 2013;20:259–266.

[101] Falkenberg KJ Johnstone RW. Histone deacetylases and their inhibitors in cancer, neurological diseases and immune disorders. Nat Rev Drug Discov. 2014;13(9):673–691.

[102] Christensen DL, Baio J, Braun KV, Bilder D, Charles J, Constantino JN, et al. Prevalence and characteristics of autism spectrum disorder among children aged 8 years—autism and developmental disabilities monitoring network, 11 sites, United States, 2012. MMWR Surveill Summ. 2016;65(3):1–23.

[103] Grafodatskaya D, Chung B, Szatmari P, Weksberg R. Autism spectrum disorders and epigenetics. J Am Acad Child Adolesc Psychiatry. 2010;49(8):794–809.

[104] Mariani J, Coppola G, Zhang P, Abyzov A, Provini L, Tomasini L, et al. FOXG1-dependent dysregulation of GABA/Glutamate neuron differentiation in autism spectrum disorders. Cell. 2015;162(2):375–390.

[105] Mikeska T, Craig JM. DNA methylation biomarkers: cancer and beyond. Genes. 2014;5:821–864.

[106] Ben-David E, Shifman S. Combined analysis of exome sequencing points toward a major role for transcription regulation during brain development in autism. Mol Psychiatry. 2013;18(10):1054–1056.

[107] Melnyk S, Fuchs GJ, Schulz E, Lopez M, Kahler SG, Fussell JJ, et al. Metabolic imbalance associated with methylation dysregulation and oxidative damage in children with autism. J Autism Dev Disord. 2012;42(3):367–377.

[108] De Rubeis S, He X, Goldberg AP, Poultney CS, Samocha K, Cicek AE, et al. Synaptic, transcriptional and chromatin genes disrupted in autism. Nature. 2014;515(7526):209–215.

[109] Loke YJ, Hannan AJ, Craig JM. The role of epigenetic change in autism spectrum disorders. Front Neurol. 2015;6:107. doi: 10.3389/fneur.2015.00107. eCollection 2015

[110] Kubota T, Mochizuki K. Epigenetic effect of environmental factors on autism spectrum disorders. Int J Environ Res Public Health. 2016;13(5)504. doi: 10.3390/ijerph13050504. PubMed PMID: 27187441; PubMed Central PMCID: PMC4881129.

[111] Fahrner JA, Bjornsson HT. Mendelian disorders of the epigenetic machinery: tipping the balance of chromatin states. Annu Rev Genomics Hum Genet. 2014;15:269–293.

[112] Berdasco M, Esteller M. Genetic syndromes caused by mutations in epigenetic genes. Hum Genet. 2013;132:359–383.

[113] Bjornsson HT. The Mendelian disorders of the epigenetic machinery. Genome Res. 2015;25:1473–1481.

[114] Schaafsma SM, Pfaff DW. Etiologies underlying sex differences in autism spectrum disorders. Front Neuroendocrinol. 2014;35(3):255–271.

[115] Davies W. Genomic imprinting on the X chromosome: implications for brain and behavioral phenotypes. Ann N Y Acad Sci. 2010;1204(Suppl):E14–E19.

[116] Singer H, Walier M, Nusgen N, Meesters C, Schreiner F, Woelfle J, et al. Methylation of L1Hs promoters is lower on the inactive X, has a tendency of being higher on autosomes in smaller genomes and shows inter-individual variability at some loci. Human Molecular Genetics. 2012;21:219–235.

[117] Gockley J, Willsey AJ, Dong S, Dougherty JD, Constantino JN, Sanders SJ. The female protective effect in autism spectrum disorder is not mediated by a single genetic locus. Mol Autism. 2015;6:25. doi: 10.1186/s13229-015-0014-3. PubMed PMID: 25973162; PubMed Central PMCID: PMC4429476.

[118] Skuse DH. Imprinting, the X-chromosome, and the male brain: explaining sex differences in the liability to autism. Pediatr Res. 2000;47(1):9–16.

[119] Donnelly SL, Wolpert CM, Menold MM, Bass MP, Gilbert JR, Cuccaro ML, et al. Female with autistic disorder and monosomy X (Turner syndrome): parent-of-origin effect of the X chromosome. Am J Med Genet. 2000;96(3):312–316.

[120] Ziats MN, Rennert OM. Sex-biased gene expression in the developing brain: implications for autism spectrum disorders. Mol Autism. 2013;4(1):10. doi: 10.1186/2040-2392-4-10.

[121] Prilutsky D, Palmer NP, Smedemark-Margulies N, Schlaeger TM, Margulies DM, Kohane IS. iPSC-derived neurons as a higher-throughput readout for autism: promises and pitfalls. Trends Mol Med. 2014;20(2):91-104. doi:10.1016/j.molmed.2013.11.004. Review. PubMed PMID: 24374161; PubMed Central PMCID: PMC4117413.

[122] Griesi-Oliveira K, Acab A, Gupta AR, Sunaga DY, Chailangkarn T, Nicol X, et al. Modeling non-syndromic autism and the impact of TRPC6 disruption in human neurons. Mol Psychiatry. 2014;20(11):1350-1365. doi: 10.1038/mp.2014.141. PubMed PMID: 25385366; PubMedCentral PMCID: PMC4427554.

[123] DeRosa BA et al. Derivation of autism spectrum disorder-specific induced pluripotent stem cells from peripheral blood mononuclear cells. Neurosci Lett. 2012;516(1):9-14. doi: 10.1016/j.neulet.2012.02.086. PubMed PMID: 22405972; PubMed Central PMCID: PMC4278654.

[124] Dandulakis MG, Meganathan K, Kroll KL, Bonni A, Constantino JN. Complexities of X chromosome inactivation status in female human induced pluripotent stem cells-a brief review and scientific update for autism research. J Neurodev Disord. 2016;8:22. doi: 10.1186/s11689-016-9155-8. eCollection 2016

[125] Gong X, Bacchelli E, Blasi F, Toma C, Betancur C, Chaste P, et al. Analysis of X chromosome inactivation in autism spectrum disorders. Am J Med Genet B Neuropsychiatr Genet. 2008;147B(6):830–835.

[126] Carrel L, Willard HF. X-inactivation profile reveals extensive variability in X-linked gene expression in females. Nature. 2005;434(7031):400–404.

[127] Carrascosa-Romero MC, Suela J, Alfaro-Ponce B, Cepillo-Boluda AJ. X-chromosome-linked ichthyosis associated to epilepsy, hyperactivity, autism and mental retardation, due to the Xp22.31 microdeletion. Rev Neurol. 2012;54(4):241–248.

[128] Howerton CL, Morgan CP, Fischer DB, Bale TL. O-GlcNAc transferase (OGT) as a placental biomarker of maternal stress and reprogramming of CNS gene transcription in development. Proceedings of the National Academy of Sciences of the United States of America. 2013;110(13):5169–5174.

[129] Bajrami E, Spiroski M. Genomic Imprinting. Open Access Maced J Med Sci. 2016; 4(1):181–184.

[130] Lee JT, Bartolomei MS. X-inactivation, imprinting, and long noncoding RNAs in health and disease. Cell. 2013;152:1308–1323.

[131] Crespi B. Genomic imprinting in the development and evolution of psychotic spectrum conditions. Biol Rev Camb Philos Soc. 2008;83(4):441–493.

[132] Pfeifer K. Mechanisms of Genomic Imprinting. Am J Hum Genet. 2000;67:777–787.

[133] Ogata T, Kagami M.J. Kagami-Ogata syndrome: a clinically recognizable upd (14) pat and related disorder affecting the chromosome 14q32.2 imprinted region. Hum Genet. 2016;61(2):87–94.

[134] van der Werf IM, Buiting K, Czeschik C, Reyniers E, Vandeweyer G, Vanhaesebrouck P, et al. Novel microdeletions on chromosome 14q32.2 suggest a potential role for non-coding RNAs in Kagami-Ogata syndrome. Eur J Hum Genet. 2016;24(12):1724–1729. doi: 10.1038/ejhg.2016.82. PubMed PMID: 27406249; PubMed Central PMCID: PMC5117931.

[135] Matsubara K, Kagami M, Nakabayashi K, Hata K, Fukami M, Ogata T, et al. Exploration of hydroxymethylation in Kagami-Ogata syndrome caused by hypermethylation of imprinting control regions. Clin Epigenetics. 2015;7:90. Epub 2015 Aug 28

[136] Kalsner L, Chamberlain SJ. Prader-Willi, Angelman, and 15q11-q13 duplication syndromes. Pediatr Clin North Am. 2015;62(3):587–606.

[137] Mabb AM, Judson MC, Zylka MJ, Philpot BD. Angelman syndrome: insights into genomic imprinting and neurodevelopmental phenotypes. Trends Neurosci. 2011; 34:293–303.

[138] Depienne C, Moreno-De-Luca D, Heron D, Bouteiller D, Gennetier A, Delorme R, et al. Screening for genomic rearrangements and methylation abnormalities of the 15q11-q13 region in autismspectrum disorders. Biol Psychiatry. 2009;66(4):349–359.

[139] Germain ND, Chen PF, Plocik AM, Glatt-Deeley H, Brown J, Fink JJ, et al. Gene expression analysis of human induced pluripotent stem cell-derived neurons carrying copy number variants of chromosome 15q11-q13.1. Mol Autism. 2014;5:44. doi: 10.1186/2040-2392-5-44. eCollection 2014

[140] Choufani S, Shuman C, Weksberg R. Molecular findings in Beckwith-Wiedemann syndrome. Am J Med Genet C. 2013;163C:131–140.

[141] Kent L, Bowdin S, Kirby GA, Cooper WN, Maher ER. Beckwith Weidemann syndrome: a behavioral phenotype-genotype study. Am J Med Genet B Neuropsychiatr Genet. 2008;147B(7):1295–1297.

[142] Eggermann T, Begemann M, Spengler S, Schröder C, Kordass U, et al. Genetic and epigenetic findings in Silver-Russell syndrome. Pediatr Endocrinol Rev. 2010;8:86–93.

[143] Arnaud P, Feil R. Epigenetic deregulation of genomic imprinting in human disorders and following assisted reproduction. Birth Defects Res C. 2005;75:81–97.

[144] Hvidtjørn D, Grove J, Schendel D, Schieve LA, Svaerke C, Ernst E, et al. Risk of autism spectrum disorders in children born after assisted conception: a population-based follow-up study. J Epidemiol Community Health. 2011;65(6):497–502.

[145] Zachor DA, Ben Itzchak E. Assisted reproductive technology and risk for autism spectrum disorder. Res Dev Disabil. 2011;32(6):2950–2956.

[146] Lehti V, Brown AS, Gissler M, Rihko M, Suominen A, Sourander A. Autism spectrum disorders in IVF children: a national case-control study in Finland. Hum Reprod. 2013;28(3):812–818.

[147] Sandin S, Nygren KG, Iliadou A, Hultman CM, Reichenberg A. Autism and mental retardation among offspring born after in vitro fertilization. JAMA. 2013;310(1):75–84.

[148] Amir RE, van den Veyver IB, Wan, M, Tran CQ, Francke U, Zoghbi HY. Rett syndrome is caused by mutations in X-linked MECP2, encoding methyl-CpG-binding protein 2. Nat. Genet. 1999;23:185–188.

[149] Wolffe AP. Histone deacetylase: a regulator of transcription. Science. 1996;272:371–372.

[150] Jones PL, Veenstra GJ, Wade PA, Vermaak D, Kass S.U, Landsbergerv N, et al. Methylated DNA and MeCP2 recruit histone deacetylase to repress transcription. Nat Genet. 1998;19:187–191.

[151] Ballestar E, Yusufzai TM, Wolffe AP. Effects of Rett syndrome mutations of the methyl-CpG binding domain of the transcriptional repressor MeCP2 on selectivity for association with methylated DNA. Biochemistry. 2000;39:7100–7106.

[152] Lilja T, Wallenborg K, Björkman K, Albåge M, Eriksson M, Lagercrantz H, et al. Novel alterations in the epigenetic signature of MeCP2-targeted promoters in lymphocytes of Rett syndrome patients. Epigenetics. 2013;8(3):246–251.

[153] Johnston M, Blue ME, Naidu S. Recent advances in understanding synaptic abnormalities in Rett syndrome. F1000Res. 2015; pii: F1000 Faculty Rev-1490. eCollection 2015. doi: 10.12688/f1000research.6987.1. Review. PubMed PMID: 26918155; PubMed Central PMCID: PMC4754036

[154] Lyst MJ, Bird A. Rett syndrome: a complex disorder with simple roots. Nat Rev Genet. 2015;16:261–275.

[155] Chao HT, Zoghbi HY, Rosenmund C. MeCP2 controls excitatory synaptic strength by regulating glutamatergic synapse number. Neuron. 2007;56:58–65.

[156] Budimirovic DB, Kaufmann WE. What can we learn about autism from studying fragile X syndrome? Dev Neurosci. 2011;33(5):379–394.

[157] Verkerk AJ, Pieretti M, Sutcliffe JS, Fu YH, Kuhl DP, Pizzuti A, et al. Identification of a gene (FMR1) containing a CGG repeat coincident with a breakpoint cluster region exhibiting length variation in fragile X syndrome. Cell. 1991;65:905–914.

[158] Sutcliffe JS, Nelson DL, Zhang F, Pieretti M, Caskey CT, Saxe D, et al. DNA methylation represses FMR-1 transcription in fragile X syndrome. Hum Mol Genet. 1992;1(6):397–400.

[159] Tabolacci E, Palumbo F, Nobile V, Neri G. Transcriptional reactivation of the FMR1 Gene. A possible approach to the treatment of the fragile X syndrome. Genes (Basel). 2016;7(8)pii: E49. doi: 10.3390/genes7080049. PubMed PMID: 27548224; PubMed Central PMCID: PMC4999837.

[160] Cukier HN, Lee JM, Ma D, Young JI, Mayo V, Butler BL, et al. The expanding role of MBD genes in autism: identification of a MECP2 duplication and novel alterations in MBD5, MBD6, and SETDB1. Autism Res. 2012;5:385–397.

[161] Laget S, Joulie M, Le Masson F et al: The human proteins MBD5 and MBD6 associate with heterochromatin but they do not bind methylated DNA. PLoS One 2010;5:e11982.

[162] Mullegama SV, Rosenfeld JA, Orellana C, van Bon BW, Halbach S, Repnikova EA,et al. Reciprocal deletion and duplication at 2q23.1 indicates a role for MBD5 in autism spectrum disorder. Eur J Hum Genet. 2014;22(1):57–63.

[163] Gregory SG, Connelly JJ, Towers AJ, Johnson J, Biscocho D, Markunas CA, et al. Genomic and epigenetic evidence for oxytocin receptor deficiency in autism. BMC Med. 2009;7:62. doi: 10.1186/1741-7015-7-62.

[164] Hu VW, Sarachana T, Sherrard RM, Kocher KM. Investigation of sex differences in the expression of RORA and its transcriptional targets in the brain as a potential contributor to the sex bias in autism. Mol Autism. 2015;6:7. doi: 10.1186/2040-2392-6-7. eCollection 2015

[165] James SJ, Shpyleva S, Melnyk S, Pavliv O, Pogribny IP. Complex epigenetic regulation of engrailed-2 (EN-2) homeobox gene in the autism cerebellum. Transl Psychiatry 2013;3:e232.

[166] Zhubi A, Chen Y, Dong E, Cook EH, Guidotti A, Grayson DR. Increased binding of MeCP2 to the GAD1 and RELN promoters may be mediated by an enrichment of 5-hmC in autism spectrum disorder (ASD) cerebellum. Transl Psychiatry.2014;4:e349. doi: 10.1038/tp.2013.123.

[167] Sheikh AM, Malik M, Wen G, Chauhan A, Chauhan V, Gong CX, et al. BDNF-Akt-Bcl2 antiapoptotic signaling pathway is compromised in the brain of autistic subjects. J Neurosci Res. 2010;88:2641–2647.

[168] Harony H, Wagner S. The contribution of oxytocin and vasopressin to mammalian social behavior: Potential role in autism spectrum disorder. Neurosignals. 2010;18:82–97.

[169] Parker KJ Garner JP, Libove RA, Hyde SA, Hornbeak KB, Carson DS, et al. Plasma oxytocin concentrations and OXTR polymorphisms predict social impairments in children with and without autism spectrum disorder. Proc Natl Acad Sci U S A. 2014;111(33):12258–12263. doi: 10.1073/pnas.1402236111

[170] Viaggi C, Gerace C, Pardini C, Corsini GU, Vaglini F.Serotonin abnormalities in Engrailed-2 knockout mice: new insight relevant for a model of autism spectrum disorder. Neurochem Int. 2015;87:34–42.

[171] Genestine M, Lin L, Durens M, Yan Y, Jiang Y, Prem S, et al. Engrailed-2 (En2) deletion produces multiple neurodevelopmental defects in monoamine systems, forebrain structures and neurogenesis and behavior. Hum Mol Genet. 2015;24(20):5805–5827.

[172] Uchino S, Waga C. SHANK3 as an autism spectrum disorder-associated gene. Brain Dev. 2013;35:106–110.

[173] Wong CC, Meaburn EL, Ronald A, Price TS, Jeffries AR, Schalkwyk LC, et al. Methylomic analysis of monozygotic twins discordant for autism spectrum disorder and related behaviouraltraits. Mol Psych. 2014;19(4):495–503.

[174] Bekinschtein P, Cammarota M, Katche C, Slipczuk L, Rossato JI, Goldin A, et al. BDNF is essential to promote persistence of long-term memory storage. Proc Nat Acad Sci. 2008;105:2711–2716.

[175] Li M, Du W, Shao F, Wang W. Cognitive dysfunction and epigenetic alterations of the BDNF gene are induced by social isolation during early adolescence. Behav Brain Res. 2016;313:177–183.

[176] Armeanu R, Mokkonen M, Crespi B. Meta-Analysis of BDNF Levels in Autism. Cell Mol Neurobiol. 2016; [Epub ahead of print] PubMed PMID: 27501933.

[177] Qin XY, Feng JC, Cao C, Wu HT, Loh YP, Cheng Y. Association of peripheral blood levels of brain-derived neurotrophic factor with autism spectrum disorderin children: a systematic review and meta-analysis. JAMA Pediatr. 2016;170(11):1079-1086. doi: 10.1001/jamapediatrics.2016.1626. PubMed PMID:27654278.

[178] Zheng Z, Zhang L, Zhu T, Huang J, Qu Y, Mu DPeripheral brain-derived neurotrophic factor in autism spectrum disorder: a systematic review and meta-analysis. Sci Rep. 2016;6:31241. doi: 10.1038/srep31241.

[179] Sullivan JM, Badimon A, Schaefer U, Ayata P, Gray J, Chung CW, et al. Autism-like syndrome is induced by pharmacological suppression of BET proteins in young mice. J Exp Med. 2015;212(11):1771–1781.

[180] Iossifov I, O'roak BJ, Sanders SJ, Ronemus M, Krumm N, Levy D, et al. The contribution of de novo coding mutations to autism spectrum disorder. Nature. 2014;515(7526):216–221.

[181] Mbadiwe T, Millis RM. Epigenetics and autism. Autism Res Treat. 2013;2013:826156. doi: 10.1155/2013/826156

[182] Vallianatos CN, Iwase S. Disrupted intricacy of histone H3K4 methylation in neurodevelopmental disorders. Epigenomics. 2015;7(3):503–519.

[183] Balan S, Iwayama Y, Maekawa M, Toyota T, Ohnishi T, Toyoshima M, et al. Exon resequencing of H3K9 methyltransferase complex genes, EHMT1, EHTM2 and WIZ, in Japanese autism subjects. Mol. Autism. 2014;5(1):49. doi: 10.1186/2040-2392-5-49. eCollection 2014.

[184] Zhu T, Liang C, Li D, Tian M, Liu S, Gao G, et al. Histone methyltransferase Ash1L mediates activity-dependent repression of neurexin-1α. Sci Rep. 2016;6:26597. doi: 10.1038/srep26597.

[185] Tanasijevic B, Rasmussen TP.X chromosome inactivation and differentiation occur readily in ES cells doubly-deficient for macroH2A1 and macroH2A2. PLoS One. 2011;6(6):e21512. doi: 10.1371/journal.pone.0021512

[186] Posavec M, Timinszky G, Buschbeck M. Macro domains as metabolite sensors on chromatin. Cell Mol Life Sci. 2013;70(9):1509–1524.

[187] Philippi A, Tores F, Carayol J, Rousseau F, Letexier M, Roschmann E, et al. Association of autism with polymorphisms in the paired-like homeodomain transcription factor 1 (PITX1) on chromosome 5q31: a candidate gene analysis. BMC Med Genet. 2007;8:74.

[188] Jones RM, Cadby G, Blangero J, Abraham LJ, Whitehouse AJ, Moses EK. MACROD2 gene associated with autistic-like traits in a general population sample. Psychiatr Genet. 2014;24(6):241–248.

[189] Kanaho Y, Funakoshi Y, Hasegawa H. Phospholipase D signalling and its involvement in neurite outgrowth. Biochim Biophys Acta. 2009;1791:898–904.

[190] Dhami GK, Ferguson SS. Regulation of metabotropic glutamate receptor signaling, desensitization and endocytosis. Pharmacol Ther. 2006;111:260–271.

[191] Mikkelsen TS, Ku M, Jaffe DB, Issac B, Lieberman E, Giannoukos G, Alvarez P,et al. Genome-wide maps of chromatin state in pluripotent and lineage-committed cells. Nature. 2007;448(7153):553–560.

[192] Vignali M, Hassan AH, Neely KE, Workman JL. ATP-dependent chromatin-remodeling complexes. Mol Cell Biol. 2000;20(6):1899–1910.

[193] Hota SK, Bruneau BG. ATP-dependent chromatin remodeling during mammalian development. Development. 2016;143(16):2882–2897.

[194] Flaus A, Martin DM, Barton GJ, Owen-Hughes T. Identification of multiple distinct Snf2 subfamilies with conserved structural motifs. Nucleic Acids Res. 2006;34:2887–2905.

[195] Shang L, Cho MT, Retterer K, Folk L, Humberson J, Rohena L, et al. Mutations in ARID2 are associated with intellectual disabilities. Neurogenetics. 2015;16(4):307–314.

[196] Vogel-Ciernia A, Matheos DP, Barrett RM, Kramar EA, Azzawi S, Chen Y, et al. The neuronspecific chromatin regulatory subunit BAF53b is necessary for synaptic plasticity and memory. Nat Neurosci. 2013;16(5):552–561.

[197] Santen GW, Aten E, Sun Y, Almomani R, Gilissen C, Nielsen M, et al. Mutations in SWI/SNF chromatin remodeling complex gene ARID1B cause Coffin-Siris syndrome. Nat Genet. 2012;44(4):379–380.

[198] Barnard RA, Pomaville MB, O'Roak BJ. Mutations and modeling of the chromatin remodeler chd8 define an emerging autism etiology. Front Neurosci. 2015;9:477. doi: 10.3389/fnins. 2015.00477. eCollection 2015.

[199] Wilkinson B, Grepo N, Thompson BL, Kim J, Wang K, Evgrafov OV. The autism-associated gene chromodomain helicase DNA-binding protein 8 (CHD8) regulates noncoding RNAs and autism-related genes. Transl Psychiatry. 2015;5:e568. doi: 10.1038/tp.2015.62

[200] Rouleau N, Domans'kyi A, Reeben M, Moilanen AM, Havas K, Kang Z, et al. Novel ATPase of SNF2-like protein family interacts with androgen receptor and modulates androgen-dependent transcription. Mol Biol Cell. 2002;13(6):2106–2119.

[201] Lee TI, Young RA. Transcription of eukaryotic protein-coding genes. Annu Rev Genet. 2000;34:77–137.

[202] Helsmoortel C, Vulto-van Silfhout AT, Coe BP, Vandeweyer G, Rooms L, van den Ende J, et al. A SWI/SNF-related autism syndrome caused by de novo mutations in ADNP. Nat Genet. 2014;46(4):380–384.

[203] Guinchat V, Thorsen P, Laurent C, Cans C, Bodeau N, Cohen D. Pre-, peri- and neonatal risk factors for autism. Acta Obstet Gynecol Scand. 2012;91(3):287–300.

[204] Hadjkacem I, Ayadi H, Turki M, Yaich S, Khemekhem K, Walha A, et al. Prenatal, perinatal and postnatal factors associated with autism spectrum disorder. J Pediatr (Rio J). 2016;S0021–S7557(16):30102–30104.

[205] Mamidala MP, Polinedi A, P T V PK, Rajesh N, Vallamkonda OR, Udani V, et al. Prenatal, perinatal and neonatal risk factors of Autism Spectrum Disorder: a comprehensive epidemiological assessment from India. Res Dev Disabil. 2013;34(9):3004–3013.

[206] Kalkbrenner AE, Schmidt RJ, Penlesky AC. Environmental chemical exposures and autism spectrum disorders: a review of the epidemiological evidence. Curr Probl Pediatr Adolesc Health Care. 2014;44(10):277–318.

[207] Vrijheid M, Casas M, Gascon M, Valvi D, Nieuwenhuijsen M. Environmental pollutants and child health-A review of recent concerns. Int J Hyg Environ Health. 2016;219(4–5):331–342.

[208] Winneke G. Developmental aspects of environmental neurotoxicology: lessons from lead and polychlorinated biphenyls. J Neurol Sci. 2011;308(1–2):9–15.

[209] Grandjean P, Herz KT. Trace elements as paradigms of developmental neurotoxicants: lead, methylmercury and arsenic. J Trace Elem Med Biol. 2015;31:130–134.

[210] Goines PE, Ashwood P. Cytokine dysregulation in autism spectrum disorders (ASD): possible role of the environment. Neurotoxicol Teratol. 2013;36:67–81.

[211] Stamou M, Streifel KM, Goines PE, Lein PJ. Neuronal connectivity as a convergent target of gene × that confer risk for autism spectrum disorders. Neurotoxicol Teratol. 2013;36:3–16.

[212] Keil KP, Lein PJ.DNA methylation: a mechanism linking environmental chemical exposures to risk of autism spectrum disorders? Environ Epigenet. 2016;2(1):dvv012. Epub 2016 Jan 30

[213] Hill DS, Cabrera R, Wallis Schultz D, Zhu H, Lu W, Finnell RH, et al. Autism-like behavior and epigenetic changes associated with autism as consequences of in utero exposure to environmental pollutants in a mouse model. Behav Neurol. 2015;2015:426263. doi: 10.1155/2015/426263

[214] Shannon M, Graef JW. Lead intoxication in children with pervasive developmental disorders. J Toxicol Clin Toxicol. 1996;34(2):177–181.

[215] Cohen DJ, Johnson WT, Caparulo BK. Pica and elevated blood lead level in autistic and atypical children. Am J Dis Child. 1976;130(1):47–48.

[216] Tian Y, Green PG, Stamova B, Hertz-Picciotto I, Pessah IN, Hansen R, Yang X, et al. Correlations of gene expression with blood lead levels in children with autism compared to typically developing controls. Neurotox Res. 2011;19(1):1–13.

[217] Albizzati A, Morè L, Di Candia D, Saccani M, Lenti C. Normal concentrations of heavy metals in autistic spectrum disorders. Minerva Pediatr. 2012;64(1):27–31.

[218] Desoto MC, Hitlan RT. Blood levels of mercury are related to diagnosis of autism: a reanalysis of an important data set. J Child Neurol. 2007;22(11):1308–1311.

[219] DeStefano F. Vaccines and autism: evidence does not support a causal association. Clin Pharmacol Ther. 2007;82(6):756–759.

[220] Miller L, Reynolds J. Autism and vaccination-the current evidence. J Spec Pediatr Nurs. 2009; 14(3):166–172.

[221] Wolstenholme JT, Rissman EF, Connelly JJ. The role of Bisphenol A in shaping the brain, epigenome and behavior. Horm Behav. 2011 Mar;59(3):296–305.

[222] Wolstenholme JT, Edwards M, Shetty SR, Gatewood JD, Taylor JA, Rissman EF, et al. Gestational exposure to bisphenol a produces transgenerational changes in behaviors and gene expression. Endocrinology. 2012;153(8):3828–3838.

[223] Sarrouilhe D, Dejean C. Autism spectrum disorders and bisphenol A: is serotonin the lacking link in the chain? Encephale. 2016; pii: S0013-7006(16)30133-6. doi: 10.1016/j.encep.2016.04.007. [Epub ahead of print] PubMed PMID: 27623126.

[224] McDermott S, Salzberg DC, Anderson AP, Shaw T, Lead J. Systematic review of chromium and nickel exposure during pregnancy and impact on child outcomes. J Toxicol Environ Health A. 2015;78(21–22):1348–1368.

[225] Ramos-Chávez LA, Rendón-López CR, Zepeda A, Silva-Adaya D, Del Razo LM, Gonsebatt ME. Neurological effects of inorganic arsenic exposure: altered cysteine/glutamate transport, NMDA expression and spatial memory impairment. Front Cell Neurosci. 2015;9:21. doi: 10.3389/fncel.2015.00021. eCollection 2015.

[226] Shafer TJ, Meyer DA, et al. Developmental neurotoxicity of pyrethroid insecticides: critical review and future research needs. Environ Health Perspect. 2005;113(2):123–136.

[227] Shelton JF, Hertz-Picciotto I, Pessah IN. Tipping the balance of autism risk: potential mechanisms linking pesticides and autism. Environ Health Perspect. 2012;120 (7):944–951.

[228] Berghuis SA, Bos AF, Sauer PJ, Roze E. Developmental neurotoxicity of persistent organic pollutants: an update on childhood outcome. Arch Toxicol. 2015;89(5):687–709.

[229] Dufour-Rainfray D, Vourc'h P, Tourlet S, Guilloteau D, Chalon S, Andres CR. Fetal exposure to teratogens: evidence of genes involved in autism. Neurosci Biobehav Rev. 2011;35(5):1254–1265.

[230] Kinast K, Peeters D, Kolk SM, Schubert D, Homberg JR. Genetic and pharmacological manipulations of the serotonergic system in early life: neurodevelopmental underpinnings of autism-related behavior. Front Cell Neurosci. 2013;7:72. doi: 10.3389/fncel.2013.00072. eCollection 2013

[231] Miyazaki K, Narita N, Narita M. Maternal administration of thalidomide or valproic acid causes abnormal serotonergic neurons in the offspring: implication for pathogenesis of autism. Int J Dev Neurosci. 2005;23(2–3):287–297.

[232] Yang EJ, Ahn S, Lee K, Mahmood U, Kim HS. Early behavioral abnormalities and perinatal alterations of pten/akt pathway in valproic acid autism model mice. PLoS One. 2016;11(4):e0153298. doi: 10.1371/journal.pone.0153298. eCollection 2016

[233] Qin L, Dai X, Yin Y. Valproic acid exposure sequentially activates Wnt and mTOR pathways in rats. Mol Cell Neurosci. 2016;75:27–35.

[234] Ghanizadeh A. Acetaminophen may mediate oxidative stress and neurotoxicity in autism. Med Hypotheses. 2012;78(2):351. doi: 10.1016/j.mehy.2011.11.009. Epub 2011 Dec 9.

[235] Thompson JM, Waldie KE, Wall CR, Murphy R, Mitchell EA. ABC study group. Associations between acetaminophen use during pregnancy and ADHD symptoms measured at ages 7 and 11 years. PLoS One. 2014;9(9):e108210. doi: 10.1371/journal.pone.0108210. eCollection 2014

[236] Bauer AZ, Kriebel D. Prenatal and perinatal analgesic exposure and autism: an ecological link. Environ Health. 2013;12:41 doi: 10.1186/1476-069X-12-41.

[237] Penella E, Sandoval J, Zaragozá R, García C, Viña JR, Torres L, et al. Molecular mechanisms of Id2 down-regulation in rat liver after acetaminophen overdose. Protection by N-acetyl-L-cysteine. Free Radic Res. 2010;44(9):1044–1053.

[238] Libbey JE, Sweeten TL, McMahon WM, Fujinami RS. Autistic disorder and viral infections. J Neurovirol. 2005;11(1):1–10.

[239] Meyer U, Feldon J, Dammann O. Schizophrenia and autism: both shared and disorder-specific pathogenesis via perinatal inflammation? Pediatr Res. 2011;69(5 Pt 2):26R–33R

[240] Measles-mumps-rubella vaccine and autistic spectrum disorder: report from the New Challenges in Childhood Immunizations Conference convened in Oak Brook, Illinois, June 12–13, 2000. Halsey NA, Hyman SL, Conference Writing Panel. Pediatrics. 2001;107(5):E84

[241] Chess S. Follow-up report on autism in congenital rubella. J Autism Child Schizophr. 1977;7(1):69–81.

[242] Markowitz PI. Autism in a child with congenital cytomegalovirus infection. J Autism Dev Disord. 1983;13(3):249–253.

[243] Ivarsson SA, Bjerre I, Vegfors P, Ahlfors K. Autism as one of several disabilities in two children with congenital cytomegalovirus infection. Neuropediatrics. 1990;21(2):102–103.

[244] Sweeten TL, Posey DJ, McDougle CJ. Brief report: autistic disorder in three children with cytomegalovirus infection. J Autism Dev Disord. 2004;34(5):583–586.

[245] Atladóttir HO, Thorsen P, Østergaard L, Schendel DE, Lemcke S, Abdallah M,Maternal infection requiring hospitalization during pregnancy and autism spectrum disorders. J Autism Dev Disord. 2010;40(12):1423–1430.

[246] Nardone S, Elliott E. The Interaction between the immune system and epigenetics in the etiology of autism spectrum disorders. Front Neurosci. 2016;10:329. doi: 10.3389/fnins.2016.00329. eCollection 2016

[247] Sauer S, Bruno L, Hertweck A, Finlay D, Leleu M, Spivakov M, et al. T cell receptor signaling controls Foxp3 expression via PI3K, Akt, mTOR. Proc Natl Acad Sci U S A. 2008;105(22):7797–7802.

[248] Miyao T, Floess S, Setoguchi R, Luche H, Fehling HJ, Waldmann H, et al. Plasticity of Foxp3(+) T cells reflects promiscuous Foxp3 expression in conventional T cells but not reprogramming of regulatory T cells. Immunity. 2012;36(2):262–275.

[249] Ahmad SF, Zoheir KM, Ansari MA, Nadeem A, Bakheet SA, Al-Ayadhi LY, et al. Dysregulation of Th1, Th2, Th17, and T regulatory cell-related transcription factor signaling in children withautism. Mol Neurobiol. 2016. [Epub ahead of print]

[250] Ashwood P, Krakowiak P, Hertz-Picciotto I, Hansen R, Pessah I, Van de Water J. Elevated plasma cytokines in autism spectrum disorders provide evidence of immune dysfunction and are associated with impaired behavioral outcome. Brain Behav Immun. 2011;25:40–45.

[251] Liu Y, Zhang Q, Ding Y, Li X, Zhao D, Zhao K, et al. Histone lysine methyltransferase Ezh1 promotes TLR-triggered inflammatory cytokine production by suppressing Tollip. J Immunol. 2015;194:2838–2846.

[252] Yamamoto Y, Verma UN, Prajapati S, Kwak YT, Gaynor RB. Histone H3 phosphorylation by IKK-α is critical for cytokine-induced gene expression. Nature. 2003;423:655–659.

[253] Bayarsaihan D. Epigenetic mechanisms in inflammation. J Dent Res. 2011;90(1):9–17.

[254] Gentile I, Zappulo E, Militerni R, Pascotto A, Borgia G, Bravaccio C. Etiopathogenesis of autism spectrum disorders: fitting the pieces of the puzzle together. Med Hypotheses. 2013;81(1):26–35.

[255] Suzuki AM, Griesi-Oliveira K, de Oliveira Freitas Machado C, Vadasz E, Zachi EC, Passos-Bueno MR, et al. Altered mTORC1 signaling in multipotent stem cells from nearly 25% of patients with nonsyndromic autism spectrum disorders. Mol Psychiatry. 2015;20(5):551–552.

[256] Wu J, de Theije CG, da Silva SL, van der Horst H, Reinders MT, Broersen LM, et al. mTOR plays an important role in cow's milk allergy-associated behavioral and immunological deficits. Neuropharmacology. 2015;97:220–232.

[257] Bourgeron T. A synaptic trek to autism. Curr Opin Neurobiol. 2009;19:231–234.

[258] Tang G, Gudsnuk K, Kuo SH, Cotrina ML, Rosoklija G, Sosunov A, et al. Loss of mTOR-dependent macroautophagy causes autistic-like synaptic pruning deficits. Neuron. 2014;83(5):1131–1143.

[259] Huber KM, Klann E, Costa-Mattioli M, Zukin RS. Dysregulation of mammalian target of rapamycin signaling in mouse models of autism. J Neurosci. 2015;35(41):13836–13842.

[260] Peça J, Feng G. Cellular and synaptic network defects in autism. Curr Opin Neurobiol. 2012;22:866–872.

[261] Wu J, de Theije CG, da Silva SL, van der Horst H, Reinders MT, Broersen LM, et al. mTOR plays an important role in cow's milk allergy-associated behavioral and immunological deficits. Neuropharmacology. 2015;97:220–232. doi: 10.1016/j.neuropharm.2015.04.035. Epub 2015 May 29

[262] McMahon JJ, Yu W, Yang J, Feng H, Helm M, McMahon E, et al. Seizure-dependent mTOR activation in 5-HT neurons promotes autism-like behaviors in mice. Neurobiol Dis. 2015;73:296–306. doi: 10.1016/j.nbd.2014.10.004. Epub 2014 Oct 12

[263] Bandini LG, Anderson SE, Curtin C, Cermak S, Evans EW, Scampini R, et al. Food selectivity in children with autism spectrum disorders and typically developing children. J Pediatr 2010;157:259–264.

[264] Hyman SL, Stewart PA, Schmidt B, Cain U, Lemcke N, Foley JT, et al. Nutrient intake from food in children with autism. Pediatrics. 2012;130(Suppl 2):S145–S153.

[265] Ranjan S, Nasser JA. Nutritional status of individuals with autism spectrum disorders: do we know enough? Adv Nutr. 2015;6(4):397–407.

[266] Newschaffer CJ, Croen LA, Daniels J, Giarelli E, Grether JK, Levy SE, et al. The epidemiology of ASD. Annu Rev Public Health. 2007;28:235–258.

[267] James SJ, Cutler P, Melnyk S, Jernigan S, Janak L, Gaylor DW, et al. Metabolic biomarkers of increased oxidative stress and impaired methylation capacity in children with autism. Am J Clin Nutr. 2004;80(6):1611–1617.

[268] James SJ, Melnyk S, Jernigan S, Cleves MA, Halsted CH, Wong DH, et al. Metabolic endophenotype and related genotypes are associated with oxidative stress in children with autism. Am J Med Genet B Neuropsychiatr Genet. 2006;141:947–956.

[269] Adams JB, Audhya T, McDonough-Means S, Rubin RA, Quig D, Geis E, et al. Nutritional and metabolic status of children with autism vs. neurotypical children, and the association with autism severity. Nutr Metab (Lond). 2011;8(1):34

[270] Hoshino Y, Yamamoto T, Kaneko M, Tachibana R, Watanabe M, Ono Y, et al. Blood serotonin and free tryptophan concentration in autistic children. Neuropsychobiology. 1984;11(1):22–27.

[271] Bursztejn C, Ferrari P, Dreux C, Braconnier A, Lancrenon S. Metabolism of serotonin in autism in children. Encephale. 1988;14(6):413–439.

[272] Yap IK, Angley M, Veselkov KA, Holmes E, Lindon JC, Nicholson JK. Urinary metabolic phenotyping differentiates children with autism from their unaffected siblings and age-matched controls. J Proteome Res. 2010;9(6):2996–3004.

[273] Bala KA, Doğan M, Mutluer T, Kaba S, Aslan O, Balahoroğlu R, et al. Plasma amino acid profile in autism spectrum disorder (ASD). Eur Rev Med Pharmacol Sci. 2016;20(5):923–929.

[274] Zheng HF, Wang WQ, Li XM, Rauw G, Baker GB. Body fluid levels of neuroactive amino acids in autism spectrum disorders: a review of the literature. Amino Acids. 2016. [Epub ahead of print]

[275] Hergüner S, Kelesoğlu FM, Tanıdır C, Cöpür M. Ferritin and iron levels in children with autistic disorder. Eur J Pediatr. 2012;171(1):143–146.

[276] Schmidt RJ, Tancredi DJ, Krakowiak P, Hansen RL, Ozonoff S. Maternal intake of supplemental iron and risk of autism spectrum disorder. Am J Epidemiol. 2014;180(9):890–900.

[277] Yasuda H, Yasuda Y, Tsutsui T. Estimation of autistic children by metallomics analysis. Sci Rep. 2013;3:1199. doi: 10.1038/srep01199. Epub 2013 Feb 4

[278] Meguid NA, Hashish AF, Anwar M, Sidhom G. Reduced serum levels of 25-hydroxy and 1,25-dihydroxy vitamin D in Egyptian children with autism. J Altern Complement Med. 2010;16:641–645.

[279] Lakshmi Priya MD, Geetha A. Level of trace elements (copper, zinc, magnesium and selenium) and toxic elements (lead and mercury) in the hair and nail of children with autism. Biol Trace Elem Res. 2011;142:148–158.

[280] Adams JB, Holloway CE, George F, Quig D. Analyses of toxic metals and essential minerals in the hair of Arizona children with autism and associated conditions, and their mothers. Biol Trace Elem Res 2006;110:193–209.

[281] W, Zhou Y, Sun C, Wang J, Wu L. A preliminary study on nutritional status and intake in Chinese children with autism. Eur J Pediatr. 2010;69(10):1201–1206.

[282] Whitehouse AJ, Holt BJ, Serralha M, Holt PG, Hart PH, Kusel MM. Maternal vitamin D levels and the autism phenotype among offspring. J Autism Dev Disord. 2013;43(7):1495-1504. doi: 10.1007/s10803-012-1676-8. PubMed PMID: 23070790.

[283] Grant WB, Soles CM. Epidemiologic evidence supporting the role of maternal vitamin D deficiency as a risk factor for the development of infantile autism. Derm Endocrinol. 2009;1:223–228.

[284] Kočovská E, Fernell E, Billstedt E, Minnis H, Gillberg C. Vitamin D and autism: clinical review. Res Dev Disabil. 201;33(5):1541–1550.

[285] Cannell JJ, Grant WB. What is the role of vitamin D in autism? Dermatoendocrinol. 2013;5(1):199–204.

[286] Sundar IK, Rahman I. Vitamin d and susceptibility of chronic lung diseases: role of epigenetics. Front Pharmacol. 2011;2:50. doi: 10.3389/fphar.2011.00050

[287] Mostafa GA, Al-Ayadhi LY. Reduced serum concentrations of 25-hydroxy vitamin D in children with autism: relation to autoimmunity. J Neuroinflammation. 2012;17(9):201

[288] Saad K, Abdel-Rahman AA, Elserogy YM, Al-Atram AA, Cannell JJ, Bjørklund G, et al. Vitamin D status in autism spectrum disorders and the efficacy of vitamin D supplementation in autistic children. Nutr Neurosci. 2015. [Epub ahead of print]

[289] Wolff T, Witkop CT, Miller T, Syed SB, Force USPST. Folic acid supplementation for the prevention of neural tube defects: an update of the evidence for the U.S. Preventive Services Task Force. Ann Intern Med. 2009;150(9):632–639.

[290] Schmidt RJ, Tancredi DJ, Ozonoff S, Hansen RL, Hartiala J, Allayee H, et al. Maternal periconceptional folic acid intake and risk of autism spectrum disorders and developmental delay in the CHARGE (Childhood Autism Risks from Genetics and Environment) case-control study. Am J Clin Nutr. 2012;96:80–89.

[291] Crider KS, Yang TP, Berry RJ,Bailey LB. Folate and DNA methylation: a review of molecular mechanisms and the evidence for folate's role. Adv Nutr. 2012;3:21–38.

[292] Amarasekera M, Martino D, Ashley S, Harb H, Kesper D, Strickland D, et al. Genome-wide DNA methylation profiling identifies a folate-sensitive region of differential methylation upstream of ZFP57-imprinting regulator in humans. FASEB J. 2014;28(9):4068–4076.

[293] Geoffroy A, Kerek R, Pourié G, Helle D, Guéant JL, Daval JL, et al. Late maternal folate supplementation rescues from methyl donor deficiency-associated brain defects by restoring Let-7 and miR-34 pathways. Mol Neurobiol. 2016. [Epub ahead of print]

[294] Castro K, Klein LD, Baronio D, Gottfried C, Riesgo R, Perry IS. Folic acid and autism: what do we know? Nutr Neurosci. 2016;19(7):310–317.

[295] Surén P, Roth C, Bresnahan M, Haugen M, Hornig M, Hirtz D, et al. Association between maternal use of folic acid supplements and risk of autism spectrum disorders in children. JAMA. 2013;309(6):570–577.

[296] Virk J, Liew Z, Olsen J, Nohr EA, Catov JM, Ritz B. Preconceptional and prenatal supplementary folic acid and multivitamin intake and autism spectrum disorders. Autism. 2016;20(6):710–718.

[297] Pu D, Shen Y, Wu J. Association between MTHFR gene polymorphism and the risk of autism spectrum disorders: a meta-analysis. Autism Res. 2013;6(5):384–392.

[298] Frye RE, Sequeira JM, Quadros EV, James SJ, Rossignol DA. Cerebral folate receptor autoantibodies in autism spectrum disorder. Mol Psychiatry. 2013;18(3):369–381.

[299] Ali A, Waly MI, Al-Farsi YM, Essa MM, Al-Sharbati MM, Deth RC. Hyperhomocysteinemia among Omani autistic children: a case-control study. Acta Biochim Pol. 2011;58:547–551.

[300] Al-Farsi YM, Waly MI, Deth RC, Al-Sharbati MM, Al-Shafaee M, Al-Farsi O, et al. Low folate and vitamin B12 nourishment is common in Omani children with newly diagnosed autism. Nutrition. 2013;29:537–541.

[301] Pasxca SP, Nemes B, Vlase L, Gagyi CE, Dronca E, Miu AC, Dronca M. High levels of homocysteine and low serum paraoxonase 1 arylesterase activity in children with autism. Life Sci. 2006;78:2244–2248.

[302] Sun C, Zou M, Zhao D, Xia W, Wu L. Efficacy of folic acid supplementation in autistic-children participating in structured teaching: an open-label trial. Nutrients. 2016;8(6) pii: E337. doi: 10.3390/nu8060337. PubMed PMID: 27338456; PubMed Central PMCID: PMC4924178.

[303] Gruber BM. B-group vitamins: chemoprevention? Adv Clin Exp Med. 2016;25(3):561–568.

[304] James SJ, Melnyk S, Fuchs G, Reid T, Jernigan S, Pavliv O, et al. Efficacy of methylcobalamin and folinic acid treatment on glutathione redox status in children with autism. Am J Clin Nutr 2009;89(1):425–430.

[305] Adams JB, George F, Audhya T. Abnormally high plasma levels of vitamin B6 in children with autism not taking supplements compared to controls not taking supplements. J Altern Complement Med. 2006;12:59–63.

[306] Xia W, Zhou Y, Sun C, Wang J, Wu L. A preliminary study on nutritional status and intake in Chinese children with autism. Eur J Pediatr. 2010;169:1201–1206.

[307] Spilioti M, Evangeliou AE, Tramma D, Theodoridou Z, Metaxas S, Michailidi E, et al. Evidence for treatable inborn errors of metabolism in a cohort of 187 Greek patients with autism spectrum disorder (ASD). Front Hum Neurosci. 2013;7:858. doi: 10.3389/fnhum.2013.00858. eCollection 2013

[308] Zeisel SH. Epigenetic mechanisms for nutrition determinants of later health outcomes. Am J Clin Nutr. 2009;89:1488S–1493S.

[309] Zeisel SH. The supply of choline is important for fetal progenitor cells. Semin Cell Dev Biol. 2011;22(6):624–628.

[310] Vance DE. Physiological roles of phosphatidylethanolamine N-methyltransferase. Biochimica et Biophysica Acta. 2013;1831(3):626–632.

[311] Zeisel SH. Choline phospholipids: signal transduction and carcinogenesis. FASEB J.1993;7(6):551–557.

[312] Selhub J, Seyoum E, Pomfret EA, Zeisel SH. Effects of choline deficiency and methotrexate treatment upon liver folate content and distribution. Cancer Res. 1991;51:16–21.

[313] Varela-Moreiras G, Selhub J, da Costa K, Zeisel SH. Effect of chronic choline deficiency in rats on liver folate content and distribution. J Nutr Biochem. 1992;3:519–522.

[314] Jacob R, Jenden D, Okoji R, Allman M, Swendseid M. Choline status of men and women is decreased by low dietary folate. FASEB J. 1998;12:A512

[315] Jacob RA, Jenden DJ, Allman-Farinelli MA, Swendseid ME. Folate nutriture alters choline status of women and men fed low choline diets. J Nutr. 1999;129:712–717.

[316] Kim YI, Miller JW, da Costa KA, Nadeau M, Smith D, Selhub J, et al. Folate deficiency causes secondary depletion of choline and phosphocholine in liver. J Nutr. 1995; 124:2197–203.

[317] Niculescu MD, Craciunescu CN, Zeisel SH. Dietary choline deficiency alters global and gene-specific DNA methylation in the developing hippocampus of mouse fetal brains. FASEB J. 2006;20(1):43–49.

[318] Hamlin JC, Pauly M, Melnyk S, Pavliv O, Starrett W, Crook TA, James SJ. Dietary intake and plasma levels of choline and betaine in children with autism spectrum disorders. Autism Res Treat. 2013;2013:578429

[319] Tran PV, Kennedy BC, Pisansky MT, Won KJ, Gewirtz JC, Simmons RA, et al. Prenatal choline supplementation diminishes early-life iron deficiency-induced reprogramming of molecular networks associated with behavioral abnormalities in the adult rat hippocampus. J Nutr. 2016;146(3):484–493.

[320] Thomas JD, Abou EJ, Dominguez HD. Prenatal choline supplementation mitigates the adverse effects of prenatal alcohol exposure on development in rats. Neurotoxicol Teratol. 2009;31(5):303–311.

[321] Wozniak JR, Fuglestad AJ, Eckerle JK, Fink BA, Hoecker HL, Boys CJ, et al. Choline supplementation in children with fetal alcohol spectrum disorders: a randomized, double-blind, placebo-controlled trial. Am J Clin Nutr. 2015;102(5):1113–1125.

[322] Janssen CI, Kiliaan AJ. Long-chain polyunsaturated fatty acids (LCPUFA) from genesis to senescence: the influence of LCPUFA on neural development, aging, and neurodegeneration. Prog Lipid Res. 2014;53:1–17.

[323] Fan C, Fu H, Dong H, Lu Y, Lu Y, Qi K. Maternal n-3 polyunsaturated fatty acid deprivation during pregnancy and lactation affects neurogenesis and apoptosis in adult offspring: associated with DNA methylation of brain-derived neurotrophic factor transcripts. Nutr Res. 2016;36(9):1013–1021.

[324] Al-Farsi YM, Waly MI, Deth RC, Al-Sharbati MM, Al-Shafaee M, Al-Farsi O, et al. Impact of nutrition on serum levels of docosahexaenoic acid among Omani children with autism. Nutrition. 2013;29(9):1142–1146.

[325] Brigandi SA, Shao H, Qian SY, Shen Y, Wu BL, Kang JX. Autistic children exhibit decreased levels of essential Fatty acids in red blood cells. Int J Mol Sci. 2015;16(5):10061–10076.

[326] Tamiji J, Crawford DA. The Neurobiology of lipid metabolism in autism spectrum disorders. Neurosignals. 2010;18(2):98–112.

[327] El-Ansary AK, Bacha AG, Al-Ayahdi LY. Impaired plasma phospholipids and relative amounts of essential polyunsaturated fatty acids in autistic patients from Saudi Arabia. Lipids Health Dis 2011;10:63

[328] Vancassel S, Durand G, Barthelemy C, Lejeune B, Martineau J, Guilloteau D, Andres C, Chalon S. Plasma fatty acid levels in autistic children. Prostaglandins. Leukot Essent Fatty Acids 2001;65:1–7.

[329] Chauhan A, Chauhan V, Brown WT, Cohen I. Oxidative stress in autism: increased lipid peroxidation and reduced serum levels of ceruloplasmin and transferrin–the antioxidant proteins. Life Sci. 2004;75:2539–2549.

[330] Maekawa M, Iwayama Y, Ohnishi T, Toyoshima M, Shimamoto C, Hisano Y, et al. Investigation of the fatty acid transporter-encoding genes SLC27A3 and SLC27A4 in autism. Sci Rep. 2015;5:16239. doi: 10.1038/srep16239

[331] Puri BK, Singh I. Normal phospholipid-related signal transduction in autism. Prog Neuropsychopharmacol Biol Psychiatry. 2002;26(7–8):1405–1407.

[332] El-Ansary A, Al-Ayadhi L. Lipid mediators in plasma of autism spectrum disorders. Lipids Health Dis. 2012;11:160. doi: 10.1186/1476-511X-11-160.

[333] Yui K, Imataka G, Nakamura H, Ohara N, Naito Y. Eicosanoids derived from arachidonic acid and their family prostaglandins and cyclooxygenase in psychiatric disorders. Curr Neuropharmacol. 2015;13(6):776–785.

[334] Wong CT, Ahmad E, Li H, Crawford DA. Prostaglandin E2 alters Wnt-dependent migration and proliferation in neuroectodermal stem cells: implications for autism spectrum disorders. Cell Commun Signal. 2014;12:19. doi: 10.1186/1478-811X-12-19

[335] Ooi YP, Weng SJ, Jang LY, Low L, Seah J, Teo S, et al. Omega-3 fatty acids in the management of autism spectrum disorders: findings from an open-label pilot study in Singapore. Eur J Clin Nutr. 2015;69(8):969–971.

[336] Mankad D, Dupuis A, Smile S, Roberts W, Brian J, Lui T, et al. A randomized, placebo controlled trial of omega-3 fatty acids in the treatment of young children with autism. Mol Autism. 2015;6:18. doi: 10.1186/s13229-015-0010-7. eCollection 2015

[337] Voigt RG, Mellon MW, Katusic SK, Weaver AL, Matern D, Mellon B, et al. Dietary docosahexaenoic acid supplementation in children with autism. J Pediatr Gastroenterol Nutr. 2014;58(6):715–722.

[338] James S, Montgomery P, Williams K. Omega-3 fatty acids supplementation for autism spectrum disorders (ASD). Cochrane Database Syst Rev 2011; 11. John Wiley & Sons, Ltd. CD007992, doi: 10.1002/14651858.CD007992.pub2.

[339] Mazahery H, Conlon C, Beck KL, Kruger MC, Stonehouse W, Camargo CA Jr, et al. Vitamin D and omega-3 fatty acid supplements in children with autism spectrum disorder: a study protocol for a factorial randomised, double-blind, placebo-controlled trial. Trials. 2016;17(1):295. doi: 10.1186/s13063-016-1428-8.

[340] Zhang YJ, Li S, Gan RY, Zhou T, Xu DP, Li HB. Impacts of gut bacteria on human health and diseases. Int J Mol Sci. 2015;16(4):7493–7519.

[341] Muszer M, Noszczyńska M, Kasperkiewicz K, Skurnik M. Human microbiome: when a friend becomes an enemy. Arch Immunol Ther Exp (Warsz). 2015;63(4):287–298.

[342] Dinan TG, Cryan JF. The impact of gut microbiota on brain and behaviour: implications for psychiatry. Curr Opin Clin Nutr Metab Care. 2015;18(6):552–558.

[343] Diaz Heijtz R. Fetal, neonatal, and infant microbiome: perturbations and subsequent effects on brain development and behavior. Semin Fetal Neonatal Med. 2016;21(6):410-417. doi: 10.1016/j.siny.2016.04.012. PubMed PMID: 27255860.

[344] Mezzelani A, Landini M, Facchiano F, Raggi ME, Villa L, Molteni M, et al. Environment, dysbiosis, immunity and sex-specific susceptibility: a translational hypothesis for regressive autism pathogenesis. Nutr Neurosci. 2015;18(4):145–161.

[345] Macfabe DF. Short-chain fatty acid fermentation products of the gut microbiome: implications in autism spectrum disorders. Microb Ecol Health Dis. 2012;23. doi: 10.3402/mehd.v23i0.19260. eCollection 2012. PubMed PMID: 23990817; PubMed Central PMCID: PMC3747729.

[346] Wang L, Conlon MA, Christophersen CT, Sorich MJ, Angley MT. Gastrointestinal microbiota and metabolite biomarkers in children with autism spectrum disorders. Biomark Med. 2014;8(3):331–344.

[347] Russo AJ, Krigsman A, Jepson B, Wakefield A. Low serum myeloperoxidase in autistic children with gastrointestinal disease. Clin Exp Gastroenterol. 2009;2:85–94.

[348] Gabriele S, Sacco R, Altieri L, Neri C, Urbani A, Bravaccio C, et al. Slow intestinal transit contributes to elevate urinary p-cresol level in Italian autistic children. Autism Res. 2016;9(7):752–759.

[349] Mussap M, Noto A, Fanos V. Metabolomics of autism spectrum disorders: early insights regarding mammalian-microbial cometabolites. Expert Rev Mol Diagn. 2016;16(8):869–881.

[350] Macfabe D. Autism: metabolism, mitochondria, and the microbiome. Glob Adv Health Med. 2013;2(6):52–66.

[351] Nankova BB, Agarwal R, MacFabe DF, La Gamma EF. Enteric bacterial metabolites propionic and butyric acid modulate gene expression, including CREB-dependent catecholaminergic neurotransmission, in PC12 cells--possible relevance to autism spectrum disorders. PLoS One. 2014;9(8):e103740. doi: 10.1371/journal.pone.0103740. eCollection 2014

[352] Zhou L, Foster JA. Psychobiotics and the gut-brain axis: in the pursuit of happiness. Neuropsychiatr Dis Treat. 2015;11:715–723.

[353] Rosenfeld CS. Microbiome disturbances and autism spectrum disorders. Drug Metab Dispos. 2015;43(10):1557–1571.

[354] Rodakis J. An n=1 case report of a child with autism improving on antibiotics and a father's quest to understand what it may mean. Microb Ecol Health Dis. 2015;26:26382. doi: 10.3402/mehd.v26.26382. eCollection 2015

[355] Ghanizadeh A, Berk M. Beta-lactam antibiotics as a possible novel therapy for managing epilepsy and autism, a case report and review of literature. Iran J Child Neurol. 2015;9(1):99–102.

[356] Ronald A, Pennell CE, Whitehouse AJ. Prenatal maternal stress associated with ADHD and autistic traits in earlychildhood. Front Psychol. 2011;1:223. doi: 10.3389/fpsyg.2010.00223. eCollection 2010

[357] Curin JM, Terzic J, Petkovic ZB, Zekan L, Terzic IM, Susnjara IM: lower cortisol and higher ACTH levels in individuals with autism. J Autism Dev Disord 2003;33:443–448.

[358] Tordjman S, Anderson GM, McBride PA, Hertzig ME, Snow ME, Hall LM, et al. Plasma beta-endorphin, adrenocorticotropin hormone, and cortisol in autism. J Child Psychol Psychiatry 1997;38:705–715.

[359] Seo MK, Ly NN, Lee CH, Cho HY, Choi CM, Nhu le H, et al. Early life stress increases stress vulnerability through BDNF gene epigenetic changes in the rat hippocampus. Neuropharmacol. 2016;105:388–397.

[360] Babenko O, Kovalchuk I, Metz GA Stress-induced perinatal and transgenerational epigenetic programming of brain development and mental health. Neurosci Biobehav Rev. 2015;48:70–91.

[361] Taurines R, Schwenck C, Westerwald E, Sachse M, Siniatchkin M, Freitag C. ADHD and autism: differential diagnosis or overlapping traits? A selective review. Atten Defic Hyperact Disord. 2012;4(3):115–139.

[362] Bergeron JD, Deslauriers J, Grignon S, Fortier LC, Lepage M, Stroh T, et al. White matter injury and autistic-like behavior predominantly affecting male rat offspring exposed to group B streptococcal maternal inflammation. Dev Neurosci. 2013;35(6):504–515.

[363] Allard MJ, Bergeron JD, Baharnoori M, Srivastava LK, Fortier LC, Poyart C,et al. A sexually dichotomous, autistic-like phenotype is induced by Group B Streptococcus maternofetal immune activation. Autism Res. 2016. doi: 10.1002/aur.1647. [Epub ahead of print]

[364] Rzehak P, Saffery R, Reischl E, Covic M, Wahl S, et al. Maternal smoking during pregnancy and dna-methylation in children at age 5.5 Years: epigenome-wide-analysis in the European childhood obesity project (CHOP)-study. PLoS One. 2016;11(5):e0155554. doi: 10.1371/journal.pone.0155554. eCollection 2016

[365] Tang S, Wang Y, Gong X, Wang G. A Meta-analysis of maternal smoking during pregnancy and autism spectrum disorder risk in offspring. Int J Environ Res Public Health. 2015;12(9):10418–10431.

[366] Hultman CM, Sandin S, Levine SZ, Lichtenstein P, Reichenberg A. Advancing paternal age and risk of autism: new evidence from a population-based study and a meta-analysis of epidemiological studies. Mol Psychiatry. 2011;16:1203–1212.

[367] Kong A, Frigge ML, Masson G, Besenbacher S, Sulem P, Magnusson G, et al. Rate of de novo mutations and the importance of father's age to disease risk. Nature. 2012;488:471–475.

[368] Frans EM, Sandin S, Reichenberg A, Langstrom N, Lichtenstein P, McGrath JJ, et al. Autism risk across generations: a populationbased study of advancing grandpaternal and paternal age. JAMA Psychiatry. 2013;70:516–521.

[369] Gardener H, Spiegelman D, Buka SL. Perinatal and neonatal risk factors for autism: a comprehensive meta-analysis. Pediatrics. 2011;128(2):344–355.

[370] Groer MW, Gregory KE, Louis-Jacques A, Thibeau S, Walker WA. The very low birth weight infant microbiome and childhood health. Birth Defects Res C Embryo Today. 2015;105(4):252–264.

[371] Pinto-Martin JA, Levy SE, Feldman JF, Lorenz JM, Paneth N, Whitaker AH. Prevalence of autism spectrum disorders in adolescents born weighing <2,000 grams. Pediatrics. 2011;128:883–891.

[372] Ouss-Ryngaert L, Álvarez L, Boissel A. Autism and prematurity: state of the art. Arch Pediatr 2012;19:970–975.

[373] Dudova I, Markova D, Kasparova M, Zemankova J, Beranova S, Urbanek T, et al. Comparison of three screening tests for autism in preterm children with birth weights less than 1,500 grams. Neuropsychiatr Dis Treat. 2014;10:2201–2208. doi: 10.2147/NDT.S72921. eCollection 2014

[374] Hack M, Taylor HG, Schluchter M, Andreias L, Drotar D, Klein N. Behavioral outcomes of extremely low birth weight children at age 8 years. J Dev Behav Pediatr. 2009;30:122–130.

[375] Johnson S, Hollis C, Kochhar P, Hennessy E, Wolke D, Marlow N. Autism spectrum disorders in extremely preterm children. J Pediatr. 2010;156:525–531.

[376] Dudova I, Kasparova M, Markova D, Zemankova J, Beranova S, Urbanek T, et al. Screening for autism in preterm children with extremely low and very low birth weight. Neuropsychiatr Dis Treat. 2014;10:277–282.

[377] Kuzniewicz MW, Wi S, Qian Y, Walsh EM, Armstrong MA, Croen LA. Prevalence and neonatal factors associated with autism spectrum disorders in preterm infants. J Pediatr. 2014;164:20–25.

[378] Buchmayer S, Johansson S, Johansson A, Hultman CM, Sparen P, Cnattingius S. Can association between preterm birth and autism be explained by maternal or neonatal morbidity? Pediatrics. 2009;124:e817–e825

[379] Rice TR. Postnatal testosterone may be an important mediator of the association between prematurity and male neurodevelopmental disorders: a hypothesis. Int J Adolesc Med Health. 2015. pii:/j/ijamh.ahead-of-print/ijamh-2015-0047/ijamh-2015-0047.xml. doi: 10.1515/ijamh-2015-0047. [Epub ahead of print]

[380] Blair LM, Pickler RH, Anderson C. Integrative review of genetic factors influencing neurodevelopmental outcomes in preterm infants. Biol Res Nurs. 2016;18(2):127–137.

[381] Behnia F, Parets SE, Kechichian T, Yin H, Dutta EH, Saade GR, et al. Fetal DNA methylation of autism spectrum disorders candidate genes: association with spontaneous preterm birth. Am J Obstet Gynecol. 2015;212(4):533.e1-9. doi: 10.1016/j.ajog.2015.02.011. Epub 2015 Feb 14

[382] Juul-Dam N, Townsend J, Courchesne E. Prenatal, perinatal, and neonatal factors in autism, pervasive developmental disorder-not otherwise specified, and the general population. Pediatrics. 2001;107(4):E63.

Chapter 9

Intracellular Pathways Associated with the Etiology of Autism

Anthony J. Russo

Additional information is available at the end of the chapter

http://dx.doi.org/10.5772/67206

Abstract

This chapter explores the relationship between the genes and proteins of the Akt and MAPK pathways and autism. This chapter presents the biology of these two pathways, their genes and cascading proteins, and then, it looks at the research that has connected these molecules to autism. Finally, it imparts current and future therapeutic modalities that might exploit abnormalities in these genes and proteins, change them and ultimately alter aberrant autistic behaviors.

Keywords: autism, Akt, MAPK, ERK

1. Introduction

In this chapter, we will review (1) the biology of intracellular pathways, with particular emphasis on the Akt and the MAPK pathways, (2) the potential association of Akt and MAPK pathway markers and autism, and (3) current and potential therapy as it might be related to these pathways.

This chapter is not a review of all pathways and biomarkers in cells, but, instead, the focus is on two prominent pathways, the Akt and MAPK, known to play a role in the etiology of autism.

2. The biology of the Akt and MAPK intracellular pathways

2.1. Structure and function of intracellular pathways associated with autism

2.1.1. Receptors and ligands

Intracellular pathways are initiated by ligands, such as growth factors, which attach to receptor proteins embedded in cell membranes (**Figure 1**). The stimulation of a pathway receptor initiates the pathway signaling that ultimately results in changes in DNA transcription and/or translation, and effects processes such as cell division, protein production, cell morphology and motility.

Two receptor proteins [epidermal growth factor receptor (EGFR) and c-Met (also called MET or hepatocyte growth factor receptor)], and their respective ligands [epidermal growth factor (EGF) and hepatocyte growth factor (HGF)] (**Figure 1**), will be reviewed here. Both of these receptor/ligand pairs have been found to initiate the Akt and MAPK pathways and have been implicated in the etiology of autism.

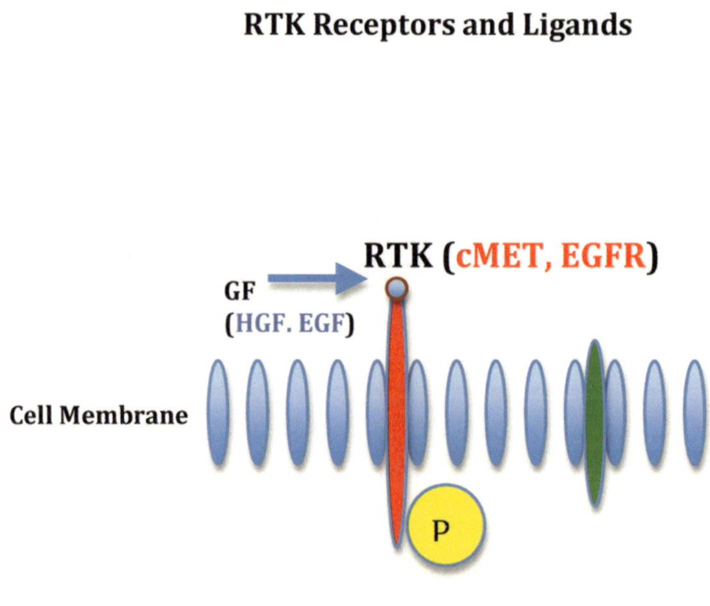

Figure 1. Membrane receptor [receptor tyrosine kinase (RTK)], either cMET or epidermal growth factor (EGFR) is signaled by growth factor (GF), either HGF or EGF, respectively. The interaction leads to phosphorylation inside the cell.

2.1.2. EGFR and EGF

EGFR is a glycoprotein that is a member of the protein kinase superfamily [1], and therefore is one of the receptor tyrosine kinases (RTKs). Binding of the receptor protein to the ligand, EGF, induces receptor dimerization, which stimulates its intracellular protein tyrosine kinase activity. As a result, there is autophosphorylation of several tyrosine (Y) residues in the C-terminal domain of EGFR [2]. This autophosphorylation causes downstream activation and signaling by several other proteins that react with the phosphorylated tyrosines.

The downstream signaling proteins initiate several signal cascades or pathways, principally the MAPK and Akt pathways [3]. These activated pathway proteins may lead to DNA synthesis, cell proliferation, cell migration, adhesion and proliferation [3].

Human EGF is a small 6045-Da protein [4] with 53 amino acid residues and three intramolecular disulfide bonds [5]. EGF acts by binding with high affinity to epidermal growth factor receptor (EGFR) on the cell surface. This stimulates ligand-induced receptor dimerization [6].

2.1.3. cMET and HGF

c-Met, or MET, is a membrane receptor protein that also possesses tyrosine kinase activity [7] and, therefore, is also a RTK. This cell surface receptor is expressed in epithelial cells of many organs, including the liver, pancreas, prostate, kidney, muscle and bone marrow, during both embryogenesis and adulthood [8]. c-MET has been shown to interact directly with the epidermal growth factor receptor (EGFR), allowing activation of c-MET after stimulation of cells with EGF [9, 10].

The ligand for c-MET is hepatocyte growth factor (HGF) [11, 12]. It is secreted as a single inactive polypeptide and is cleaved by serine proteases into a 69-kDa alpha-chain and a 34-kDa beta-chain. A disulfide bond between the alpha and beta chains produces the active, heterodimeric molecule [13].

HGF, through its signaling of c-MET, has been found to regulate cell growth, cell motility and morphogenesis through its activation of the c-Met receptor [14].

2.1.4. Downstream MAPK and AKT pathways

Stimulation of RTKs by EGF or HGF begins the downstream cascade of activated pathway proteins. The cascade starts when a signaling molecule (i.e., EGF or HGF) binds to the RTK on the cell surface. The pathways are chains of proteins that activate each other in a cascade fashion. A protein in the pathway is inactive, until it is phosphorylated by another protein in the cascade. Once it is activated, it can then catalyze the next substrate (protein) in the pathway. Overall, the proteins communicate a signal from the receptor on the membrane to the DNA in the nucleus. The DNA, through protein translation, orchestrates a change in the cell, such as increasing or decreasing cell division, cell morphology or cell motility.

2.1.5. Downstream MAPK pathway

The mitogen-activated protein kinases (MAPK) pathway (**Figure 2**) may begin with binding of EGF to EGFR. This activates the tyrosine kinase activity of the portion of the receptor in the cytoplasm. Docking proteins such as GRB2 (growth factor receptor-bound protein 2) contain an SH2 domain that binds to the phosphotyrosine residues of the activated receptor [15]. GRB2 then binds to the guanine nucleotide exchange factor Son of Sevenless (SOS) by way of the two SH3 domains of GRB2. When the GRB2-SOS complex docks to phosphorylated EGFR, SOS becomes activated [16]. (SOS was inactivated until it binds to activated EGFR, hence the cascade begins.) Activated SOS then promotes the removal of GDP from a member of the Ras subfamily (most notably H-Ras (transforming protein p21) or K-Ras (V-Ki-ras2 Kirsten rat sarcoma viral oncogene homolog). Ras can then bind guanosine-5′-triphosphate (GTP) and become active. Activated Ras activates the protein kinase activity of RAF (proto-oncogene serine/threonine-protein kinase) kinase [17]. RAK kinase then phosphorylates MEK1 and MEK2 (mitogen-activated protein kinase kinase). MEK then phosphorylates and activates mitogen-activated protein kinase (MAPK), also known as extracellular signal-regulated kinases (ERK).

MAPK regulates the activities of several transcription factors. It can phosphorylate factor MYK, which plays a role in cell cycle progression, apoptosis and cellular transformation [18], and it can phosphorylate and activate MNK (interacting protein kinases), which, in turn, phosphorylates cAMP response element-binding protein (CREB). CREB has a well-documented role in neuronal plasticity and long-term memory [19] (**Figure 2**).

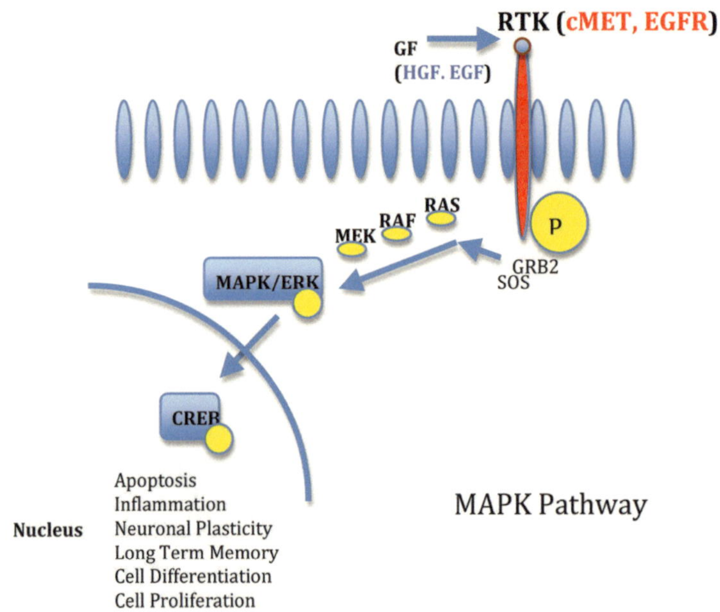

Figure 2. The MAPK pathway may begin with a growth factor (EGF or HGF) binding to the membrane RTK (cMET or EGFR). A cascade of activation ensues when the cytoplasmic portion of the RTK is phosphorylated, which, in turn, reacts with GRB2. At the end of the cascade, a transcription such as CREB affects protein production.

2.1.6. Downstream AKT pathway

The Akt pathway also starts with stimulation by a growth factor (i.e., EGF). This causes activation of a cell surface receptor (i.e., EGFR) and phosphorylation of phosphatidylinositol 3-kinase (PI3K) (**Figure 3**). Activated PI3K then phosphorylates lipids on the plasma membrane, forming second messenger PIP_3 (phosphatidylinositol (3,4,5)-trisphosphate). Akt, a serine/threonine kinase, is recruited to the membrane by interaction with these docking sites, so that it can be fully activated [20] (**Figure 3**).

Activated Akt causes downstream activation, which, by phosphorylating a range of intracellular proteins, ultimately results in changes in cell survival, growth, proliferation, cell migration and/or angiogenesis.

http://dx.doi.org/10.5772/67206

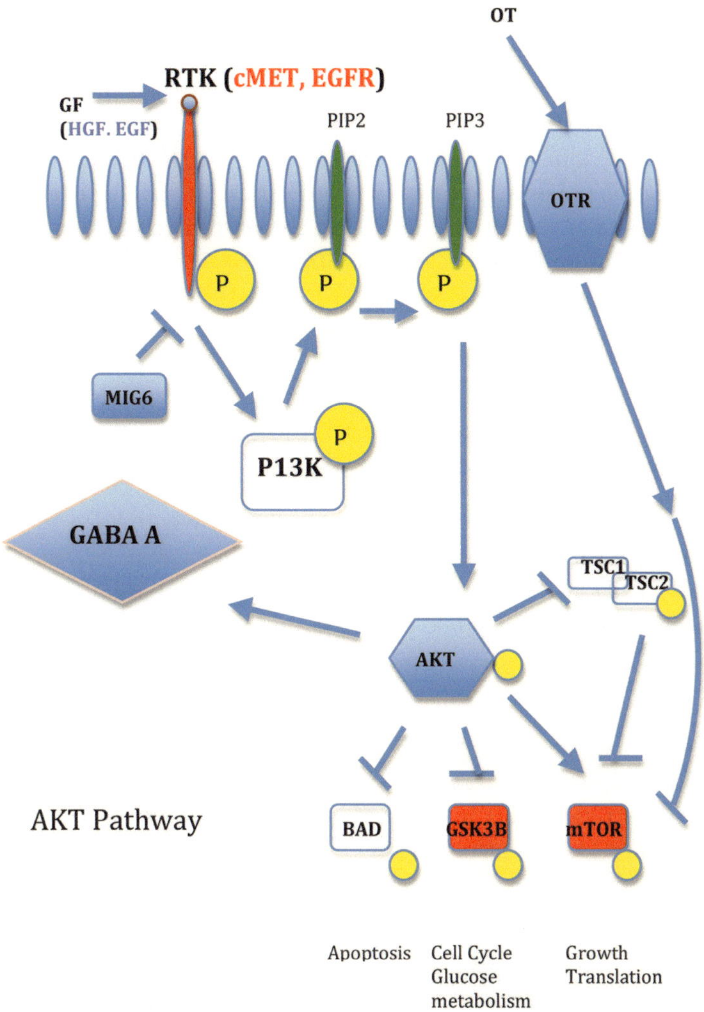

Figure 3. The Akt pathway may begin with a growth factor (EGF or HGF) binding to the membrane RTK (cMET or EGFR). A cascade of activation ensues when the cytoplasmic portion of the RTK is phosphorylated, which, in turn, reacts with P13K. At the end of the cascade, pathway proteins such as mTOR and GSK3 are affected.

The downstream effects of the Akt pathway are thoroughly regulated. The pathway is negatively regulated by phosphatase and tensin homolog (PTEN), which antagonizes PI3K. Demonstrated by the fact that loss of PTEN function leads to over-activation of Akt [21], the Akt pathway, in turn, regulates PTEN levels by activating transcription factors such as nuclear factor kappa-light-chain-enhancer of activated B cells (NF-κB). These factors activate PTEN agonists, such as tumor necrosis factor alpha (TNFα), which, in turn, suppress PTEN [22].

Once it is activated, Akt interacts with its many substrates. As examples, Akt can phosphorylate Bcl-2-associated death promoter (BAD) causing it to lose its pro-apoptotic function, and promote cell survival [23]. Under various circumstances, activation of Akt has been shown to overcome cell cycle arrest in the G1 [24] and G2 [25] phases. Once activated, it can also affect cell division by activating the transcription factor CREB [26], inhibiting the enzyme inhibitor p27 (cyclin-dependent kinase inhibitor 1B) [27], localizing the transcription factor, forkhead box class O (FOXO) in the cytoplasm [27], activating the membrane lipid, phosphatidylinositol (PtdIns)-3ps [28], and activating the kinase mechanistic target of rapamycin (mTOR) [25], which can affect transcription of p70 or eukaryotic initiation factor 4E binding protein 1 (4EBP1) [27]. Glycogen synthase kinase 3 (GSK-3) is inhibited upon phosphorylation by Akt. This results in an increase in glycogen synthesis [29]. Akt also enhances pathological angiogenesis and tumor growth associated with abnormalities in skin and blood vessels [25, 30].

2.2. Other biomarkers related to MAPK or Akt pathways

2.2.1. Oxytocin

There is evidence suggesting that oxytocin (OXT) is a regulator of the PI3K/Akt/mTORC1 pathway in gut cells and may, therefore, modulate translation in these cells [31].

The MAPK pathway is thought to be upregulated in the paraventricular (PVN) nuclei during lactation, and many of OXT's effects in peripheral and brain tissue are mediated through a MAPK/ERK pathway. Data also suggest an enhanced activation of the MAPK/ERK pathway in OXT neurons, specifically during late pregnancy in both the SON and PVN [32].

2.2.2. GABA

There is also evidence suggesting a relationship between the Akt pathway and GABA transmission. This relationship may be important in glucose metabolism and B cell proliferation. In human islets, GABA activates a calcium-dependent signaling pathway through both GABA-A and GABA-B receptors. This, in turn, activates the P13K-Akt and CREB-IRS-2 signaling pathways that convey GABA signals responsible for β-cell proliferation and survival [33].

The MAPK pathway may be a negative modulator of GABA-A receptor function [34]. Also, baicalin, a flavone glycoside, which modulates MAPK, has been found to have neuroprotective properties as a sedative associated with altering GABAergic signaling [35].

3. Association between pathway genes, proteins and autism

3.1. Genes associated with autism

Twin studies suggest that autism is highly heritable [36, 37], but there has not been just one gene associated with the etiology of the disorder(s). This could be because the majority of genes linked to autism are related to a specific symptom. Instead, not one, but many genes that are known to play a role in brain development are candidates for conferring susceptibility to autism.

According to the Simons Foundation Autism Research Initiative (SFARI) (Updated June, 2016), there are more than 800 genes implicated in autism, with annotations and links to published papers [38, 39]. The SAFARI gene-scoring module offers critical evaluation of the strength of the evidence for each gene's association with autism, with at least 50 high-ranking candidate risk genes so far identified.

We will be focusing here on only a few of the high-ranking autism-associated gene candidates, with particular emphasis on genes related to the Akt and MAPK pathways.

3.2. Pathway genes

MET (met proto-oncogene) encodes the hepatocyte growth factor receptor. MET, which has tyrosine kinase activity. Positive associations between MET and autism have been found in the Caucasian, Japanese and Italian populations as well as in Autism Genetic Resource Exchange (AGRE) family cohorts from multiple studies [40–42]. Interestingly, a positive association has also been found between MET and schizophrenia [43]. There is evidence to suggest that MET variances and MET/AKT interaction may affect facial emotion perception, implicating that the MET/AKT cascade plays a significant role in facial emotion perception [44].

Phosphatase and tensin homolog (PTEN) gene encodes a phosphatidylinositol-3,4,5-trisphosphate 3-phosphatase, which contains a tensin-like domain, as well as a catalytic domain similar to that of the dual specificity protein tyrosine phosphatases. Several studies have found rare single variations in the PTEN gene associated with autism [45–47], including in Cowden syndrome [48], where some individuals with the syndrome develop autism.

Engrailed homeobox 2 (EN2) is a homeobox gene that is critical to the development of the midbrain and cerebellum [49]. It regulates the combined processes of cell division, differentiation and organ development. Four candidate gene studies have explored the relationship between EN2 and autism—three found a positive association.

Reelin (RELN) gene produces an extracellular matrix protein with serine protease activity [50], which is responsible for correct lamination of the brain during the embryonic period and cell signaling and synaptic plasticity in adult life [51]. Deficits in brain levels of Reelin mRNA and protein have been found in subjects with schizophrenia and bipolar disorder [52], as well as major depression [53] and autism [54]. Genetic studies show an association of polymorphisms in the RELN gene in autism [55, 56]. Reelin has recently been shown to activate Akt, as well as Src family kinases, suggesting a relationship between Reelin and the Akt pathway [57].

GABA-A receptor, BETA-3 polypeptide (GABRB3) encodes the GABA receptor. GABA is the main inhibitory neurotransmitter in the adult brain. During neurotransmission, GABA activates the GABA-A receptor. Data suggest that rare variants of GABRB3 might be associated with autism, and increased GABRB3 expression may contribute to the pathogenesis of autism in some patients [58]. Insulin-induced translocation of GABA-ARs to the cell surface requires activation of Akt, a primary target of insulin signaling downstream of PI3K. Akt phosphorylates a conserved phosphorylation site present in all three b subunits of GABA-ARs, which increases cell surface expression of these receptors [59, 60].

Fragile X mental retardation 1 (FMR1) mutations are associated with a substantial degree of increased risk of autism and are consistently associated with additional features not required for an ASD diagnosis [61]. The fragile X mental retardation protein (FMRP), the gene product of FMR1, is an RNA-binding protein that negatively regulates translation in neurons. The Akt pathway is affected by this protein, which is demonstrated by the data that show that mTOR phosphorylation and activity are elevated in the hippocampus of juvenile FMR1 knockout mice [62].

Neurfibromin 1 (NF1): Genetic association has been found between the NF1 gene and autism. In particular, positive association was found with a NF1 polymorphism in the Japanese population [63]. The NF1-encoded protein, neurofibromin, functions as a Ras-GTPase activating protein, and the Akt/mTOR pathway is tightly regulated by neurofibromin [64]. Neurofibromatosis type 1 (NF1) is an autosomal dominant neurocutaneous syndrome, resulting from functional inactivation of the NF1 gene. Identification of SPRED1 gene mutations in individuals with mild NF1-like syndrome, and the direct involvement of these proteins in the RAS-MAPK pathway, potentially links the action of the NF1 gene to this pathway [65].

Tuberous sclerosis 1 (TSC1): This gene has been associated with syndromic autism, where a subpopulation of individuals with tuberous sclerosis syndrome develop autism [66]. This gene encodes a growth inhibitory protein thought to play a role in the stabilization of tuberin, and the protein has been implicated as a tumor suppressor. Akt and protein kinase B (PKB) both regulate and are regulated by the TSC1-TSC2 complex by interacting with and regulating mTOR [67].

Tuberous sclerosis 2 (TSC2): In addition to this gene's association with TSC1, its association with autism has also been found in an AGRE cohort [68], and a rare mutation in TSC2 has been identified in an individual with ASD [69].

Protein tyrosine kinase 7 (PTK7) is a gene strongly enriched for variants likely to affect ASD risk [70]. This gene encodes a member of the receptor protein tyrosine kinase family of proteins that transduce extracellular signals across the cell membrane. This protein may be associated with inhibition of cell proliferation, invasion and migration by inactivation of AKT and ERK [71].

Forkhead box P1 (FOXP1): Studies have found that rare mutations in this gene are associated with autism [72], and there is considerable evidence that FOXP1 protein expression is regulated by a PI3K/Akt/p70S6K signaling cascade [73].

SH3 and multiple ankyrin repeat domains 3 (SHANK3): Several studies have found rare single-gene variations in the SHANK3 gene in autism [74, 75]. However, Italian IMGSAC and Chinese Han studies claimed to find no genetic association or rare variations in the SHANK3 gene in autistic patients [76]. Pharmacological activation of Akt, and inhibition of CLK2, relieves synaptic deficits in SHANK3-deficient, as well as PMDS patient-derived, neurons. This suggests a strong relationship between SHANK3 and the Akt pathway [77].

Ubiquitin-protein ligase E3A (UBE3A) produces ubiquitin-protein ligase (E6AP) that is involved in targeting proteins for degradation within cells [78]. Mutations in the UBE3A gene are found in patients with Angelman syndrome (AS) [79]. AS is characterized by impaired motor and cognitive development, sleep disturbance, clumsy gait, seizures and irregular behaviors such as flapping and bursts of laughter. There is a phenotypic overlap between autism and AS, and dysregulation of UBE3A may play a role in the causation of autism [80]. UBE3A functions as a co-activator to regulate PI3K-Akt signaling pathway [81].

NHE9 (SLC9A9) is an endosomal cation/proton antiporter with orthologues in yeast and bacteria. Rare, missense substitutions in NHE9 are genetically linked to autism, but have not been functionally evaluated. Loss-of-function mutations in NHE9 may contribute to autistic phenotype by modulating synaptic membrane protein expression and neurotransmitter clearance [82]. In addition, endosomal NHE9 is mechanistically involved in the pathophysiology of autism [83]. Specifically, in glioblastoma cells, altered NHE9 blocks proton leakage from endosomes, causing them to become more acidic. This changes the transportation dynamics of proteins in the cell [98]. Epidermal growth factor receptor (EGFR) signaling is a potent driver of glioblastoma, a malignant and lethal form of brain cancer. Data demonstrate that endolysosomal pH is critical for receptor sorting and turnover. By functioning as a leak pathway for protons, the Na+/H+ exchanger NHE9 limits luminal acidification to circumvent EGFR turnover and prolongs downstream signaling pathways [84].

MECP2 Rett syndrome (RTT), a neurodevelopmental disorder that commonly involves autism, is caused by mutations in this gene. The expressed protein, MECP2, is important for nerve cell maturation and both activates and represses transcription [85].

It should be recognized that the genes represented here are a small representation of the hundreds of de novo and familial risk genes, copy number variants, and epigenetic modifiers have been identified through linkage analysis, genome-wide association studies and exon and whole-genome sequencing of individuals with autism over the past few years [86–89].

3.3. Biomarkers associated with autism

3.3.1. Growth factors

3.3.1.1. EGF

An increased frequency of EGF single-nucleotide polymorphisms has been reported in children with autism [90]. Lower plasma EGF levels have been found in adults with autism [91], as well as in children [92, 93]. But these data appear to be uncertain, as one report of younger children with autism showed increased levels of EGF [94]. Our lab found reduced levels of EGF in an autistic group, and these decreased levels were associated with the inflammatory marker HMGB1 and severity of hyperactivity in individuals with autism [94].

3.3.1.2. HGF

Decreased serum levels of HGF were found in male adults with high-functioning autism [95]. Our lab found HGF decreased in the serum of older autistic children with co-occurring GI disease when compared to non-autistic children with GI disease, autistic children without GI disease and healthy controls (non-autistic children without GI disease) [96]. The c-Met promoter variant rs1858830 reflects a common single-nucleotide polymorphism that increases the risk of ASD and is distinctively associated with ASD in individuals with co-occurring GI dysfunction [97]. These data strongly suggest that decreased MET function is due to the

ASD-associated common genetic variant rs1858830, which predisposes a subset of ASD individuals that exhibit GI problems. These results may be one reason for the association between gastrointestinal issues and autism [98].

3.3.2. Receptors

3.3.2.1. EGFR

Our lab measured soluble EGFR in individuals with autism. We found that EGFR levels were significantly higher in the autism group. These receptor levels also correlated significantly with the inflammatory marker HMGB1 and several autism behavioral symptoms, including hyperactivity [99]. We found that EGF levels (described above) also correlated significantly with HMGB1 and hyperactivity severity. This helps to confirm a possible etiological relationship between the receptor (EGFR) and its ligand (EGF). In glioblastoma cells, when researchers administered drugs that countered NHE9 proteins (above), as well as drugs that countered EGFR proteins, the cells were more readily killed, compared to cells that were only treated with EGFR-countering medication [84]. This suggests a relationship between NHE9 and EGFR, and, also, if EGFR is elevated, in autism, and this elevation is associated with the etiology of autism, it might represent an important way to lower EGFR levels.

3.3.2.2. cMET

c-MET/HGF signaling is directly related to HGF expression via a positive feedback mechanism A polymorphism in the upstream region of the hepatocyte growth factor receptor, c-Met, identified in a study involving 1231 autistic children plus appropriate controls [100], shows a deficiency in c-Met protein level which corresponds to reduced transcription rate, as well as a downregulation of HGF production [101, 102]. Also, MET receptor protein expression is decreased in the postmortem brain of individuals with the MET 'C' allele [103], which further substantiates its association with the etiology of autism.

3.3.3. MAPK and Akt pathway proteins

3.3.3.1. MAPK proteins

Recent advances in autism genetics and progress in the study of animal models have provided evidence suggesting that Akt and MAPK pathway proteins are adversely affected in individuals with autism [104]. Genome-wide association studies [105] and genomic copy number variant (CNV) analyses have identified enrichment in gene sets involved in RAS (rat sarcoma)/MAPK signaling and kinase activation in ASD individuals [106]. It has been suggested in an animal model that activation of this pathway in peripheral lymphocytes may serve as a marker for central nervous system (CNS) ERK activity, and possibly autistic behavior [107], and there is evidence of developmental abnormalities in neurogenesis and behavioral impairment associated with the 16p11.2 chromosomal deletion, which is associated with ERK dysregulation [108]. Therefore, disruption of the ERK (MAPK) signaling pathway may be an important mediator of abnormal social behavior in individuals with autism.

http://dx.doi.org/10.5772/67206

In a mouse model, researchers found a significant association between juvenile social behavior and phosphorylated mitogen-activated protein kinase (p-Mek) and p-Erk levels in the prefrontal cortex, but not in the cerebellum [105]. Others found that neuronal cell differentiation and maturation, and unchanged apoptosis, are associated with the presence of amplified Mapk/Erk, although these data have since been retracted [109]. However, other studies have demonstrated that decreased Mapk/Erk activation can also disrupt stem cell proliferation [110–112] and may be associated with autistic behavior. This conflict suggests that dysregulation of the MAPK/ERK pathway may be associated with separate autism subpopulations, such that some populations have over-activation of MAPK, and others are characterized by lower activation.

The Kyoto Encyclopedia of Genes and Genomes (KEGG) Pathway Database lists an array of highly associative genes associated with the MAPK/ERK pathway that are likely major contributors to ASD pathophysiology [113].

3.3.4. Akt proteins

3.3.4.1. Akt

Akt and mTOR, as well as related pathway proteins, have been found to be decreased in autistic groups [114]. Full-length PI3K, Akt and phosphorylated and total mTOR were reduced in the fusiform gyrus of a small group of autistic individuals [115]. Our lab has found significantly decreased levels of phosphorylated Akt in individuals with autism, and these low Akt levels correlated significantly with high EGFR and low GABA [116]. The low Akt levels in this study also correlated with high symptom severity. Our results suggest that the Akt pathway, starting with aberrant EGFR signaling, and followed by dysfunctional downstream Akt, may be involved in the etiology of autism.

3.3.4.2. PTEN

The gene for PTEN, the phosphatase that suppresses P13K/AKT signaling, is mutated in a small percentage of autistic individuals. In one study, all PTEN mutations from cases of PHTS (hamartoma tumor syndrome) appeared to disrupt the ability to inhibit AKT signaling, at the same time that PTEN expression was significantly reduced [117]. Inherited dominant PTEN mutations have been identified in patients with Cowden syndrome and Bannayan-Riley-Ruvalcaba syndrome, conditions that are often grouped together as PTEN hamartoma tumor syndrome (PHTS) [118], and inhibition of mTORC1 with the inhibitor rapamycin suppresses anatomical and behavioral abnormalities in PTEN knockout mice, suggesting a strong relationship between mTOR and PTEN [119], as well as an association with the etiology of autism.

3.3.4.3. MECP2

This protein, which is deficient in RETTs, may regulate PTEN expression with the help of a specific miRNA, miR-137. Conversely, PTEN can indirectly regulate MECP2 via the transcription factor, CREB and miR-132 [120].

3.3.4.4. mTOR

Significant decreases in protein expression and phosphorylation of mTOR, as well as components of its downstream signaling pathways, have been found in autism [121]. When mTOR is disrupted or decreased, downstream, effectors of protein translation are also reduced [122]. Mutations in TSC1, TSC2, NF1 and PTEN lead to an over-activated PI3K-mTOR pathway, as well as autism-relevant behaviors, tuberous sclerosis, neurofibromatosis and/or macrocephaly [123]. PI3K-mTOR signaling is also over-activated at synapses of fragile X syndrome (FXS) mice [124] and in humans with FXS [125]. mTOR signaling and protein synthesis are also impaired in a mouse model of Rett syndrome [126, 127]. Our lab found significantly high mTOR levels in individuals with autism, and these high levels correlated significantly with decreased oxytocin [128]. These data, collectively, suggest that mTOR may serve as a good marker for subgroups of individuals with autism.

3.3.4.5. TSC1 and TSC2

Tuberous sclerosis complex (TSC) is an autosomal dominant disorder caused by mutations in either the TSC1 or TSC2 gene [122, 129]. Tsc1+/− and Tsc2+/− mice, both male and female, exhibit deficient social interaction, which is reversed by pharmacological inhibition of mTOR with rapamycin [130], demonstrating the strong relationship between TSC and mTOR.

4. Potential therapy for autism associated with Akt and MAPK pathway alteration of genes and/or proteins

4.1. Akt pathway

As outlined above, mutations in PTEN, NF1 or in the TSC 1 and 2, cause an over-activation of the PI3K/Akt/mTOR pathway, leading to autism-related behavior. Furthermore, fragile X syndrome (FXS), a common inherited form of mental retardation and the leading cause of autism, has been associated with over-activation of the PI3K-mTOR pathway. On the other hand, low levels of PI3K/Akt/mTOR activity are linked with Rett syndrome (RTT), a rare form of autism-associated disease. These data suggest that therapy designed to alter these pathway genes and/or proteins may be affective at altering autistic behaviors.

On the basis of observations that mTOR signaling, synaptic plasticity and protein translation are over-activated in these disorders, compounds that can potentially inhibit the mTOR pathway represent promising therapeutic candidates.

However, under-activation of this pathway has been reported in RTT. So, when developing therapy for RETTs, it may be important to use therapy that will raise mTOR levels.

Because mTOR has been found to be both high and low, depending on the syndrome, it is possible that altered mTOR levels may be associated with certain ASD behaviors and/or subpopulations, and therefore may provide a means for subgrouping those in the autistic spectrum.

For mTOR over-activation, the mTORC1 inhibitor rapamycin has shown promising results in PTEN KO mice [119] and TSC2 mice [131]. Other inhibitors of mTOR have been tried.

For instance, treatment of Fmr1 (protein of fragile X syndrome) knockout mice with temsirolimus, an mTOR inhibitor, prevented object recognition memory deficits and reduced audiogenic seizure susceptibility in mice [132].

Elevated phosphorylation of translational control molecules and exaggerated protein synthesis in fragile X mice were corrected through the targeting of S6K1 (ribosomal protein S6 kinase beta-1 (S6K1), also known as p70S6 kinase (p70S6K)), a serine/threonine kinase that acts downstream of PIP3 and targets the S6 ribosomal protein. Deletion of S6K1 prevents a broad range of fragile X phenotypes, including exaggerated translation and abnormal dendritic spine morphology [133]. Also, targeting downstream mTOR signaling, such as eukaryotic translation initiation factor 4E (eIF4E), reversed autism [122]. Thus, interventions that target mTOR signaling should be at the leading edge of future translational research for autism.

GSK3 (isoforms GSK3α and GSK3β) is a serine/threonine kinase that is controlled by inhibitory serine phosphorylation induced by both Akt and MAPK pathways [134]. In Fmr1 knockout mice, GSK3 phosphorylation was reduced in several brain regions, resulting in elevated GSK3 signaling [135]. Lithium is a GSK3 inhibitor that both increases the inhibitory serine phosphorylation of GSK3 and directly inhibits GSK3 activity [136, 137]. Particularly with chronic administration, in Fmr1 knockout mice, lithium was found to be able to correct abnormal behavior, such as hyperactivity [138]. Also, specific GSK3 inhibitors SB216763 141, TDZD-8 and VP0.7 corrected hippocampus-dependent learning deficits in fragile X mice [139, 140].

RTT is characterized by loss of function of the X-linked MECP2 gene [141]. Multiple studies, using different knockout mouse models, indicate that the pathological deficit in RTT is associated with the structure and function of synapses, synaptic transmission and plasticity [142, 143]. BDNF, the gene encoding the BDNF protein, is one of the first recognized direct targets of MECP2 transcriptional regulation [144]. BDNF, through the receptor tropomyosin-related kinase B (TrkB), activates intracellular signaling cascades, Akt and MAPK, critical for neuronal development, synaptic maturation, and learning and memory [145]. Therefore, one direction of potential therapy for MECP2 deficiency is the trial and use of drugs that boost BDNF. Compounds that boost BDNF levels such as fingolimod and glatiramer acetate (copaxone), both FDA-approved drugs for the treatment of multiple sclerosis, lead to an increase in BDNF expression and activation of TrkB/Akt downstream signaling pathways [146].

Insulin growth factor-1 (IGF-1) binds to the IGF-1 receptor and also activates intracellular signaling cascades, similar to those triggered by BDNF activation of TrkB receptors, by modulating synaptic plasticity and neuronal maturation through PI3K-Akt and MAPK pathways [147]. Unlike BDNF, IGF-1 permeability through the blood-brain barrier makes it an attractive compound for therapy. Based on these promising leads, a phase 2 double-blind placebo-controlled clinical trial is underway to treat 3- to 10–year-old RTT patients with full-length IGF-1 [148].

4.2. MAPK pathway

ERK levels, for the most part, are decreased in autism. Different classes of antidepressants rapidly increase ERK [149] and CREB [150] activity. This supports the involvement of the MAPK pathway in autism and may suggest the need to develop alternative therapies that increase ERK levels.

Supplemental zinc, which has been found to increase ERK levels, has an antidepressant-like effect. This zinc activity may be dependent on the activation of ERK and PI3K/GSK3β pathways [151].

4.3. Neurotransmitters

Multiple studies have documented low levels of neurotransmitters (dopamine, 5-HT, noradrenaline) in autopsy RTT brains and in MECP2-deficient mice [152]. Desipramine, an antidepressant that blocks the uptake of noradrenaline and has been shown to reverse the depletion of tyrosine hydroxylase in the brainstem, helps the regulation of breathing and extending the life span of male MECP2 knockout mice [153].

The NMDA-type of glutamate receptor is altered in MECP2 knockout mice [154], and the FDA-approved NMDA receptor antagonist ketamine has been useful in improving RTT-like phenotypes in MECP22 knockout mice [155].

Studies have shown that GABAergic signaling is also impaired in MECP2-deficient mice [156], and selective deletion of MECP2 in GABAergic neurons has led to impaired GABAergic transmission, cortical hyperexcitability and several neurological features of RTT and autism [157]. Vigabatrin is an antiepileptic drug that irreversibly inhibits GABA transaminase, inhibits GABA catabolism and thereby increases GABA levels. The drug is already FDA approved for use in epilepsy syndromes. Our lab has shown that decreased Akt levels are associated with low GABA [116], suggesting that therapy designed to increase Akt levels may also increase GABA.

4.4. Oxytocin

The neuropeptide oxytocin (OXT), a natural brain peptide produced in the hypothalamus, has been implicated in the pathophysiology and possibly the etiology of autism [158]. There is a significant association of a sequence variant in the OXT receptor gene with Asperger's syndrome [159]. However, the molecular mechanisms underlying the role of OXT in autism remain unclear. Recent studies have shown that OXT plays an important role in reducing behavioral deficits in an ASD-like mouse model, mediated by inhibiting the ERK signaling pathway and its downstream proteins [160]. OXT increases the salience of social stimuli, promotes parental nurturing and social bonds and, therefore, has received considerable attention as a potential treatment for social deficits in autism. Recent studies in mice have demonstrated that a mutation in Cntnap2 (the gene that encodes contactin-associated protein-like 2), which, in humans, may result in autism, displays robust social deficits and reduced brain OXT. In this model, daily intranasal OXT treatment improved later social engagement [161].

Acute intranasal OXT may temporarily enhance social cognition, empathy and reciprocity in individuals with autism [160]. In a recent small double-blind study, those taking OXT spray therapy had significantly reduced autism core symptoms specific to social reciprocity [162]. However, other recent clinical trials have yielded mixed results [161, 163].

Recent studies suggest that, in addition to its role in the brain, OXT may also have an important neuromodulatory role in the gut by activating the PI3K/Akt pathway in a dose- and time-dependent manner [164]. Our lab has found decreased plasma oxytocin in individuals

http://dx.doi.org/10.5772/67206

with autism, and these oxytocin levels correlated with high mTOR, suggesting a possible relationship between oxytocin and aberrant Akt pathway signaling [128].

In summary, because of the diversity of autism symptoms and behaviors, it is likely that drugs, based on altering genes or proteins of the Akt and/or MAPK pathways, will be most effective after biomarker screening. Marker screening may also provide an opportunity to identify and study subgroups of individuals with autism.

Acknowledgements

I would like to thank the Autism Research Institute, the Pfeiffer Medical Center, Health Research Institute and the Hartwick College for their support.

Author details

Anthony J. Russo

Address all correspondence to: dr.a.j.russo@gmail.com

Hartwick College, Oneonta, NY, USA

Pfeiffer Medical Center, Health Research Institute, Warrenville, IL, USA

References

[1] Herbst RS. Review of epidermal growth factor receptor biology. Int J Radiat Oncol Biol Phys. 2004;59: 21–26.

[2] Downward J, Parker P, Waterfield MD. Autophosphorylation sites on the epidermal growth factor receptor. Nature. 1984;311: 483–485.

[3] Oda K, Matsuoka Y, Funahashi A, Kitano H. A comprehensive pathway map of epidermal growth factor receptor signaling. Mol Syst Biol. 2005;1: 2005–2010.

[4] Harris RC, Chung E, Coffey RJ. EGF receptor ligands. Exp Cell Res. 2003;284 (1): 2–13.

[5] Carpenter G, Cohen S. Epidermal growth factor receptor. J Biol Chem. 1990;265 (14): 7709–7712.

[6] Dawson JP, Berger MB, Lin CC, Schlessinger J, Lemmon MA, Ferguson KM. Epidermal growth factor receptor dimerization and activation require ligand-induced conformational changes in the dimer interface. Mol Cell Biol 2005;25 (17): 7734–7742.

[7] Cooper CS. The met oncogene: from detection by transfection to transmembrane receptor for hepatocyte growth factor. Oncogene. 1992;7 (1): 3–7.

[8] Comoglio PM, Giordano S, Trusolino L. Drug development of MET inhibitors: targeting oncogene addiction and expedience. Nat Rev Drug Discov. 2008;7: 504–516.

[9] Jo M, Stolz DB, Esplen JE, Dorko K, Michalopoulos GK, Strom SC. Cross-talk between epidermal growth factor receptor and c-Met signal pathways in transformed cells. J Biol Chem. 2000;275: 8806–8811.

[10] Puri N, Salgia R. Synergism of EGFR and c-Met pathways, cross-talk and inhibition, in non-small cell lung cancer. J Carcinog. 2008;7: 9.

[11] Weidner KM, Arakaki N, Hartmann G, Vandekerckhove J, Weingart S, Rieder H, et al. Evidence for the identity of human scatter factor and human hepatocyte growth factor. Proc Natl Acad Sci USA. 1991;88: 7001–7005.

[12] Nakamura T, Nishizawa T, Hagiya M, Seki T, Shimonishi M, Sugimura A, et al. Molecular cloning and expression of human hepatocyte growth factor. Nature. 1989;342: 440–443.

[13] Entrez Gene: HGF hepatocyte growth factor (hepapoietin A; scatter factor)

[14] Basilico C, Arnesano A, Galluzzo M, Comoglio PM, Michieli P. A high affinity hepatocyte growth factor-binding site in the immunoglobulin-like region of Met. J Biol Chem. 2008;283: 21267–21277.

[15] Schulze WX, Deng L, Mann M. Phosphotyrosine interactome of the ErbB- receptor kinase family. Mol Syst Biol. 2005;1: 2005.0008.

[16] Zarich N, Oliva JL, Martínez N, et al. Grb2 Is a Negative Modulator of the Intrinsic Ras-GEF Activity of hSos1 Mol Biol Cell. 2006;17 (8): 3591–3597.

[17] Avruch J, Khokhlatchev A, Kyriakis JM, et al. Ras activation of the Raf kinase: tyrosine kinase recruitment of the MAP kinase cascade. Recent Progr Hormone Res. 2001;56 (1): 127–155.

[18] Finver SN, Nishikura K, Finger LR, Haluska FG, Finan J, Nowell PC, Croce CM. Sequence analysis of the MYC oncogene involved in the t(8;14)(q24;q11) chromosome translocation in a human leukemia T-cell line indicates that putative regulatory regions are not altered. Proc Natl Acad Sci USA. 1988;85 (9): 3052–3056.

[19] Silva AJ, et al. CREB and Memory (PDF). Annu Rev Neurosci. 2010;21: 127–148.

[20] Osaki M, Oshimura M, Ito H. The PI3K-Akt pathway: its functions and alterations in human cancer. Apoptosis. 2004;9 (6): 667–676.

[21] Georgescu MM. PTEN tumor suppressor network in PI3K-Akt pathway control. Genes Cancer 1. 2010;12: 1170–1177.

[22] Carracedo A, Pandolfi PP. The PTEN-PI3K pathway of feedbacks and cross-talks. Oncogene. 2008;27 (41): 5527–5541.

[23] Lodish H, Berk A, Zipursky LS, Matsudaira P, Baltimore D, Darnell J. Figure 23-50: BAD interaction with Bcl-2. Mol Cell Biol, New York: Scientific American Books, 2000 ISBN 0-7167-3136-3.

[24] Kandel ES, Skeen J, Majewski N, Di Cristofano A, Pandolfi PP, Feliciano CS, Gartel A, Hay N. Activation of Akt/protein kinase B overcomes a G(2)/m cell cycle checkpoint induced by DNA damage. Mol Cell Biol. 2002;22 (22): 7831–7841.

[25] Chen J, Somanath PR, Razorenova O, Chen WS, Hay N, Bornstein P, Byzova TV. Akt1 regulates pathological angiogenesis, vascular maturation and permeability in vivo. Nat Med. 2005;11 (11): 1188–1196.

[26] Peltier J, O'Neill A, Schaffer DV. PI3K/Akt and CREB regulate adult neural hippocampal progenitor proliferation and differentiation. Dev Neurobiol. 2007;67 (10): 1348–1361.

[27] Rafalski VA, Brunet A. Energy metabolism in adult neural stem cell fate. Progr Neurobiol. 2011;93 (2): 182–203.

[28] Man HY, Wang Q, Lu WY, Ju W, Ahmadian G, Liu L, d'Souza S, Wong TP, Taghibiglou C, Lu J, Becker LE, Pei L, Liu F, Wymann MP, MacDonald JF, Wang YT. Activation of PI3-kinase is required for AMPA receptor insertion during LTP of mEPSCs in cultured hippocampal neurons. Neuron. 2003;38 (4): 611–624.

[29] Fang X, et al. Phosphorylation and inactivation of glycogen synthase kinase 3 by protein kinase A. PNAS. 2000;97: 11960–11965.

[30] Somanath PR, Razorenova OV, Chen J, Byzova TV. Akt1 in endothelial cell and angiogenesis. Cell Cycle. 2006;5 (5): 512–518.

[31] Klein BY, et al. Oxytocin modulates mTORC1 pathway in the gut. Biochem Biophys Res Commun. 2013;432(3):466–471.

[32] Chandaka GK, et al. Late pregnancy is a critical period for changes in phosphorylated MAPK/ERK1/2 in oxytocin neurons. J Neuroendocrinol. 2016;28: 1–7.

[33] Purwana I, et al. GABA promotes human β-cell proliferation and modulates glucose homeostasis. Diabetes. 2014;(12):4197–4205. doi:10.2337/db14-0153

[34] Bell-Horner CL, et al. ERK/MAPK pathway regulates GABAA receptors. J Neurobiol. 2006;66(13):1467–1474.

[35] Dai J, et al. Activations of GABAergic signalling, HSP70 and MAPK cascades are involved in baicalin's neuroprotection against gerbil global ischemia/reperfusion injury. Brain Res Bull. 2013;90:1–9.

[36] Alarcon M, Cantor RM, Liu J, Gilliam TC. Evidence for a language quantitative trait locus on chromosome 7q in multiplex autism families. Am J Hum Genet. 2002;70: 60–71.

[37] Auranen M, Vanhala R, Varilo T, Ayers K, Kempas E, Ylisaukko-Oja T, Sinsheimer JS, Peltonen L, Jarvela I. A genomewide screen for autism-spectrum disorders: evidence for a major susceptibility locus on chromosome 3q25-27. Am J Hum Genet. 2002;71:777–790.

[38] Abrahams BS, Arking DE, Campbell DB, Mefford HC, Morrow EM, Weiss LA, Menashe I, Wadkins T, Banerjee-Basu S, Packer A. SFARI Gene 2.0: a community-driven knowledge-base for the autism spectrum disorders (ASDs). Mol Autism. 2013;4:36–40.

[39] Banerjee-Basu S, Packer A. SFARI gene: an evolving database for the autism research community. Dis Model Mech. 2010;3: 133–135.

[40] Campbell DB, et al. Genetic evidence implicating multiple genes in the MET receptor tyrosine kinase pathway in autism spectrum disorder. Autism Res. 2008;3: 159–168.

[41] Thanseem I, et al. Further evidence for the role of MET in autism susceptibility. Neurosci Res. 2010;2: 137–141.

[42] Lambert N, et al. A familial heterozygous null mutation of MET in autism spectrum disorder. Autism Res. 2014;5: 617–622.

[43] Burdick KE, et al. Association of genetic variation in the MET proto-oncogene with schizophrenia and general cognitive ability. Am J Psychiatry. 2010;4:436–443.

[44] Lin MT, et al. MET and AKT genetic influence on facial emotion perception. PLoS One. 2012;7: e36143.

[45] D'Gama AM, et al. Targeted DNA sequencing from autism spectrum disorder brains implicates multiple genetic mechanisms. Neuron. 2015;88: 910–917.

[46] Frazier TW, et al. Molecular and phenotypic abnormalities in individuals with germline heterozygous PTEN mutations and autism. Mol Psychiatry. 2015;9: 1132–1138.

[47] Iossifov I, et al. Low load for disruptive mutations in autism genes and their biased transmission. Proc Natl Acad Sci USA. 2015;41:E5600–E5607.

[48] Goffin A, et al. PTEN mutation in a family with Cowden syndrome and autism. Am J Med Genet. 2001;105:521–524.

[49] James SJ, et al. Complex epigenetic regulation of Engrailed-2 (EN-2) homeobox gene in the autism cerebellum. Transl Psychiatry. 2013;3: e232.

[50] Quattrocchi CC, et al. Reelin is a serine protease of the extracellular matrix. J Biol Chem. 2002;277(1):303–309.

[51] Costa E, et al. REELIN and schizophrenia: a disease at the interface of the genome and the epigenome. Mol. Intervent. 2006;2:47–57.

[52] Impagnatiello F, et al. A decrease of reelin expression as a putative vulnerability factor in schizophrenia. Proc Natl Acad Sci (USA). 1998;95: 15718–15723.

[53] Fatemi SH, et al. Reduction in Reelin immunoreactivity in hippocampus of subjects with schizophrenia, bipolar disorder and major depression. Mol Psychiatry. 2000;5: 654–663.

[54] Fatemi SH, et al. Dys-regulation of reelin and Bcl-2 proteins in autistic cerebellum. J Aut Devel Dis. 2001; 31: 529–535.

[55] Persico AM, et al. Reelin gene alleles and haplotypes as a factor predisposing to autistic disorder. Mol Psychiatry. 2001; 6: 150–159.

[56] Zhang H, et al. Reelin gene alleles and susceptibility to autism spectrum disorders. Mol Psychiatry. 2002;7: 1012–1017.

[57] Ballif BA, et al. Tyrosine phosphorylation of Disabled-1 is essential for Reelin-stimulated activation of Akt and Src family kinases. Mol Brain Res. 2003;117: 152–159.

[58] Chen CH, et al. Genetic analysis of GABRB3 as a candidate gene of autism spectrum disorders. Mol Autism. 2014;25:36–38.

[59] Wang Q, Liu L, Pei L, Ju W, Ahmadian G, Lu J, Wang Y, Liu F, Wang YT. Control of synaptic strength, a novel function of Akt. Neuron. 2003;38: 915–928.

[60] Luscher B, et al. GABAA receptor trafficking-mediated plasticity of inhibitory synapses. Neuron. 2011;70: 385–409.

[61] Vincent JB, et al. Point mutation analysis of the FMR-1 gene in autism. Mol Psychiatry. 1996;3: 227–231.

[62] Sharma A, et al. Dysregulation of mTOR signalling in fragile X syndrome. J Neurosci. 2010;30:694–702.

[63] Marui T, et al. Association between the neurofibromatosis-1 (NF1) locus and autism in the Japanese population. Am J Med Genet B Neuropsychiatr Genet. 2004;131: 43–47.

[64] Johannessen CM, et al. The NF1 tumor suppressor critically regulates TSC2 and mTOR. Proc Natl Acad Sci USA. 2005;102: 8573–8578.

[65] Bennet E, et al. Neurofibromatosis type 1: its association with the Ras/MAPK pathway syndromes. J Pediatric Neurol. 2009;7: 105–115.

[66] Smalley SL. Autism and tuberous sclerosis. J Autism Dev Disord. 1998;28: 407–414.

[67] Huang J, Manning BD. A complex interplay between Akt, TSC2 and the two mTOR complexes. Biochem Soc Trans. 2009;1:217–222.

[68] Serajee FJ, et al. Association of INPP1, PIK3CG, and TSC2 gene variants with autistic disorder: implications for phosphatidylinositol signalling in autism. J Med Genet. 2003;11: e119.

[69] O'Roak BJ, et al. Sporadic autism exomes reveal a highly interconnected protein network of de novo mutations. Nature. 2012;485:246–250.

[70] Sanders SJ, et al. Insights into autism spectrum disorder genomic architecture and biology from 71 risk loci. Neuron. 2015;87: 1215–1233.

[71] Kim JH, et al. Protein tyrosine kinase 7 plays a tumor suppressor role by inhibiting ERK and AKT phosphorylation in lung cancer. Oncology Reports. 2014;31:2708–2712.

[72] O'Roak BJ, et al. Exome sequencing in sporadic autism spectrum disorders identifies severe de novo mutations. Nat Genet. 2011;43: 585–589.

[73] Halacli SO, Dogan AL. FOXP1 regulation via the PI3K/Akt/p70S6K signalling pathway in breast cancer cells. Oncol Lett. 2015;9: 1482–1488.

[74] Durand CM, et al. Mutations in the gene encoding the synaptic scaffolding protein SHANK3 are associated with autism spectrum disorders. Nat Genet. 2007;39: 25–27.

[75] Shao S, et al. A commonly carried genetic variant, rs9616915, in SHANK3 gene is associated with a reduced risk of autism spectrum disorder: replication in a Chinese population. Mol Biol Rep. 2014;41: 1591–1595.

[76] Liu Y, et al. Lack of association between NLGN3, NLGN4, SHANK2 and SHANK3 gene variants and autism spectrum disorder in a Chinese population. PLoS One. 2013;8: e56639.

[77] Bidinosti M, et al. CLK2 inhibition ameliorates autistic features associated with SHANK3 deficiency. Science. 2016;351: 1199–1203.

[78] Anan T, Nagata Y, Koga H, Honda Y, Yabuki N, Miyamoto C, Kuwano A, Matsuda I, Endo F, Saya H, Nakao M. Human ubiquitin-protein ligase Nedd4: expression, subcellular localization and selective interaction with ubiquitin-conjugating enzymes. Genes Cells. 1998;3: 751–763.

[79] Nawaz Z, Lonard DM, Smith CL, Lev-Lehman E, Tsai SY, Tsai MJ, O'Malley BW. The Angelman syndrome-associated protein, E6-AP, is a coactivator for the nuclear hormone receptor superfamily. Mol Cell Biol. 1999;19: 1182–1189.

[80] Peters SU, et al. Autism in Angelman syndrome: implications for autism research. Clin Genet. 2004;66:530–536.

[81] Khan O, Fu G, Ismail A, Srinivasan S, Cao X, Tu Y, Lu S, Nawaz Z. Multifunction steroid receptor coactivator, E6-associated protein, is involved in development of the prostate gland. Mol Endocrinol 2006; 20: 544–559.

[82] Kondapalli KC, et al. Functional evaluation of autism-associated mutations in NHE9. Nat Commun. 2013;4: 2510.

[83] Schwede M, et al. Genes for endosomal NHE6 and NHE9 are misregulated in autism brains. Mol Psychiatry. 2014;19: 277–279.

[84] Kondapalli KC, et al. A leak pathway for luminal protons in endosomes drives oncogenic signalling in glioblastoma. Nat. Commun. 2015;6: 6289. doi:10.1038/ncomms7289

[85] Chahrour M, et al. MECP2, a key contributor to neurological disease, activates and represses transcription. Science. 2008;320: 1224–1249.

[86] Bourgeron T. From the genetic architecture to synaptic plasticity in autism spectrum disorder. Nat Rev. 2015;16: 551–563.

[87] Lossifov I, et al. The contribution of de novo coding mutations to autism spectrum disorder. Nature. 2014;515: 216–221.

http://dx.doi.org/10.5772/67206

[88] De Rubeis S, et al. Synaptic, transcriptional and chromatin genes disrupted in autism. Nature. 2014;515: 209–215.

[89] Geschwind DH, State MW. Gene hunting in autism spectrum disorder: on the path to precision medicine. Lancet Neurol. 2015;14: 1109–1120.

[90] Suzuki K, Hashimoto K, Iwata Y, et al., Decreased serum levels of epidermal growth factor in adult subjects with high-functioning autism. Biol Psychiatry. 2007;62: 267–269.

[91] Toyoda T, Nakamura K, Yamada K, et al., SNP analyses of growth factor genes EGF, TGFβ-1, and HGF reveal haplotypic association of EGF with autism. Biochem Biophys Res Commun. 2007;360: 715–720.

[92] Onore C, et al. Decreased levels of EGF in plasma of children with autism spectrum disorder. Autism Res Treat. 2012;12: 205362.

[93] Russo AJ. Decreased epidermal growth factor (EGF) associated with HMGB1 and increased hyperactivity in children with autism. Biomarker Insights. 2013;8: 35–41.

[94] İseri E, et al. Increased serum levels of epidermal growth factor in children with autism. J Autism Dev Disorders. 2011;41(2): 237–241.

[95] Sugihara G, Hashimoto K, Iwata Y, Nakamura K, Tsujii M, Tsuchiya KJ, Sekine Y, Suzuki K, Suda S, Matsuzaki H, Kawai M, Minabe Y, Yagi A, Takei N, Sugiyama T, Mori N. Decreased serum levels of hepatocyte growth factor in male adults with high-functioning autism. Prog Neuropsychoph Biol Psychiatry. 2007;31: 412–415.

[96] Russo AJ, et al. Decreased serum hepatocyte growth factor (HGF) in autistic children with severe gastrointestinal disease. Biomark Insights. 2009;4:181–190.

[97] Campbell DB, Buie TM, Winter H, et al. Distinct genetic risk based on association of MET in families with co-occurring autism and gastrointestinal conditions. Pediatrics. 2009;123: 1018–1024.

[98] Hsiao E. Gastrointestinal issues in autism spectrum disorder. Harvard Rev Psychiatry. 2014;22: 104–111.

[99] Russo AJ. Increased epidermal growth factor receptor (EGFR) associated with hepatocyte growth factor (HGF) and symptom severity in children with autism spectrum disorders (ASDs). J Cent Nerv Syst Dis. 2014; 6: 79–83.

[100] Campbell DB, Sutcliffe JS, Ebert PJ, Militerni R, Bravaccio C, Trillo S, Elia M, Schneider C, Melmed R, Sacco R, Persico AM, Levitt P. A genetic variant that disrupts MET transcription is associated with autism. Proc Natl Acad Sci USA. 2006;103: 16834–16839.

[101] Yo Y, Morishita R, Yamamoto K, Tomita N, Kida I, Hayashi S, Moriguchi A, Kato S, Matsumoto K, Nakamura T, Higaki J, Ogihara T. Actions of hepatocyte growth factor as a local modulator in the kidney: potential role in pathogenesis of renal disease. Kidney Int. 1998;53: 50–58.

[102] Elliott BE, Hung WL, Boag AH, Tuck AB. The role of hepatocyte growth factor (scatter factor) in epithelial-mesenchymal transition and breast cancer. Can J Physiol Pharmacol. 2002;80: 91–102.

[103] Campbell DB, D'Oronzio R, Garbett K, Ebert PJ, Mirnics K, Levitt P, et al. Disruption of cerebral cortex MET signalling in autism spectrum disorder. Ann Neurol. 2007; 62: 243–250.

[104] Samuels IS, Saitta SC, Landreth GE. MAP'ing CNS development and cognition: an ERKsome process. Neuron. 2009;61: 160–167.

[105] Anney RJ, Kenny EM, O'Dushlaine C, Yaspan BL, Parkhomenka E, Buxbaum JD, Sutcliffe J, Gill M, Gallagher L. Gene-ontology enrichment analysis in two independent family-based samples highlights biologically plausible processes for autism spectrum disorders. Eur J Hum Genet. 2011;19: 1082–1089.

[106] Pinto D, Pagnamenta AT, Klei L, Anney R, Merico D, Regan R, Conroy J, Magalhaes TR, Correia C, Abrahams BS, Almeida J, Bacchelli E, Bader GD, Bailey AJ, Baird G, Battaglia A, Berney T, Bolshakova N, Bölte S, Bolton PF, Bourgeron T, Brennan S, Brian J, Bryson SE, Carson AR, Casallo G, Casey J, Chung BH, Cochrane L, Corsello C. Functional impact of global rare copy number variation in autism spectrum disorders. Nature. 2010;466: 368–372.

[107] Faridar A, et al. Mapk/Erk activation in an animal model of social deficits shows a possible link to autism. Mol Autism. 2014;5:57–62.

[108] Pucilowska J, et al. The 16p11.2 deletion mouse model of autism exhibits altered cortical progenitor proliferation and brain cytoarchitecture linked to the ERK MAPK pathway. J Neurosci. 2015;35: 3190–3200.

[109] Yang K, Cao F, Sheikh AM, Malik M, Wen G, Wei H, Ted Brown W, Li X. Up-regulation of Ras/Raf/ERK1/2 signalling impairs cultured neuronal cell migration, neurogenesis, synapse formation, and dendritic spine development. Brain Struct Funct. 2012;5: 5–8.

[110] Menard C, Hein P, Paquin A, Savelson A, Yang XM, Lederfein D, Barnabé-Heider F, Mir AA, Sterneck E, Peterson AC, Johnson PF, Vinson C, Miller FD. An essential role for a MEK-C/EBP pathway during growth factor-regulated cortical neurogenesis. Neuron. 2002;36: 597–610.

[111] Li XY, Newbern JM, Wu YH, Morgan-Smith M, Zhong J, Charron J, Snider WD. MEK is a key regulator of gliogenesis in the developing brain. Neuron. 2012;75: 1035–1050.

[112] Pucilowska J, Puzerey PA, Karlo JC, Galán RF, Landreth GE. Disrupted ERK signalling during cortical development leads to abnormal progenitor proliferation, neuronal and network excitability and behavior, modeling human neuro-cardio-facial-cutaneous and related syndromes. J Neurosci. 2012;32: 8663–8677.

[113] Wen Y, et al. Pathway network analyses for autism reveal multisystem involvement, major overlaps with other diseases and convergence upon MAPK and calcium signaling. PLoS One. 2016;11: e0153329.

[114] Sheikh AM, et al. BDNF-Akt-Bcl2 antiapoptotic signalling pathway is compromised in the brain of autistic subjects. J Neurosci Res. 2010;88:2641–2647.

[115] Nicolini C, et al. Decreased mTOR signalling pathway in human idiopathic autism and in rats exposed to valproic acid. Acta Neuropathol Commun. 2015; 3: 3–6.

[116] Russo AJ. Decreased phosphorylated protein kinase B (Akt) in individuals with autism associated with high epidermal growth factor receptor (EGFR) and low gamma-aminobutyric acid (GABA). Biomark Insights. 2015;10:89–94.

[117] Spinelli L, et al. Functionally distinct groups of inherited PTEN mutations in autism and tumour syndromes. J Med Genet. 2015;52:128–134.

[118] Bubien V, Bonnet F, Brouste V, Hoppe S, Barouk-Simonet E, David A, Edery P, Bottani A, Layet V, Caron O, Gilbert-Dussardier B, Delnatte C, Dugast C, Fricker JP, Bonneau D, Sevenet N, Longy M, Caux F. French Cowden Disease N. High cumulative risks of cancer in patients with PTEN hamartoma tumour syndrome. J Med Genet. 2013;50:255–263.

[119] Zhou J, et al. Pharmacological inhibition of mTORC1 suppresses anatomical, cellular, and behavioral abnormalities in neural-specific Pten knock-out mice. J Neurosci. 2009;29, 1773–1783.

[120] Lyu JW, et al. Reciprocal regulation of autism-related genes MeCP2 and PTEN via microRNAs. Sci Rep. 2008;6: 20392–20398.

[121] European Chromosome 16 Tuberous Sclerosis Consortium. Identification and characterization of the tuberous sclerosis gene on chromosome 16. Cell 1993;75:1305–1315.

[122] Gkogkas CG, Khoutorsky A, Ran I, Rampakakis E, Nevarko T, Weatherill DB, et al. Autism-related deficits via dysregulated eIF4E-dependent translational control. Nature. 2013;493: 371–377.

[123] Kwon CH, Luikart BW, Powell CM, Zhou J, Matheny SA, Zhang W, Li Y, Baker SJ, Parada LF. Pten regulates neuronal arborization and social interaction in mice. Neuron. 2006;50: 377–388.

[124] Sharma A, Hoeffer CA, Takayasu Y, Miyawaki T, McBride SM, Klann E, Zukin RS. Dysregulation of mTOR signalling in fragile X syndrome. J Neurosci. 2010;30: 694 –702.

[125] Hoeffer CA, Sanchez E, Hagerman RJ, Mu Y, Nguyen DV, Wong H, Whelan AM, ZukinRS, KlannE, Tassone F. Altered mTOR signalingand enhanced CYFIP2 expression levels in subjects with fragile X syndrome. Genes Brain Behav. 2012;11:332–341.

[126] Ricciardi S, Boggio EM, Grosso S, Lonetti G, Forlani G, Stefanelli G, Calcagno E, Morello N, Landsberger N, Biffo S, Pizzorusso T, Giustetto M, Broccoli V. Reduced AKT/mTOR signaling and protein synthesis dysregulation in a Rett syndrome animal model. Hum Mol Genet. 2011;20:1182–1196.

[127] Jiang M, Ash RT, Baker SA, Suter B, Ferguson A, Park J, Rudy J, Torsky SP, ChaoHT, Zoghbi HY, Smirnakis SM. Dendriticarborizationand spine dynamics are abnormal in the mouse model of MECP2 duplication syndrome. J Neurosci. 2013;33:19518–19533.

[128] Russo AJ, Anubrolu L. Decreased oxytocin associated with high mTOR in individuals with autism. JLSB. 2016;3: 119–126.

[129] van Slegtenhorst M, et al. Identification of the tuberous sclerosis gene TSC1 on chromosome 9q34. Science. 1997;277: 805–808.

[130] Sato A, et al. Rapamycin reverses impaired social interaction in mouse models of tuberous sclerosis complex. Nat Commun. 2012;3: 1292–1298.

[131] Ehninger D, Han S, Shilyansky C, Zhou Y, Li W, Kwiatkowski DJ, Ramesh V, Silva AJ Reversal of learning deficits in a Tsc2+/− mouse model of tuberous sclerosis. Nat Med 2008;14: 843–848.

[132] Busquets-Garcia A, Gomis-González M, Guegan T, Agustín-Pavón C, Pastor A, Mato S, et al.. Targeting the endocannabinoid system in the treatment of fragile X syndrome. Nat Med. 2013;19: 603–607.

[133] Bhattacharya A, Kaphzan H, Alvarez-Dieppa AC, Murphy JP, Pierre P, Klann E. Genetic removal of p70 S6 kinase 1 corrects molecular, synaptic and behavioral phenotypes in fragile X syndrome mice. Neuron. 2012;76: 325–337.

[134] Sugden PH, Fuller SJ, Weiss SC, Clerk A. Glycogen synthase kinase 3 (GSK3) in the heart: a point of integration in hypertrophic signalling and a therapeutic target? A critical analysis. Br J Pharmacol. 2008;153: S137–S153.

[135] Yuskaitis CJ, Mines MA, King MK, Sweatt JD, Miller CA, Jope R S. Lithium ameliorates altered glycogen synthase kinase-3 and behavior in a mouse model of fragile X syndrome. Biochem Pharmacol. 2010;79: 632–646.

[136] Chiu CT, Chuang DM. Molecular actions and therapeutic potential of lithium in preclinical and clinical studies of CNS disorders. Pharmacol Ther. 2010;128: 281–304.

[137] Mines MA, Jope RS. Glycogen synthase kinase-3: a promising therapeutic target for fragile x syndrome. Front Mol Neurosci. 2011;4:35.

[138] Min WW, Yuskaitis CJ, Yan Q, Sikorski C, Chen S, Jope RS, et al. Elevated glycogen synthase kinase-3 activity in fragile X mice: key metabolic regulator with evidence for treatment potential. Neuropharmacology. 2009;56: 463–472.

[139] Guo W, Murthy AC, Zhang L, Johnson EB, Schaller EG, Allan AM, et al. Inhibition of GSK3beta improves hippocampus-dependent learning and rescues neurogenesis in a mouse model of fragile X syndrome. Hum Mol Genet. 2012;21: 681–691.

[140] Franklin AV, King MK, Palomo V, Martinez A, McMahon LL, Jope RS. Glycogen synthase kinase-3 inhibitors reverse deficits in long-term potentiation and cognition in fragile X mice. Biol Psychiatry. 2014;75: 198–206.

[141] Amir RE, Van den Veyver IB, Wan M, Tran CQ, Francke U, Zoghbi HY. Rett syndrome is caused by mutations in X-linked MECP2, encoding methyl-CpG-binding protein 2. Nat Genet. 1999;23: 185–188.

[142] Guy J, Gan J, Selfridge J, Cobb S, Bird A. Reversal of neurological defects in a mouse model of Rett syndrome. Science. 2007;315: 1143–1147.

[143] Guy J, Hendrich B, Holmes M, Martin JE, Bird A. A mouse Mecp2-null mutation causes neurological symptoms that mimic Rett syndrome. Nat Genet. 2001;27: 322–326.

[144] Chen WG, Chang Q, Lin Y, Meissner A, West AE, Griffith EC, et al. Derepression of BDNF transcription involves calcium-dependent phosphorylation of MeCP2. Science. 2003;302: 885–889.

[145] Segal RA, Greenberg ME. Intracellular signalling pathways activated by neurotrophic factors. Annu Rev Neurosci. 1996;19:463–489.

[146] Deogracias R, Yazdani M, Dekkers MP, Guy J, Ionescu MC, Vogt KE, et al. Fingolimod, a sphingosine-1 phosphate receptor modulator, increases BDNF levels and improves symptoms of a mouse model of Rett syndrome. Proc Natl Acad Sci USA. 2012;109: 14230–14235.

[147] Zheng WH, Quirion R. Comparative signalling pathways of insulin-like growth factor-1 and brain-derived neurotrophic factor in hippocampal neurons and the role of the PI3 kinase pathway in cell survival. J Neurochem. 2001;89: 844–852.

[148] Khwaja OS, Ho E, Barnes KV, O'Leary HM, Pereira LM, Finkelstein Y, et al. Safety, pharmacokinetics and preliminary assessment of efficacy of mecasermin (recombinant human IGF-1) for the treatment of Rett syndrome. Proc Natl Acad Sci USA. 2014;111: 4596–4601.

[149] Hisaoka K, et al. Antidepressants increase glial cell line-derived neurotrophic factor production through monoamine-independent activation of protein tyrosine kinase and extracellular signal-regulated kinase in glial cells. J Pharmacol Exp Ther. 2007;32: 148–157.

[150] Hisaoka K, et al. Antidepressants induce acute CREB phosphorylation and CRE-mediated gene expression in glial cells: a possible contribution to GDNF production. Brain Res. 2008: 53–58.

[151] Manosso L, et al. Antidepressant-like effect of zinc is dependent on signalling pathways implicated in BDNF modulation. Progr Neuro-Psychopharmacol Biol Psychiatry. 2015;59:59–67.

[152] Roux JC, Dura E, Villard L. Tyrosine hydroxylase deficit in the chemoafferent and the sympathoadrenergic pathways of the Mecp2 deficient mouse. Neurosci Lett. 2008;447: 82–86.

[153] Roux JC, Dura E, Moncla A, Mancini J, Villard L. Treatment with desipramine improves breathing and survival in a mouse model for Rett syndrome. Eur J Neurosci. 2007;25: 1915–1922.

[154] Blue ME, Kaufmann WE, Bressler J, Eyring C, O'driscoll C, Naidu S, et al. Temporal and regional alterations in NMDA receptor expression in Mecp2-null mice. Anat Rec (Hoboken). 2011;294: 1624–1634.

[155] Kron M, Howell CJ, Adams IT, Ransbottom M, Christian D, Ogier M, et al. Brain activity mapping in Mecp2 mutant mice reveals functional deficits in forebrain circuits, including key nodes in the default mode network, that are reversed with ketamine treatment. J Neurosci. 2012;32: 13860–13872.

[156] Calfa G, Li W, Rutherford JM, Pozzo-Miller L. Excitation/inhibition imbalance and impaired synaptic inhibition in hippocampal area CA3 of Mecp2 knockout mice. Hippocampus 2015;25: 159–168.

[157] Chao HT, Chen H, Samaco RC, Xue M, Chahrour M, Yoo J, et al. Dysfunction in GABA signalling mediates autism-like stereotypies and Rett syndrome phenotypes. Nature 2010;468: 263–269.

[158] Ruggieri VL, Arberas CL. Therapeutic approaches in autism spectrum disorders. Rev Neurol. 2015;1: 45–49.

[159] Napoli DA, et al. Genetic variation in the oxytocin receptor (OXTR) gene is associated with Asperger syndrome. Mol Autism. 2014;5: 48–52.

[160] Wang Y, Zhao S, Wu Z, Feng Y, Zhao C, Zhang C. Oxytocin in the regulation of social behaviours in medial amygdala-lesioned mice via the inhibition of the extracellular signal-regulated kinase signalling pathway. Clin Exp Pharmacol Physiol. 2015;42: 465–474.

[161] Anagnostou E, Soorya L, Brian J, Dupuis A, Mankad D, Smile S, Jacob S. Intranasal oxytocin in the treatment of autism spectrum disorders: a review of literature and early safety and efficacy data in youth. Brain Res. 2014;1580: 188–198.

[162] Watanabe T, et al. Clinical and neural effects of six-week administration of oxytocin on core symptoms of autism. Brain. 2015;3: 249–253.

[163] Guastella AJ, et al. The effects of a course of intranasal oxytocin on social behaviors in youth diagnosed with autism spectrum disorders: a randomized controlled trial. J Child Psychol Psychiatry. 2015;56: 444–452.

[164] Klein BY, Tamir H, Welch MG. PI3K/Akt responses to oxytocin stimulation in Caco2BB gut cells. J Cell Biochem. 2011;112: 3216–3226.

Section 5

Development and Behaviour of Persons with Autism

Chapter 10

Proprioceptive and Kinematic Profiles for Customized Human-Robot Interaction for People Suffering from Autism

Pauline Chevalier, Brice Isableu, Jean-Claude Martin,

Christophe Bazile and Adriana Tapus

Additional information is available at the end of the chapter

http://dx.doi.org/10.5772/67339

Abstract

In this chapter, we presented a method to define individual profiles in order to develop a new personalized robot-based social interaction for individual with autistic spectrum disorder (ASD) with the hypothesis that hyporeactivity to visual motion and an overreliance on proprioceptive information would be linked to difficulties in integrating social cues and in engaging in successful interactions. We succeed to form three groups among our 19 participants (children, teenagers, and adults with ASD), describing each participant's response to visual and proprioceptive inputs. We conducted a first experiment to present the robot Nao as a social companion and to avoid fear or stress toward the robot in future experiment. No direct link between the behavior of the participants toward the robot and their proprioceptive and visual profiles was observed. Still, we found encouraging results going in the direction of our hypothesis. In addition, almost all of our participants showed great interest to Nao. Defining such individual profiles prior to social interactions with a robot could provide promising strategies for designing successful and adapted human-robot interaction (HRI) for individuals with ASD.

Keywords: autism, personalized interaction, socially assistive robotics, proprioception, kinematics

1. Introduction

Autism spectrum disorders (ASDs) are characterized by deficits in communication and social skills and the presence of restricted and repetitive patterns of behaviors, interests, or activities, as described in the DSM-V [1]. The ASD literature describes widely the impairments in communication, interaction, emotion recognition, joint attention, and imitation [2]. Children with ASD show a great affinity for robots, computers, and mechanical components [3]. In the field of socially assistive robotics (SAR), robots are used as tools in socialization therapies for children with ASD in order to enhance social engagement, imitation, and joint attention skills [4–7].

In Ref. [8], the authors suggest that individuals with ASD show an overreliance on proprioceptive information. *Proprioception* can be defined as the sense of an individual of the relative position of body segment (i.e., joint position sense) and the strength of efforts to produce movements. This sense is derived from complex somatosensory signals provided to the brain by different sensors in the body: multiple muscles [9–11], joints [12], and skin receptors [13]. Individuals with ASD show normal to exacerbated integration of proprioceptive cues compared to typically developed (TD) individuals [14]. TD individuals have been repeatedly shown to rely more heavily on vision in various perceptivo-cognitive and sensorimotor tasks, followed by a progressive age-related decline of visual dependency [15, 16]. Proprioceptive integration in ASD is studied so as to better understand how the contribution of these cues influences interactive and social capacities. In Ref. [8], the authors observed the link between the proprioception and social and imitation skills in children with ASD. Results showed that more the children had a high reliance on proprioception cues, the more they exhibited impairments in social functions and imitation.

Moreover, children with ASD show impaired visual processing skills that would lead to difficulties in managing social interactions [17]. Indeed, vision is an important component in communication and social skills. In individuals with ASD, the visual processing impairment may lead to unusual eye contact, difficulty in following the gaze of others or supporting joint attention, and difficulty in interpreting facial and bodily expressions of emotions [17]. In addition, visual field-dependent individuals are considered to show more social skills than visual field-independent individuals [18, 19].

Our project aim is to develop a new personalized human-robot interaction model for individuals with ASD. This would come as a complement to standard therapy. We based our work on the interindividual sensory differences between individuals with ASD. Indeed, there are strong interindividual differences in ASD [1], and adapted interaction is a need in ASD therapies. We built our work on the hypothesis that an individual's own integration of proprioceptive and visual cues will affect the way he/she interacts with a humanoid robot [8, 18–20]. We hypothesize that *a hyporeactivity to visual motion and an overreliance on proprioceptive information are linked in individuals with ASD to their difficulties in integrating social cues and engaging in successful interactions* (H1). The chapter is structured as follow: Section 2 presents the related work in the atypical integration of cues in ASD and SAR for individuals with ASD; Section 3 presents the participants of our study; Section 4 presents our method to define participants' perceptivo-cognitive and sensorimotor profile with respect to the integration of visual inputs; Section 5 describes the first interaction between the robot Nao and our participants; finally, Section 6 concludes our work.

2. Related work

2.1. Atypical integration of proprioceptive and visual integration of cues in ASD

Motor, sensory, and visual processing impairments are present in autism and were taken into account recently with the publication of the DSM-V [1, 14, 17]. However, these deficits have an influence on the quality of life of individuals suffering from ASD and on their social development. In Ref. [21], the authors showed that children with motor impairments are more likely to have solitary play and less interaction with peers in comparison with TD children. They do not explore their physical and social environment, which leads to social and emotional difficulties. Visual deficiencies are known to lead to difficulties in social behaviors and have been widely documented in the literature.

An overreliance on proprioceptive information in ASD is suggested [8, 14, 22–25]. Individuals with autism show normal to exacerbated integration of proprioceptive cues compared to TD individuals [14]. More specifically, in Refs. [22] and [23], the authors observed abnormal postural behavior in autism. They found that individuals with ASD show less age-related postural behaviors and are less stable than TD individuals. Results in Ref. [22] suggest that postural hyporeactivity to visual information is present in the tested individuals with autism (individuals suffering from ASD with IQs comparable to those of TD individuals). Furthermore, Gepner et al. [24] pointed out that individuals with ASD show very poor postural response to visual motion and have movement perception impairments. This result was also observed in Ref. [25]. Proprioceptive integration in ASD has been studied to better understand how the contribution of these cues influences interactive and social capacities. In Ref. [8], the authors observed a stronger than normal association between self-generated motor commands and proprioceptive feedback in the autistic brain. This would confirm that individuals with ASD have an overreliance on proprioceptive cues. Furthermore, they observed that the more the children with ASD rely on proprioception, the more they exhibit impairments in social function and imitation.

2.2. Robots in ASD therapy

Over the past decade, SAR has been a growing research area, with a great interest for therapy for individuals with ASD. Indeed, robots have been shown to be appealing, attracting, and engaging for individuals with ASD. In addition to their mechanical system that is known to attract people with ASD [3, 5], they propose simple, repetitive, and predictable behaviors, which can be reassuring for individuals with ASD. SAR focuses on different topics [26]: the design of adapted robots for individuals with ASD, the design of autonomous interaction between the children and the robots, and the evaluations of the therapy proposed for children with ASD.

Numerous studies relate the positive effects of robots on children with ASD. In Ref. [27], the authors observed an increased collaborative behavior with a human partner after an intervention of dyadic interactions through play between children with ASD and a robot. In Ref. [5], the authors observed that a robot was a successful social bridge with a human partner for children with ASD in triadic interactions. In therapy designed for children with autism [7], the authors found that children with ASD engaged spontaneously in dyadic play with the robot Keepon. This study was also expanded to a triadic interaction between a robot, an adult, and a child. In Ref. [27], the authors used the robot Probo as a social story telling agent for children with ASD. The authors observed that in specific situations, the social performance of children with ASD improves more significantly when it was the robot Probo telling the stories than when it was a human reader. In light of these encouraging findings, many challenges in SAR for individuals with ASD must be addressed. Because of small subject pools and/or short-term experiments, generalized results in the improved skills are often questionable [28]. In addition, there is a great variability in the human-robot interaction (HRI) setups that may influence the findings in SAR for individuals with ASD [29]. The new challenge of SAR will be to identify how to reduce the variability in HRI therapies for individuals with ASD. In particular, in Ref. [30], the authors propose a new step in robot-assisted therapy: robotic-assisted therapeutic scenarios should develop more substantial levels of autonomy, which would allow the robot to adapt to the individual needs of children over longer periods of time.

3. Participants

We conducted our research in collaboration with three care facilities for people suffering from ASD: *IME MAIA* (France) and *IME Notre Ecole* (France), associations for children and teenagers with ASD, and *FAM La Lendemaine* (France) a medical house for adults with ASD. Informed consent for participation was obtained from the parents or by the participants themselves when able. The experimental protocol was approved by the EA 4532 local university ethics committee.

Our subject pool is composed of 12 children and teenagers with ASD (11.7 ± 2.6 years old) and seven adults with ASD (26.8 ± 7.9 years old) from these three care facilities. There are 14 male and five female participants. For confidentiality reasons, we coded the participants' identities as follows: CH#, with # from 1 to 12 for children and teenagers and AD#, with # from 1 to 7 for adults. In **Table 1**, we give a short description of each participant.

ID#	Gender	Age	Comments
CH3	M	12	–
CH5	F	11	Nonverbal; West syndrome (uncommon to rare epileptic disorder [31]).
CH8	M	15	–
CH10	M	10	–
CH11	M	17	–
AD2	F	25	Diagnosed with creatine transporter deficiency
AD4	F	21	–
AD6	M	25	Suffers of echolalia (i.e., defined as the unsolicited repetition of vocalizations made by another person)
CH1	M	11	–
CH4	M	13	High level of cognition. Asked to be part of the program to meet Nao.
CH7	M	8	–
CH9	F	12	–
CH12	M	9	–
AD1	F	25	–
AD3	M	44	Asperger syndrome
CH2	M	9	Suffers of echolalia
CH6	M	13	–
AD5	M	27	Suffers of epilepsy
AD7	M	21	–

Table 1. Participants' description.

4. Defining proprioceptive and kinematic profiles

4.1. Methods

The first step of our work was to determine how to define participants' perceptivo-cognitive and sensorimotor profiles. We used two methodologies: (1) the perceptivo-cognitive adolescents/adults sensory profiles (AASP) developed by Dunn and Brown [31] and (2) an experimental sensorimotor setup dedicated to assess the individual's reliance on visual over proprioceptive inputs to control postural balance while confronted to a moving virtual visual room.

The AASPs were completed by all participants. We selected this questionnaire because it has been successfully used in ASD [32–34]. As described in Ref. [35], it enabled us to assess an individual's sensory processing preferences described in terms of the quadrants in Dunn's model of sensory processing [35]:

- Low registration: tendency to miss or take a long time to respond to stimuli.
- Sensation seeking: tendency to try to create additional stimuli or to look for environment that provides sensory stimuli.
- Sensory sensitivity: tendency to answer quickly to stimuli.
- Sensation avoiding: tendency to be overwhelmed or bothered by sensory stimuli and to be actively involved to reduce the stimuli in their environment.

As most of our participants do not have the cognitive level to fill themselves the questionnaire, it was filled with the help of their caregivers who know well their habits and response to everyday life sensory stimuli. In the instruction of the questionnaire, it is specified that the questions can be filled (1) by the person himself/herself; (2) with the help of a caregiver or parent; and (3) by a caregiver or parent. Indeed, this questionnaire targets also individuals with intellectual deficiencies. We asked the caregivers to fill the questionnaire as we had a direct contact with them and were able to inform them well about the conditions and forms of the questionnaire. We assessed movement, visual, touch, and auditory processing using 29 of the 60 items of the AASP. We eliminated the taste/smell processing and activity level and questions, which were not relevant for the purpose of our study or suitable for individual with invasive ASD's behavior. We designed a sensorimotor experimental setup to assess the sensory integration of each participant. The setup has been used in several studies [36, 37]. It evaluates (1) the effect of a moving virtual visual room on postural control and (2) one's capability to use proprioceptive information to reduce visual dependency [36, 37]. It has been shown that the integration of proprioceptive cues differs among individuals in unstable posture [38–40]. A visual-dependent individual integrates less proprioceptive cues than other individuals, and when they are exposed to visual motion in an unstable posture, their body sway follow the visual stimulus [41].

To assess the visual dependence of our participants with ASD, they were asked to stand quietly in two postural conditions: (1) normal and (2) tandem Romberg (i.e., one foot in front of the other one), in front of a virtual room, static (SVR) or rolling (RVR) at 0.25 Hz with an inclination of ±10°. We chose a rolling frequency of 0.25 Hz: virtual room setups frequently use rolling frequency between 0.1 and 0.5 Hz [24, 25, 42]. It has been found that a frequency of 0.2 Hz produces the strongest, most synchronized body sway, and that frequencies above 0.5 Hz produce little body sway [43].

They were asked to stand on a force platform in front of the virtual room, static or rolling in three conditions (see **Figure 1**):

- C1—stable position with SVR: the participant stands on the force platform, straight, feet separated by the length of the hips. The VR stays still. The recording lasts 30 seconds.
- C2—stable position with RVR: the participant stands on the force platform, straight with feet separated by the length of the hips. The VR has a sinusoidal movement. The recording lasts 50 seconds.
- C3—tandem Romberg position with RVR: the participant stands on the force platform, straight, one foot in front of the other one. The VR has a sinusoidal movement. The recording lasts 50 seconds.

http://dx.doi.org/10.5772/67339

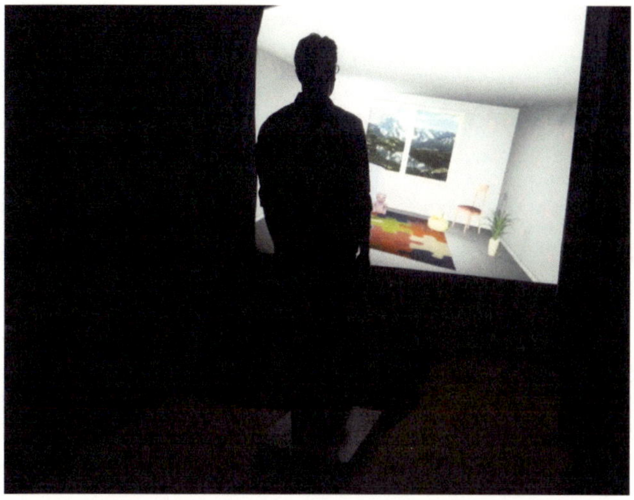

Figure 1. Experimental setup for adult participants in condition C3.

The virtual room consisted of a 3D environment (see **Figure 2**) created with Blender, a free 3D rendering software. It was designed as a child bedroom and was decorated with child toys and furniture, as we aimed to create a friendly environment. We placed in the line of sight of the participants with ASD a toy plane in order to help them to focus on the task, and not to be distracted away: we instructed them to focus on this plane [24, 25]. The virtual room was projected to a white wall with a short focal projector in a dark room. For the adult group setup, the dimension of the projection was 2.4 m large × 1.8 m high and the participants stood at 1.3 m of the point of observation. For the children group setup, the dimension was 1.75 m large × 1.30 m high and the participants stood at 1 m. This permitted us to maintain the angular diameter around 31° in horizontal and 41° in vertical in both setup.

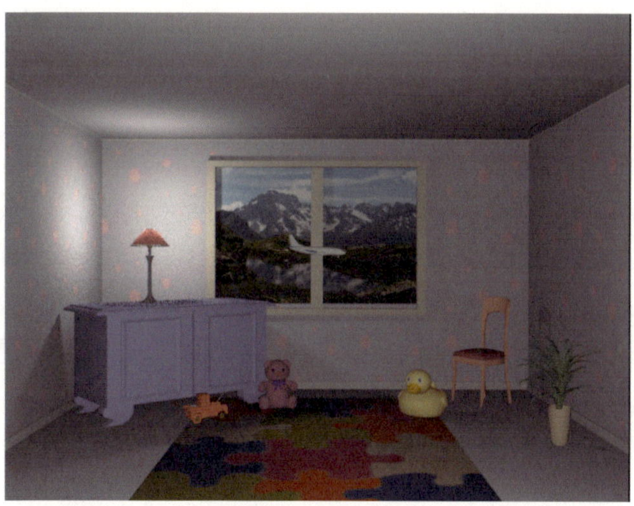

Figure 2. Screenshot of the virtual room used in the experiment, developed with Blender.

We investigated if the age of our participants had an influence on their center of pressure (CoP) behavior. Indeed, in TD individuals, children show more dramatic postural reactions to visual sway than adults [44]. However, as shown in Ref. [25], children with ASD showed less response to visual stimulus in virtual room experiments in stable position than TD children.

We expect that:

(1) children participants will show more swaying than adults in stable position and without visual stimulus (C1);

(2) as we work in a population with ASD, the postural reaction to visual sway will not be influenced by age;

(3) the effect of the RVR should be maximum in the unstable postural condition (C3); and

(4) the effect of (3) should not be larger in adults than in children.

4.2. Data analysis

We used an AMTI OR6-5-1000 force platform to record the displacement of the CoP of our participants. The sampling frequency was of 1 KHz. To reduce noise, a Butterworth filter with a cut-off frequency of 10 Hz on the recorded data was used. The root mean square (RMS) of the displacement of the CoP in mediolateral directions was computed as an indicator of an individual's stability. Indeed, as described in Ref. [45], the RMS provided the information about the variability of the CoP in space. The frequency power at 0.25 Hz (Fpo) of the CoP was computed to evaluate the postural response to the visual stimulus. The more an individual is coupled with the visual stimulus, the more the Fpo. We observed the CoP behavior in mediolateral direction as it is the direction of our visual stimulus. RMS and Fpo should be correlated if our participants with ASD follows the RVR movement:

(1) If the RMS and the Fpo are correlated, then we can expect these coupling capabilities with contextual cues promise higher social interaction capabilities.

(2) If the RMS and the Fpo are not correlated (no coupling), then one can conclude that the visual stimulus is integrated as noise, inducing disorientation and instability.

We performed repeated measures analysis on the RMS and the Fpo for the age groups (adults; children) and the conditions (C1; C2; C3). The significance threshold was set to $p < 0.05$. We used Statistica version 13 to perform the analyses.

Except for the clustering analysis, we excluded four participants (AD6, CH6, CH7, and CH12) of the statistical analysis, as they showed distress, nervousness, and/or agitation during the recording, resulting to dramatic changes in their CoP behavior during some recording.

4.3. Results

4.3.1. Displacements and root mean square (RMS)

As we expected, we found a significant main effect of the participants' age on their RMS (F (1; 13) = 6.92; $p < 0.05$) across all conditions. The mediolateral RMS of the adults was smaller ($M = 0.84$; SD = 0.57) than those of the children ($M = 1.70$; SD = 1.12), indicating that the children were globally more variable than the adults (see **Figure 3**). The conditions (C1 vs. C2 vs. C3) did not impact the displacements of the CoP of the participants. The conditions × age interaction was not significant on the RMS.

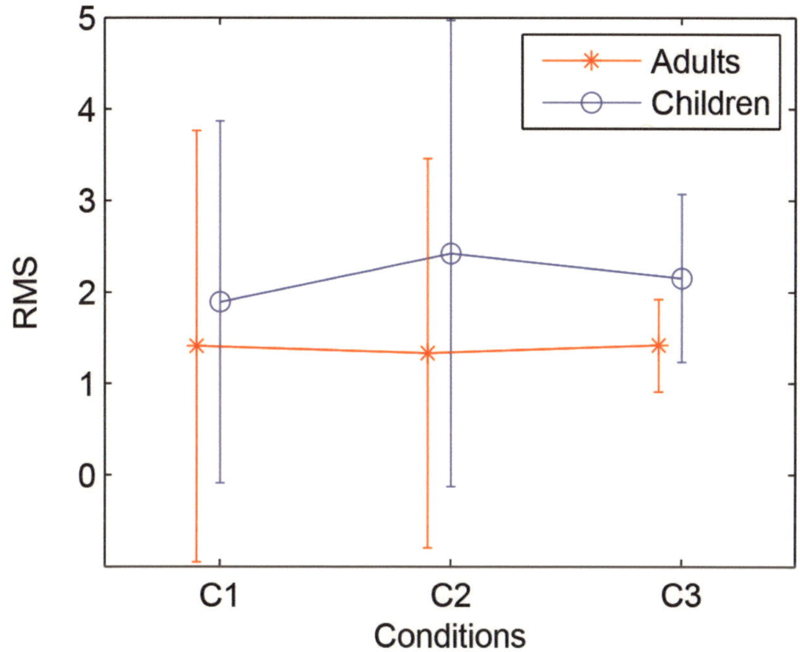

Figure 3. Mean RMS for the adults and children in the three conditions.

4.3.2. Displacements and frequency power response at 0.25 Hz (Fpo)

As we expected, the main effect of conditions was significant on the Fpo (F (2; 26) = 13.11; $p < 0.05$). In condition C1 ($M = 0.17$; SD = 0.16), participants had the smallest Fpo, followed by condition C2 ($M = 0.34$; SD = 0.38) and condition C3 ($M = 0.67$; SD = 0.31) had the highest Fpo. This suggests that the participants' displacements of the CoP were coupled with the movement of the visual room when they were exposed to it, and that this coupling is maximized in the more difficult stance. In addition, the Fpo was positively correlated with the RMS in condition C3 ($R = 0.73$; $p < 0.01$), indicating that the larger displacement of the CoP are possibly coupled with the RVR (i.e., the visual stimulus). We found a significant main effect of the participants' age (F (1; 13) = 5.37; $p < 0.05$). The Fpo of adults was smaller (M = 0.29; SD = 0.33) than those of children (M = 0.46; SD = 0.36) across all conditions. This suggests a higher coupling between postural response to the RVR and the displacements of the CoP in children than in adults. However, the age × conditions interaction for the Fpo was not significant. In **Figure 4**, we can observe that children's and adults' postural response to the visual stimulus is similar in condition C3, indicating that children with ASD do not respond in a higher way to visual cues in comparison with adults with ASD. The frequency of 0.25 Hz is present in natural swaying [43] and the RMS was higher in children than in adults. As the age × conditions interaction for the Fpo was not significant, we can assume that the higher Fpo on the whole experiment was induced by the greater variability of the displacements of the CoP of the children. This result suggests that our participants' postural behavior was not driven by age as we expected. We found that our participants' postural coupling to the virtual room was driven by the conditions (C1; C2; C3).

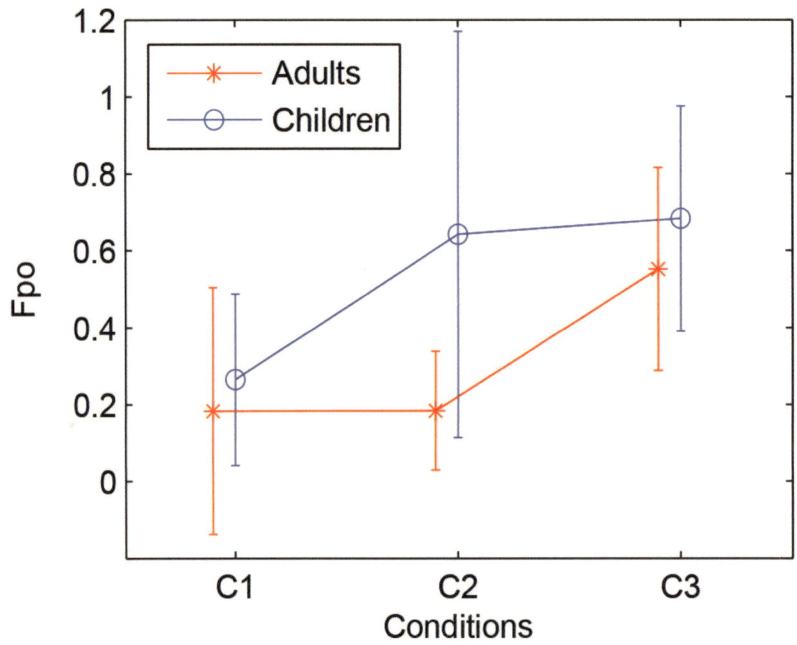

Figure 4. Mean Fpo for the adults and children in the three conditions.

4.3.3. Grouping the participants

We performed a clustering analysis (dendrogram, Ward method) on the AASP items on movement and visual sensory preferences, the RMS, and the Fpo of all the 19 participants (12 children and seven adults with ASD) (see **Table 2** to see the specific items selected). We sought to identify if the postural response to the visual stimulus and AASP scores were able to discriminate our participants, as we aimed to use theses profiles to propose personalized interactions with robots. The dendrogram gave us three groups, see **Figure 5**:

Movement low registration
Visual low registration
Movement sensation seeking
Visual sensation seeking
Movement sensory sensitivity
Visual sensory sensitivity
Movement sensation avoiding
Visual sensation avoiding
Mediolateral RMS for condition C1, C2, and C3
Fpo for conditions C1, C2, and C3 in mediolateral direction

Table 2. AASP items and CoP behavior selected for the dendrogram analysis.

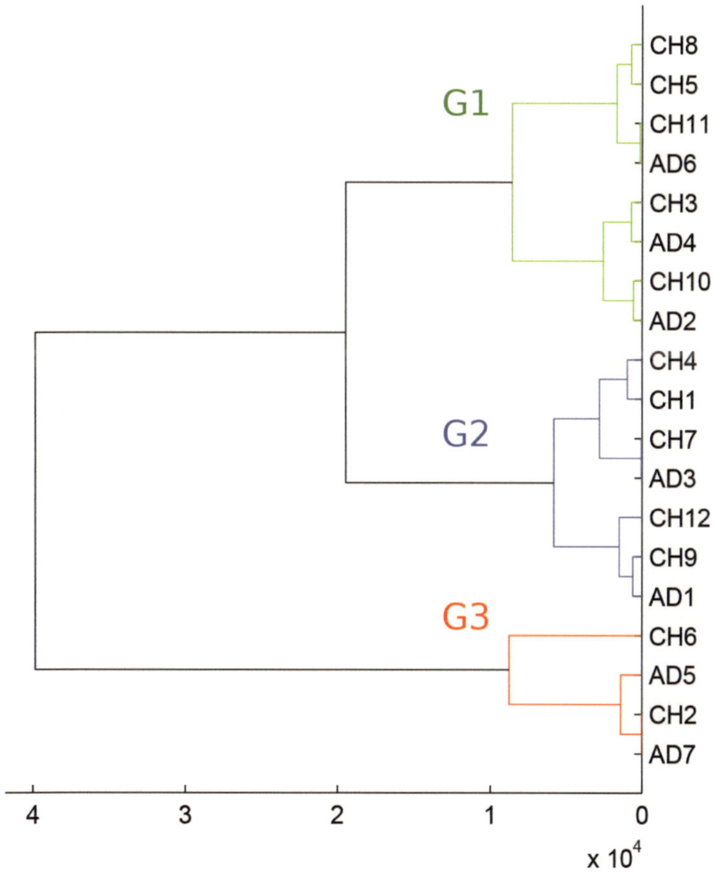

Figure 5. Dendrogram analysis.

- G1: 8 participants CH3; CH5; CH8; CH10; CH11; AD2; AD4; AD6.
- G2: 7 participants CH1; CH4; CH7; CH9; CH12; AD1; AD3.
- G3: 4 participants CH2; CH6; AD5; AD7.

The RMS in all conditions for the three groups detected is shown in **Figure 6**. **Figure 7** shows Fpo in condition C3. In **Figure 8**, the mean AASP score (movement sensory sensitivity (MSS), visual sensory sensitivity (VSS), and visual sensation avoiding (VSA)) for each group is illustrated.

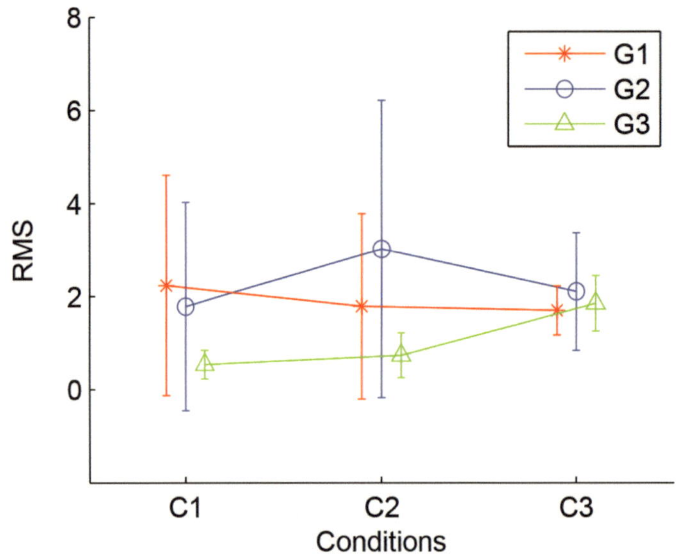

Figure 6. Histogram of the mean RMS for the groups defined by clustering analysis for the three conditions.

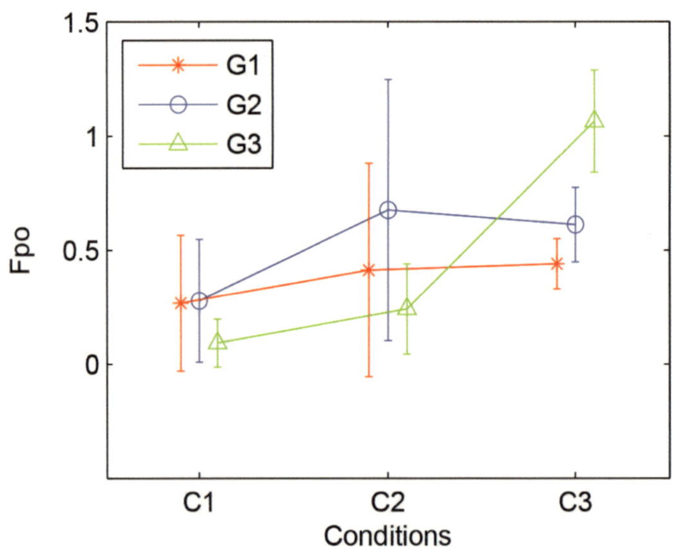

Figure 7. Histogram of frequency power at 0.25 Hz in all conditions of the three groups.

http://dx.doi.org/10.5772/67339

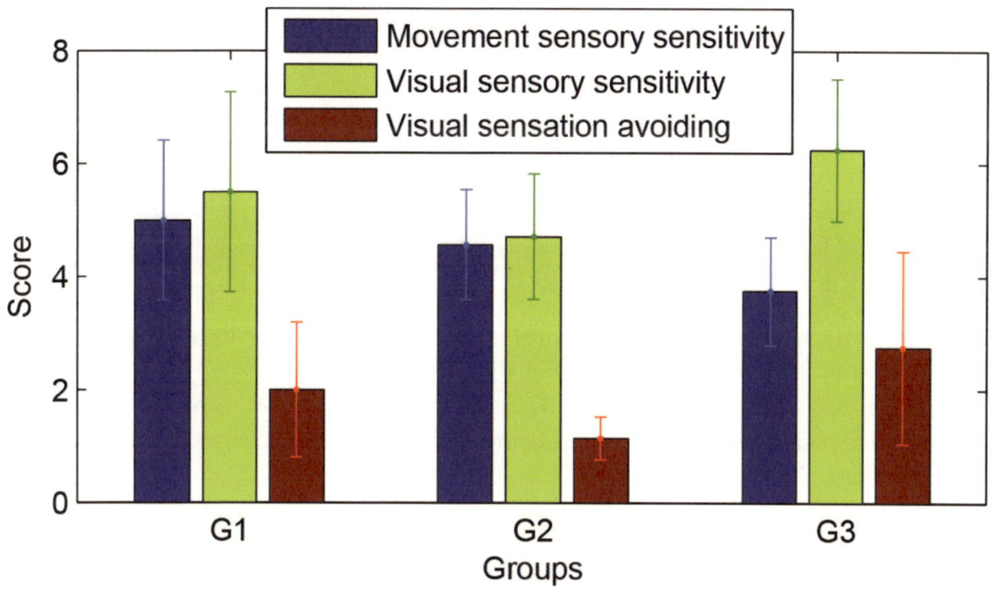

Figure 8. Histograms for three relevant AASP items scores of the groups.

Repeated measures analysis was applied on the RMS and the Fpo for the groups (G1; G2; G3) and the conditions (C1; C2; C3). We found no main effect of the groups on the RMS and on the Fpo of the participants. However, we found significant interaction effect between groups over the conditions on the RMS (F (4; 24) = 3.55; $p < 0.05$), see **Figure 6**. Participants from groups G1 and G2 showed great CoP variability in all conditions, unlike participants from group G3 that showed a greater CoP variability only in condition C3. **Figure 6** also informs us that participants in group G1 had their RMS that decrease from C1 to C3, whereas participants in group G3 had their RMS that increased from C1 to C3. This indicates that participants from group G1 maximized the use of proprioception to reduce the effect of the visual stimulus in unstable position. Identically, we found significant interaction effect between the groups and the conditions on the Fpo (F (4; 24) = 9.79; $p < 0.001$), see **Figure 7**. This indicates us that each group has a different postural response toward the visual stimulus. **Figure 7** suggests that in condition C1, participants from groups G1 and G2 showed a higher coupling with the frequency of the visual stimulus than participants from group G3. As in this condition, the participants are not exposed to the RVR, this result shows the higher instability of these participant in comparison to participants from G3. The coupling with the rolling visual stimulus is similar in conditions C2 and C3 for participants from groups G1 and G2, indicating that the difficulty of postural task (stable or unstable) did not increase the strength of the coupling with the rolling virtual room: being in a stable or unstable posture did not affected them in their response to the visual stimulus. Participants from G3 showed a greater coupling to the visual stimulus in condition C3 than in other conditions, indicating that they responded more strongly to the visual stimulus in an unstable posture and thus they are more visual dependent (see **Figure 7**). Furthermore, we also examined the correspondence between the scores of different items of the AASP and the data obtained from the CoP recording, listed in **Table 2**:

- High score in MSS (i.e., tendency to answer quickly to movement stimuli) was inversely correlated to Fpo in mediolateral direction for condition C3 ($R = 0.53$; $p < 0.05$), indicating that participants who showed by the AASP questionnaire to have a tendency to answer quickly to movement stimuli were less driven by the visual stimulus in unstable position.
- High score in VSS (i.e., tendency to answer quickly to visual stimuli) was positively correlated to mediolateral RMS for condition C3 ($R = 0.61$; $p < 0.05$). This suggests that participants who showed by the AASP questionnaire to have a tendency to answer quickly to visual stimuli were more unstable when exposed to the visual stimulus in unstable position.
- High score in VSA (i.e., tendency to be overwhelmed or bothered by visual sensory stimuli) was positively correlated to mediolateral RMS for condition C3 ($R = 0.59$; $p < 0.05$), indicating that participants who showed by the AASP questionnaire to have a tendency to be overwhelmed or bothered by visual stimuli were more unstable when exposed to the visual stimulus in unstable position.

Three of the selected items of the AASP showed to be correlated with the postural response variability to a visual stimulus in an unstable position (C3), confirming that these AASP items match with the behavioral response of the participants.

4.4. Conclusion

Thanks to this experiment, we succeeded to form three groups between our participants, describing each participant's response to visual and proprioceptive inputs:

- ***Group G1*** (participants: CH3; CH5; CH8; CH10; CH11; AD2; AD4; AD6) includes participants with high scores in MSS, low scores in VSS, and low score in VSA. Participants showed strong visual independence to the RVR, suggesting an overreliance on proprioceptive cues and hyporeactivity to visual cues.
- ***Group G2*** (participants: CH1; CH4; CH7; CH9; AD1; AD3) includes participants with high scores in MSS, low scores in VSS, and low score in VSA. Participants showed moderate reactivity to the RVR, suggesting that they rely evenly on visual and proprioceptive cues.
- ***Group G3*** (participants: CH2; CH6; AD5; AD7) includes participants with low scores in MSS, high scores in VSS, and high score in VSA. Participants showed hypereactivity to the RVR, suggesting a hyporeactivity to proprioceptive cues and an overreliance on visual cues.

We found that overall children had greater variability of their CoP than adults which was expected (due to biomechanical, anthropometrical, sensory integration factors and maturation of these processes). The different conditions of posture and exposure to the visual stimulus (C1; C2; C3) did not impact the variability of the CoP of our participants. However, the participants' displacements of the CoP showed to be more coupled with the frequency of the visual stimulus in condition C3 than in conditions C1 and C2. We observed that the coupling to the frequency of the visual stimulus was higher in children than in adults on the whole experiment, but not inside the conditions. As the children were experiencing more variability to their CoP and as the frequency 0.25 Hz (i.e., the frequency of our visual stimulus) is present in natural swaying [43],

http://dx.doi.org/10.5772/67339

we posit that this higher coupling to this frequency on the whole experiment by the children was induced by the greater variability of the displacements of their CoP. This result suggests that our participants' postural behavior was not driven by age as we expected.

In TD individuals, children show more dramatic postural reaction to visual stimulus [44]. In children with ASD, it is suggested that sensory integration differs from TD individuals [8, 14, 24, 25]. We found in this experiment that the age of the participants with ASD did not impact the strength of the postural coupling with the visual stimulus, differently to TD individuals. Similarly to TD individuals, children with ASD had more variability in the displacement of their CoP in comparison to adults with ASD.

We also observed a great variability in our participants' postural behavior. In our results, we found three groups with different sensory integration among our participants. As in Refs. [46] and [47], we found in our participants individuals(mixing children and adults) with a weak proprioceptive integration and strong visual dependency. In Ref. [46], the authors found an impairment of the proprioception input in autism: children with ASD used more visual cues to reduce sway and maintain balance. In Ref. [47], the authors found that unlikely to typically developed individuals, individuals with ASD have an impaired proprioception development. Their sensory motor signal appears to remain at the kinesthetic stage of typically developed 3–4 years old children and have to rely on visual inputs. They also conjectured that the impaired proprioception of physical micromovements of the individuals with ASD impedes as well their visual perception of micromovements in others during real-time interactions, impairing their abilities to interact with people. And, as in Refs. [8] and [25], we found in our participants individuals relying more on proprioceptive inputs and weak visual dependency.

With these results and our hypothesis H1, we are able to make assumptions on the behaviors that each individual will have during human-robot interaction sessions. Therefore, we posit that individuals from group G1 will have less successful social interactions than the ones from groups G2 and G3, and that individuals from group G3 will have the most successful social interactions.

5. Greetings with Nao

5.1. Objectives

A first analysis of the behavior of the participants toward the Nao robot was conducted. Nao is a minihumanoid robot, developed by SoftBank Robotics (former Aldebaran Robotics). The purpose of the interaction was to present the robot to the children and adults with ASD for a short duration (up to 2 minutes). Indeed, some of the individuals with ASD are reluctant to unusual events and changes in their daily routine. The robot was smoothly introduced so as to avoid fear toward the robot. In addition, in Ref. [48], the authors observed that children who saw the robot act in a social-communicative way and were more likely to follow its gaze than those who did not. Hence, we believe that introducing them smoothly the robot as a social partner by showing them the Nao robot in the context of a short greeting task may help the participants to interact with the robot in further experiments.

We also wanted to verify that the behavior of our participants was linked to their proprioceptive and visual profiles as described in Section 4. To do so, we video analyzed the interaction with Nao robot and annotated our participants' social behavior following the items described in **Table 3**.

Smiles, laughter
Speech to Nao by his/her initiative
Speech to Nao after being encouraged by his/her caregiver
Social gesture toward Nao (waving back)
Gaze of the participant toward:
1. The robot
2. His/her caregiver
3. Other (somewhere else)

Table 3. Description of the tracked social behaviors.

5.2. Method

The scenario of this first interaction with the robot was in two phases. First, the greetings: the participant was seated in front of the robot and Nao said "Hello, I am Nao. You and I, we are going to be friends" while waving to him/her (**Figure 9**). Then, if the participant was verbal, the robot asked his/her name, and repeated it. Second, the dance: the robot asked if the participant wanted it to dance, and then danced (**Figure 10**). During the interaction with the robot, all participants were with their caregiver. The caregivers were instructed to encourage the participants to look and answer to the robot.

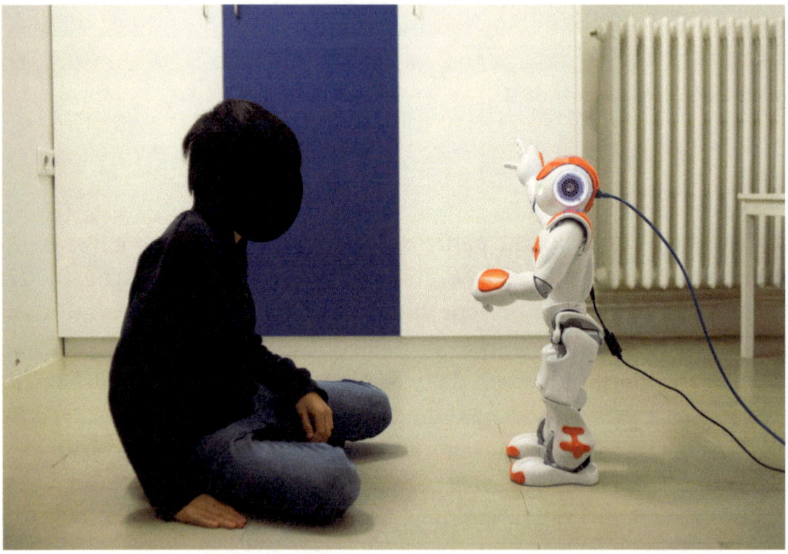

Figure 9. Nao greets a child.

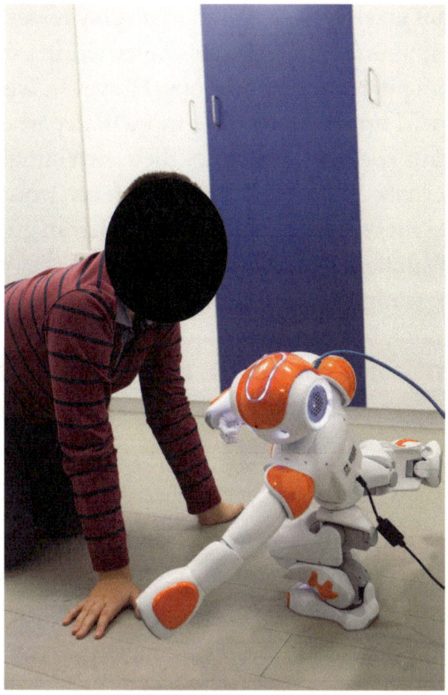

Figure 10. Nao dances for a child.

5.3. Data analysis

We analyzed the videos of the interaction with the robot and observed the parameters described in **Table 3** for each participant. A first coder (first author) annotated all of the videos of the interaction. A second coder, unaware of the hypotheses of the setup, annotated a 21% of the videos, randomly selected. The intraclass correlation coefficient (ICC) was used to ensure intercoder reliability. The ICC score was of 0.99, indicating a very good reliability.

AD3 was removed from the statistical analysis as he was becoming more withdrawn from social interaction since few weeks, and unwilling to participate into the tasks. CH5 was removed from the statistical analysis on speech data as this participant is nonverbal. For the gaze and smile behavior analyses, we performed a one-way ANOVA among the groups. We performed Fisher's exact test on the speech and gesture behaviors. The significance threshold was set to $p < 0.05$. We used Statistica version 13 to perform the analyses.

5.4. Results

The participants' behaviors are described in **Tables 4** and **5**. Overall, except from AD6 (G1) and AD3 (G2), participants from all groups looked more than 60% of the time to the robot. No statistical evidence was found about the gazing behavior of our participants and its relations with the groups. However, we can still observe in **Figure 11** the frequency/percentage distribution of the participants' gaze toward the robots among the groups. Participants from group G3 appeared to show more interest (gaze more frequently) toward the robot than the two other groups, and participants from group G1 appeared to display fewer gaze toward the robot than the two other groups. Participants from all groups smiled during the interaction. No statistical evidence was found on smiling behavior and groups. However, we can still notice in **Figure 11** that participants from group G1 appeared to smile more than participants from groups G2 and G3. The number of participants speaking to Nao by their own initiative was significantly different among groups ($p < 0.05$). Only one participant out of seven from group G1 responded by its own initiative to the robot, when five out of six participants from group G2 and three out of four participants from group G3 spoke to Nao by their own initiative. We can see that participants CH8, CH11, and AD2 from group G1 were the only participants not to respond to the robot with or without encouragement. No statistical evidence was found between social gesture and groups. However, we observed that participants from group G1 did not show social gesture toward the robot, but two participants from group G2 and two participants from group G3 did.

Groups	ID#	Gaze toward			Smiles, laughter	Speech to Nao		Social gesture toward Nao (waving back)
		Nao	Caregiver	Other		By his/her initiative	After being encourage by his/ her caregiver	
G1	CH3	63.1%	18.17%	18.73%	19.93%	0	1	0
G1	CH5	81.90%	2.76%	15.34%	0%	–	–	0
G1	CH8	100%	0%	0%	100%	0	0	0
G1	CH10	88.52%	5.35%	6.13%	43%	0	2	0
G1	CH11	83.28%	0%	16.72%	0%	0	0	0
G1	AD2	61.73%	34.13%	4.13%	71.22%	0	0	0
G1	AD4	83.05%	14.15%	2.81%	91.47%	4	1	0
G1	AD6	23.14%	0%	76.86%	8.99%	0	1	0
G2	CH1	74.61%	1.59%	23.8%	0%	0	1	0
G2	CH4	88.31%	0%	11.69%	0%	2	0	0
G2	CH7	85.13%	4.21%%	10.66%	58.61%	1	2	0
G2	CH9	71.68%	0%	28.32%	6.54%	1	1	0
G2	CH12	81.24%	7.74%	11.02%	4.85%	2	2	2
G2	AD1	94.47%	2.33%	3.20%	46.37%	4	0	2
G2	AD3	18.87%	2.04%	79.1%	3.26%	0	2	0
G3	CH2	91.86%	0.79%	7.35%	0%	1	1	1
G3	CH6	99.09%	0%	0.91%	22.09%	2	0	3
G3	AD5	99.12%	0%	0.88%	61.81%	1	0	0
G3	AD7	66.70%	5.58%	27.72%	12.34%	2	0	0

Table 4. Participants' behavior during the interaction with the robot.

Groups	ID#	Comments
G1	CH3	He was really amazed by the robot, and switched his gaze to his caregiver to show his amazement
G1	CH5	Her caregiver was really impressed of the concentration she showed for the robot
G1	CH8	–
G1	CH10	–
G1	CH11	His caregiver was impressed that he looked that much the robot.
G1	AD2	She was more talking and looking at the caregiver than to Nao but was enthusiast to participate to the task
G1	AD4	She was really amazed by the robot and the task was corresponding of one of her routine: asking the name of the person near her
G1	AD6	–
G2	CH1	–
G2	CH4	He was really excited and impressed to see the robot (this boy asked to participate to the project)
G2	CH7	First, he was impressed by the robot and stand back. He finally approached it and gave it a kiss at the end of the interaction
G2	CH9	She was impressed by the robot and stand back. She moved several time across the room, without giving that much attention to the robot
G2	CH12	–
G2	AD1	She was scared of the robot when its arms were moving toward her
G2	AD3	It has been reported that he was more withdrawn since few weeks, and unwilling to participate to tasks
G3	CH2	–
G3	CH6	He was particularly enthusiast to see the robot moving and talking to him (saying his name, waving)
G3	AD5	He showed some reluctance toward the robot, by saying "we should put it in the garbage"
G3	AD7	He was reported by his caregiver by being really shy toward new things

Table 5. Descriptive comments on the behavior of the participants during the interaction.

5.5. Conclusion

The presentation of the Nao robot to the ASD participants permitted us to introduce it as a social partner. Most of the participants answered to it and some showed social gesture toward it. This introduction to the robot may help the participants to interact easier with the robot in further experiments, as found in Ref. [48]. We also removed the "surprise" and "novelty" effect of the robot. Some participants showed to be slightly afraid and impressed by the robot. These participants seemed to be reassured at the end of the interaction. Participants showed numerous smiles, and looked toward the robot a great amount of time. The statistical analysis only showed a relation between the participants' groups and their answer to Nao, when initiated by their own. Participants from group G3 showed more free speech to Nao than the two other groups, and participants from group G1 showed less free speech than the others. Still, we can observe that the participants from group G3 appeared to show more gaze at the robot and social gesture than participants from group G1, and that participants from group G1 showed fewer gazes to the robot and social gesture than participants from groups G2 and G3. However, participants from G1 appeared to show more smiles than participants from groups G2 and G3. Unfortunately, this first experiment did not permit us to validate that the behavior of the participants was linked to their proprioceptive and visual profiles. However, we have some encouraging results going in the direction of our hypothesis.

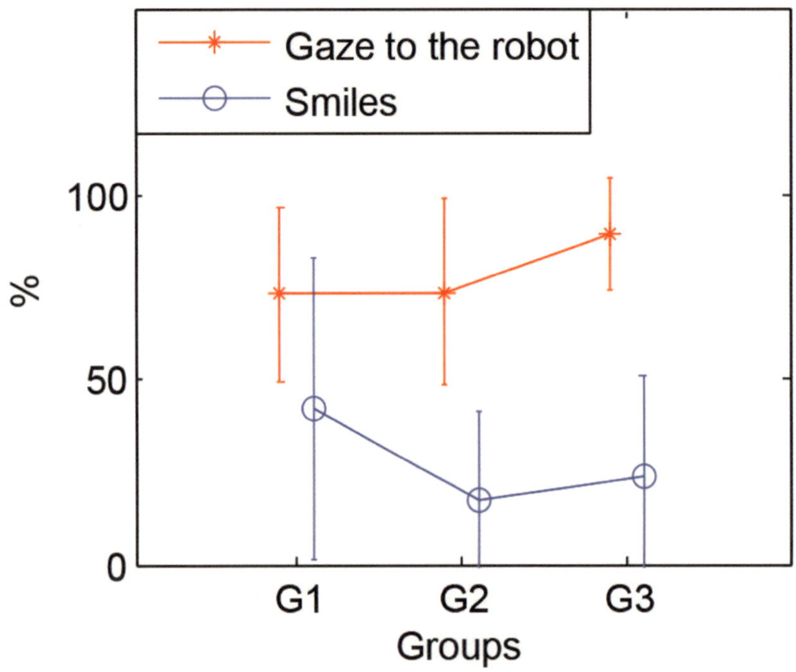

Figure 11. Plot of the percentage of participants' gaze toward the robot and smiles.

6. General conclusion and discussion

The long-term goal of our work is to define individual profiles in order to develop a new personalized robot-based social interaction for individual with ASD. We hypothesized that hyporeactivity to visual motion and an overreliance on proprioceptive information would be linked to difficulties in integrating social cues and in engaging in successful interactions. We worked with 19 children, teenagers, and adults with ASD from three care facilities.

Our first experiment enabled us to form three groups between our participants, describing each participant's response to visual and proprioceptive inputs. Based on our hypothesis,

http://dx.doi.org/10.5772/67339

we made assumptions on the behaviors each individual will have during the human-robot interaction sessions. With these results and our hypothesis H1, we were able to make assumptions on the behaviors that each individual will have during human-robot interaction sessions. Therefore, we posit that *individuals from group G1 will have less successful interactions than the ones from groups G2 and G3, and that individuals from group G3 will have the most successful interactions.*

A first interaction with the robot was conducted. The robot Nao was presented to our 19 participants. The purpose of this experiment was to present the robot Nao as a social companion and to avoid fear or stress toward the robot in future experiment. We did not observe a direct link between the behavior of the participants toward the robot and their proprioceptive and visual profiles, but we still found encouraging results going in the direction of our hypothesis. As it was already seen in SAR almost all of our participants (children, teenagers, and adults) showed great interest to their new mechanical companion.

Defining such individual profiles prior to social interactions with a robot could provide promising strategies for designing successful and adapted HRI for individuals with ASD. The behavior of our participants toward emotion recognition [49] and joint attention [50] has already been studied. We are currently planning to investigate these issues in repetitive interaction involving imitation, where the behavior of the robot is adapted to the profile of the participants.

Author details

Pauline Chevalier[1, 2, 3, 4], Brice Isableu[5], Jean-Claude Martin[4], Christophe Bazile[6] and Adriana Tapus[1]*

*Address all correspondence to: adriana.tapus@ensta-paristech.fr

1 Robotics and Computer Vision Lab, ENSTA-ParisTech, Palaiseau, France

2 CIAMS, Paris-Sud Univ, Paris-Saclay Univ, Orsay Cedex, France

3 CIAMS, Orléan Univs, Orléans, France

4 LIMSI, CNRS, Paris-Sud Univ, Paris-Saclay Univ, Orsay Cedex, France

5 Aix-Marseille Univ, PSYCLE, Aix-en-Provence, France

6 Grouping of the Partner Associations of Social Action (GAPAS), France

References

[1] American Psychiatric Association and Others. Diagnostic and Statistical Manual of Mental Disorders (DSM-5). American Psychiatric Association: Pub; 2013.

[2] Charman, T, Swettenham, J, Baron-Cohen, S, Cox, A, Baird, G, and Drew, A. Infants with autism: an investigation of empathy, pretend play, joint attention, and imitation. Developmental Psychology. 1997;**33**(5):781.

[3] Hart, M. Autism/excel study. Proceedings of the 7th International ACM SIGACCESS Conference on Computers and Accessibility. 2005:136–141.

[4] Tapus, A, Peca, A, Aly, A, Pop, C, Jisa, L, Pintea, S, Rusu, AS, and David, DO. Children with autism social engagement in interaction with Nao, an imitative robot-A series of single case experiments. Interaction Studies. 2012;**13**(3):315–347.

[5] Kim, ES, Berkovits, LD, Bernier, EP, Leyzberg, D, Shic, F, Paul, R, and Scassellati, B. Social robots as embedded reinforcers of social behavior in children with autism. Journal of Autism and Developmental Disorders. 2013;**43**(5):1038–1049.

[6] Wainer, J, Dautenhahn, K, Robins, B, and Amirabdollahian, F. Collaborating with Kaspar: Using an autonomous humanoid robot to foster cooperative dyadic play among children with autism. 10th IEEE-RAS International Conference on Humanoid Robots (Humanoids), 2010. 2010:631–638.

[7] Kozima, H, Nakagawa, C, and Yasuda, Y. Interactive robots for communication-care: A case-study in autism therapy. IEEE International Workshop on Robot and Human Interactive Communication, 2005. ROMAN 2005. 2005:341–346.

[8] Haswell, CC, Izawa, J, Dowell, LR, Mostofsky, SH, and Shadmehr, R. Representation of internal models of action in the autistic brain. Nature Neuroscience. 2009;**12**(8):970–972.

[9] Goodwin, GM, McCloskey, DI, and Matthews, PBC. Proprioceptive illusions induced by muscle vibration: Contribution by muscle spindles to perception? Science. 1972; **175**(4028):1382–1384.

[10] Burke, D, Hagbarth, K-E, Löfstedt, L, and Wallin, BG. The responses of human muscle spindle endings to vibration of non-contracting muscles. The Journal of Physiology. 1976;**261**(3):673–693.

[11] Roll, JP, and Vedel, JP. Kinaesthetic role of muscle afferents in man, studied by tendon vibration and microneurography. Experimental Brain Research. 1982;**47**(2):177–190.

[12] Ferrell, WR, Gandevia, SC, and McCloskey, DI. The role of joint receptors in human kinaesthesia when intramuscular receptors cannot contribute. The Journal of Physiology. 1987;**386**(1):63–71.

[13] Edin, BB. Cutaneous afferents provide information about knee joint movements in humans. The Journal of Physiology. 2001;**531**(1):289–297.

[14] Gowen, E, and Hamilton, A. Motor abilities in autism: A review using a computational context. Journal of Autism and Developmental Disorders. 2013;**43**(2):323–344.

[15] Bagust, J, Docherty, S, Haynes, W, Telford, R, and Isableu, B. Changes in rod and frame test scores recorded in schoolchildren during development-A longitudinal study. PloS One. 2013;**8**(5):e65321.

[16] Assaiante C. Development of locomotor balance control in healthy children. Neuroscience & Biobehavioral Reviews. 1998;**22**(4):527–532.

[17] Simmons, DR, Robertson, AE, McKay, LS, Toal, E, McAleer, P, and Pollick, FE. Vision in autism spectrum disorders. Vision Research. 2009;**49**(22):2705–2739.

[18] Liu, W, and Chepyator-Thomson, JR. Field dependence-independence and physical activity engagement among middle school students. Physical Education and Sport Pedagogy. 2009;**14**(2):125–136.

[19] Saracho, O. Matching teachers' and students' cognitive styles. Early Child Development and Care. 2003;**173**(2–3):161–173.

[20] Coates, S, Lord, M, and Jakabovics, E. Field dependence-independence, social-non-social play and sex differences in preschool children. Perceptual and Motor Skills. 1975;**40**(1):195–202.

[21] Bar-Haim, Y, and Bart, O. Motor function and social participation in kindergarten children. Social Development. 2006;**15**(2):296–310.

[22] Greffou, S, Bertone, A, Hahler, E-M, Hanssens, J-M, Mottron, L, and Faubert, J. Postural hypo-reactivity in autism is contingent on development and visual environment: a fully immersive virtual reality study. Journal of Autism and Developmental Disorders. 2012;**42**(6):961–970.

[23] Kohen-Raz, R, Volkman, FR, and Cohen, DJ. Postural control in children with autism. Journal of Autism and Developmental Disorders. 1992;**22**(3):419–432.

[24] Gepner, B, Mestre, D, Masson, G, and de Schonen, S. Postural effects of motion vision in young autistic children. NeuroReport. 1995;**6**(8):1211–1214.

[25] Gepner, B, and Mestre, DR. Brief report: postural reactivity to fast visual motion differentiates autistic from children with Asperger syndrome. Journal of Autism and Developmental Disorders. 2002;**32**(3):231–238.

[26] Feil-Seifer, D, and Mataric, M. Defining socially assistive robotics. 9th International Conference on Rehabilitation Robotics, 2005. ICORR 2005. 2005:465–468.

[27] Dautenhahn, K, Nehaniv, CL, Walters, ML, Robins, B, Kose-Bagci, H, Mirza, NA, and Blow, M. KASPAR-A minimally expressive humanoid robot for human-robot interaction research. Applied Bionics and Biomechanics. 2009;**6**(3–4):369–397.

[28] Scassellati, B, Admoni, H, and Mataric, M. Robots for use in autism research. Annual Review of Biomedical Engineering. 2012;**14**:275–294.

[29] Salter, T, Michaud, F, and Larouche, H. How wild is wild? A taxonomy to characterize the 'wildness' of child-robot interaction. International Journal of Social Robotics. 2010;**2**(4):405–415.

[30] Thill, S, Pop, CA, Belpaeme, T, Ziemke, T, and Vanderborght, B. Robot-assisted therapy for autism spectrum disorders with (partially) autonomous control: Challenges and outlook. Paladyn, Journal of Behavioral Robotics. 2012;**3**(4):209–217.

[31] Brown, C, and Dunn, W. Adolescent-Adult Sensory Profile: User's Manual. Therapy Skill Builders, Tucson, AZ; 2002.

[32] Jones, CRG, Happe, F, Baird, G, Simonoff, E, Marsden, AJS, Tregay, J, Phillips, RJ, Goswami, U, Thomson, JM, and Charman, T. Auditory discrimination and auditory sensory behaviours in autism spectrum disorders. Neuropsychologia. 2009;**47**(13):2850–2858.

[33] Ferguson, H, Myles, BS, and Hagiwara, T. Using a personal digital assistant to enhance the independence of an adolescent with Asperger syndrome. Education and Training in Developmental Disabilities. 2005;**40**(1):60–67.

[34] Crane, L, Goddard, L, and Pring, L. Sensory processing in adults with autism spectrum disorders. Autism. 2009;**13**(3):215–228.

[35] Dunn, W. The Sensory Profile: User's Manual. Psychological Corporation, San Antonio, TX; 1999.

[36] Bray, A, Subanandan, A, Isableu, B, Ohlmann, T, Golding, JF, and Gresty, MA. We are most aware of our place in the world when about to fall. Current Biology. 2004; **14**(15):R609–R610.

[37] Isableu, B, Fourre, B, Vuillerme, N, Giraudet, G, Amorim, M-A. Differential integration of visual and kinaesthetic signals to upright stance. Experimental Brain Research. 2011;**212**(1):33–46.

[38] Kluzik, J, Peterka, RJ, and Horak, FB. Adaptation of postural orientation to changes in surface inclination. Experimental Brain Research. 2007;**178**(1):1–17.

[39] Isableu, B, and Vuillerme, N. Differential integration of kinaesthetic signals to postural control. Experimental Brain Research. 2006;**174**(4):762–768.

[40] Isableu, B, Ohlmann, T, Cremieux, J, Vuillerme, N, Amblard, B, and Gresty, MA. Individual differences in the ability to identify, select and use appropriate frames of reference for perceptuo-motor control. Neuroscience. 2010;**169**(3):1199–1215.

[41] Ravaioli, E, Oie, KS, Kiemel, T, Chiari, L, and Jeka, JJ. Nonlinear postural control in response to visual translation. Experimental Brain Research. 2005;**160**(4):450–459.

[42] Greffou, S, Bertone, A, Hanssens, J-M, and Faubert, J. Development of visually driven postural reactivity: A fully immersive virtual reality study. Journal of Vision. 2008;**8**(11):15.

[43] Van Asten, WNJC, Gielen, CCAM, and van der Gon, JJD. Postural adjustments induced by simulated motion of differently structured environments. Experimental Brain Research. 1988;**73**(2):371–383.

[44] Schmuckler, MA. Children's postural sway in response to low-and high-frequency visual information for oscillation. Journal of Experimental Psychology: Human Perception and Performance. 1997;**23**(2):528.

[45] Chiari, L, Rocchi, L, and Cappello, A. Stabilometric parameters are affected by anthropometry and foot placement. Clinical Biomechanics. 2002;**17**(9):666–677.

[46] Molloy, CA, Dietrich, KN, and Bhattacharya, A. Postural stability in children with autism spectrum disorder. Journal of Autism and Developmental Disorders. 2003;**33**(6):643–652.

[47] Torres, EB, Brincker, M, Isenhower, RW, Yanovich, P, Stigler, KA, Nurnberger, JI, Metaxas, DN, and José, JV. Autism: The micro-movement perspective. Frontiers in Integrative Neuroscience. 2013;**7**:32.

[48] Meltzoff, AN, Brooks, R, Shon, AP, and Rao, RPN. "Social" robots are psychological agents for infants: A test of gaze following. Neural Networks. 2010;**23**(8):966–972.

[49] Chevalier, P, Martin, J-C, Isableu, B, Bazile, C, and Tapus, A. Impact of sensory preferences of individuals with autism on the recognition of emotions expressed by two robots, an avatar, and a human. Autonomous Robots. 2016;**40**(5):1–23.

[50] Chevalier, P, Martin, J-C, Isableu, B, Bazile, C, Iacob, DO, and Tapus, A. Joint attention using human-robot interaction: Impact of sensory preferences of children with autism. 25th IEEE International Symposium on Robot and Human Interactive Communication (RO-MAN). New York; 2016; 849–854.

Chapter 11

Joint Attention Impairment in Autism: Clinical Picture, Rationale and Functional MRI Findings

Marwa Saleh and Aya Adel

Additional information is available at the end of the chapter

http://dx.doi.org/10.5772/65662

Abstract

Joint attention is a keystone in social cognitive development and a skill acquired early in life. It is the triadic coordination of attention between two people and an object or event in which they are commonly interested. Language development follows in its tracks and is dependent on this early acquired skill. Its deviation from typical development is considered one of the earliest signs of autism. Consequently, its remediation has gained intensive focus in therapy. In this review, the development of joint attention skill in initiating (IJA) and responding (RJA), and its atypical development in autism and related spectrum disorders would be discussed. This would include existing problems in pointing, sharing attention with the participant, and facial recognition; and the rationale behind these deviations as covert attention. Related fMRI findings would also be reviewed, outlining the integration between the posterior involuntary parietal and superior temporal cortices (RJA) and the anterior volitional prefrontal and orbital frontal areas (IJA) in typical development, and the long-distance underconnectivity and local overconnectivity in autism. Several cortical regions are implicated in autism, revealing the heterogeneity of the findings, but general conclusions could be drawn.

Keywords: autism, initiating joint attention, responding to joint attention, functional MRI, social development

1. Introduction

Joint attention is a triadic organization of attention and communication between two persons sharing an object or event, and turning occasionally to look at each other to communicate what they are experiencing. This coordinated joint attention can be initiated, 'Initiating Joint Attention'

(IJA), or responded to, 'Responding to Joint Attention' (RJA). Pointing, shifting of eye gaze, and displaying facial expression are essential components of joint attention.

The typical form of joint attention is that of two people engaged in an activity, following a performance, or watching another person or picture or object, nevertheless, turning every now and then to look at each other. This momentary sharing of attention during the course of activity is very meaningful. It conveys to the other partner that his/her presence is recognized, checks his/her reactions, and registers with him/her the responses of the first partner.

If two persons are just engaged in watching a common object without looking at each other, their attention would be 'parallel,' not 'coordinated.' Joint attention means that attention is not exclusively on the object; as in this condition, 'the sense of sharing' would be missed. Attention is divided between the object and a person interested in this object. This human communication model is imprinted from early on in life through brain communication circuits and social emotional brain areas. The acquired outcome is 'cognitive' from the object and 'social/ cognitive' from the person.

That is why joint attention is a pivotal skill in a child's social/communicative path, paving the way toward language development [1]. Impairment of joint attention before 1 year is one of the earliest indicators of autism [2]. Furthermore, joint attention intervention in autism is reported to produce better language acquisition and outcome [3].

The aim of this chapter is to review the clinical presentation of deficient joint attention in autism, the proposed rationale behind it, and the related radiological picture in functional MRI (fMRI) of autistic children

2. Body

2.1. Clinical picture and rationale

Early home videos in the first 2 years of life in children, later diagnosed as having autism, show deviation in the typical development of joint attention [4–7]. There is deficient facial expression, social interaction, orientation to name, and pointing to/showing of objects. So, what's the typical development of joint attention and how are those children not following the expected path?

Pointing is a cornerstone in joint attention development; giving the social reference of: 'Look this way, I want to show you something!' Children's behavior during the first 6 months of meaningful words' acquisition is soaked in pointing. It becomes evident as a declarative tool at 12 months of age [8]. They want to show the parents what they are exploring as they go around. This is, however, preceded by months of social exploration, not of the surroundings, but of the facial expression of adults.

As early as 2 months of age, infants focus on facial expressions of caregivers. They learn to identify emotional states from facial expressions and spend a lot of time doing that during the first year of life. Facial expressions and vocalizations characterize early human communication, especially before 6 months of age [9].

As infants become mobile and begin to attend more to objects in the environment, the caregiver starts to label and comment on objects at which the infant's attention is focused [10]. The joint attention becomes 'supported' with the caregiver being the director of communication and then 'coordinated' with the caregiver and infant sharing in the communicative game by alternating looking at each other and at the object of interest.

Supported joint attention appears by the middle of the first year and remains prevalent in communication between 18 and 30 months of age. Coordinated joint attention emerges gradually between 9 and 15 months of age. At 18 months, children sustain well-timed glances between them and the caregiver during a coordinated joint attention play activity [11].

Initiating joint attention (IJA) is a voluntary skill; while responding to it occurs automatically. The child uses gestures and eye contact to direct others to objects, events, and to themselves. The propensity to initiate joint attention develops across 9 months to one and a half years, while the natural tendency to respond to joint attention (RJA) increases during that period. The frequency of both is, however, unrelated. Mundy [12] finds responding to joint attention to be highly related to vocabulary development in typically developing children.

Although both IJA and RJA have similar social roles, yet they have different motivational origins. RJA is possibly maintained by extrinsic reinforcement (as tangible rewards) [13], while IJA is maintained an intrinsic drive (social sharing) [14]. Joint attention becomes gradually symbol-infused. Although adults speak during their first encounter with a newborn, infants begin to understand and produce symbolic acts late in their first year, and with a greater variety in their second year. The initial period of joint attention is thus nonsymbol infused and becomes symbol infused when language skills emerge [15].

Joint attention is related to both language development and social development. Nonlinguistic interactions between the child and the mother encourage early language development. These interactions provide the child with a predictable referential context that makes the language of the mother meaningful. The underlying mechanism that works in these mother-child interactions is joint attention [16]. Tomasello et al. [17] found positive correlation between joint attention at 15 months of age and vocabulary size at 21 months.

In social development, joint attention is related to both pretend/symbolic play and theory of mind. These two social cognitive abilities are later developing and specifically impaired in individuals with autism. Whereas joint attention first develops before 1 year of age, pretend play is not seen until the second year of life, while theory of mind emerges in preschool years [18]. Theory of mind, when developed, allows the child to understand that other people have their own feelings, thoughts, and beliefs that differ from one's own [19].

In symbolic play, the theme of pretence evolves from playing with toys functionally as in constructing a building to playing with toys symbolically as pretending that a banana is a telephone [20]. In comparison with typically developing children at the same mental age, autistic children have significant delay in development of symbolic play [21]. Children with autism handle and manipulate toys in a rigid and stereotyped manner [22] and are less likely to start symbolic play activities [23] or get involved with people sharing the activity with them. They are object focused [24].

Holmes and Willoughby [25] have likewise observed solitary or parallel functional play in seventeen 4- to 8-year-old autistic children in the classroom. Keen et al. [26] studied eight children with autism and found that except for few instances of commenting, they mainly communicated for the purpose of requesting objects or protesting. Unfortunately, it was observed that teachers infrequently acknowledged the children's communicative trials, as a result of their atypical nature [27].

The atypical development of this trend of nonverbal communication, termed joint attention, continues as a barrier to proper social development in autistic individuals. There is little motivation in autistic children to look at people's facial expression, because it does not provide them with information about the emotional states, motives, or intentions of others [28]. They are unable to shift attention/eye gaze from a person to object, to point to initiate joint attention, or to use the eye direction of other people as a guide [29]. When they use pointing, it is for the sake of regulating other persons' behavior by indicating that they want something (protoimperative), rather than for the purpose of sharing interest with others (protodeclarative) [30]. Generally, autistic patients are more likely to respond to joint attention bids than to initiate joint attention [31].

Investigation of the nature of aberrant joint attention has led to multiple rationales. Experiments show that attention in autism is covert (without head and eye movement [32]). Overt attention involves directed eye movements (namely, saccades) toward a certain target, while in covert attention, the focus on the object is mental, without significant eye movement. As people look toward things that interest them, the direction of eye gaze reveals people's goals and focus of attention. Typically, people tend to reflexively orient to where other people are gazing, especially if the gaze shows an eye movement or shift of eye gaze without a head movement. The deficit in gaze following in autism may result from a focus on details and features rather than a more holistic integration of eye direction, head position, body posture, and pointing cues [33].

Autistics tend to orient only if another person's gaze is predictive [34]. They respond significantly more accurately than nonautistics if another person's gaze is informative, whereas nonautistics reflexively orient their attention in the direction of the other person's gaze, even if that direction is not expected. They want to find out where/what the gaze leads to.

Posner et al. [35] pioneered in measuring covert attention using signal detection on a screen. Participants are seated in front of the screen and instructed to fixate their eyes on the central point of the screen, marked by a dot. An arrow appears to the right or to the left of the central dot. It is followed by a target stimulus, usually a shape. In 80% of trials, the target is on the same side of the arrow, while in 20%, it is on the opposite side. The participant should immediately respond when the target appears and the response time is measured. Data show that autistics show more covert attention than age-matched nonautistic controls [36].

http://dx.doi.org/10.5772/65662

Autistic children have atypical prolonged resistance to distraction [37]. They do not disengage their attention from their immediate focus with ease and consequently cannot readily follow eye gaze of other people. This underlies the lack of the automatic social response of eye gaze following, especially if there is no predicted target in the direction of the eye gaze [2]. Bayliss et al. [38] described autistics as "possessing a stronger ability to inhibit the influence of non-informative social cues." This is in contrast to non-autistics who "suffer greater interference" and cannot ignore another person's gaze, even if the direction of the gaze seems to be irrelevant.

Autistics also have enhanced visual processing. They have a three times more powerful recognition of a visual object in a complex visual background [39]. This atypical visual perception is one of the most intriguing puzzles in the diverse world of autism. If asked to search for a target element among a display of 25 elements, as a white cube among white balls and colored cubes, autistics are nearly twice as fast as nonautistics to find the target. They perceive in parallel; they do not inspect the presented picture, item by item [40].

Defective imitation abilities in autism were described as early as the 1970s by DeMeyer et al. [41]. There is a lower rate of spontaneous imitation of gestures in children with autism when compared with age-matched typically developing children. Other studies have focused on home videos during the first 2 years of life, of children later diagnosed as having autism and revealed lower rates of spontaneous imitation [5]. This defective imitation was viewed by some authors as a form of motor dyspraxia, meaning that the autistic child is unable to execute the components of the movement of pointing or looking where another person is pointing [42].

The atypical response of autistic children to conventional bids for joint attention has been related to multiple rationales, namely, difficult volitional action execution; ability to attend covertly not overtly, to perceive the environment fluidly, and to resist distraction or interruption. So, the proposed rationale behind joint attention deficit in autism has scanned both the sensory perception and the motor execution abilities. A simultaneous sensorimotor dysfunction paradigm could be coexisting to a variable degree in autistic patients.

2.2. fMRI studies related to joint attention in autism

By fMRI, joint attention was found to be the outcome of the integration between two attention regulation systems: a posterior involuntary, related to RJA and operated by parietal and superior temporal cortices, and an anterior volitional, related to IJA and operated by prefrontal association cortex, orbital frontal cortex, and anterior cingulate [43].

The aforementioned posterior involuntary system is a perceptual system that starts to develop in the first 3 months of life. It orients the infant toward biologically meaningful stimuli [44]. The parietal and superior temporal areas serve the development of representation; imitation; perception of other people's head and eye movements; as well as the perception of spatial position of self, others, and the environment. The following quote summarizes the cognitive message gained from this system: "where others' eyes go, their behaviors follow [45]."

The anterior attention system related to IJA is later developing and gives the following cognitive message: "where my eyes go, my behavior follows." This system is volitional, goal-directed, and reward affected. It also supervises integration of activity between the anterior and posterior attention systems. Starting from 4 to 6 months of age, the anterior attention system integrates the internal control of one's gaze direction together with goal-directed behavior, with the external monitoring of the gaze direction of others and their behavior. This integration yields the specific form of human attention called joint attention [46]. Also, this comparative monitoring between the external looking behavior in the form of overt attention and the attention to internal self-representations is a very important substrate for cognitive development. Joint attention, after all, is a social cognitive skill, and practice with joint attention in the first 9 months of life is a major contributor to the development of social cognition [47].

The decreased brain connectivity in ASD implicated in fMRI studies, specifically between frontal and posterior-temporal cortical regions, affects social and emotional information processing [48]. Local overconnectivity and long-distance underconnectivity are, however, the recent understanding of the cortical neural dysfunction in autism. This model addresses the heterogeneity of the disorder and the pervasive nature in general [49]. There is more tendency in autistic individuals to process tasks in a manner that relies less on anterior frontal gray matter centers (theory of mind, face, and social processing) and more on those of posterior temporal gray matter (visual processing). The white matter alteration of structure, as defective myelination, is implicated in this lack of fast synchronous communication between these gray matter areas [50]. This disrupted connective circuitry in the brain was proposed by Just et al. [51] in the cortical underconnectivity theory, describing a lower communication bandwidth between frontal and posterior temporal areas in autistic compared to control participants. On the other hand, McFadden and Minshew [52] pointed to local overconnectivity in the form of consistent finding of excess interstitial neurons that reflects failure of appropriate developmental apoptosis and leads to improper brain connective function.

In an fMRI study of joint attention in 2005 [53], activity was detected in association with joint attention in ventromedial frontal cortex, the left superior frontal gyrus (BA10), cingulate cortex, and caudate nuclei. Both the ventromedial frontal cortex and BA10 are related to mental activity and cognitive integration tasks. Authors concluded that a developmental defect in the left anterior frontal lobe could be an underlying factor in autism spectrum disorders (ASD).

On the other hand, a review of fMRI findings in autism spectrum disorders (ASD) described hypoactivation of the 'social brain' in prefrontal cortex, posterior superior temporal gyrus, amygdala, and fusiform gyrus; decreased anterior-posterior functional connectivity during resting states; and anomalous mesolimbic responses to social rewards [54]. It should be put in mind, however, that there is heterogeneity in fMRI findings. Findings are complex, because as Geschwind and Levitt [55] described, there are 'many autisms'.

Faces are social stimuli that infants attend to from very early in life [56]. Defective face processing and discrimination, as reduced face emotion recognition, exist in autism [57]. In neurotypical individuals, activation of fusiform gyrus, in addition to superior temporal sulcus, amygdala, and orbitofrontal cortex, occurs in response to face viewing [58]. Most fMRI studies in autism implicate hypoactivation of fusiform gyrus in response to faces and facial expressions [59]. However, the predicted fusiform activation has been reported to occur in autistic individuals when there are familiar faces [60] or unfamiliar faces in the presence of an attentional cue [61].

Atypical amygdala activation has been implicated in tasks of judging emotional state from eyes [62], or from facial expression [63], as Amygdala functions in identification of emotional situation based on the facial expression [64]. Reduced activity in the inferior frontal region in ASD has been described by Bookheimer et al. [65] during face processing tasks, as matching faces presented in upright versus inverted positions. The typical response of increased activation for inverted faces was lacking, due to the absence of the social significance of the stimulus.

A neurological human skill that is related to theory of mind, called Empathy, was also studied by functional brain imaging. Empathy is the ability to understand the emotional state of others by mapping of the feelings of others onto our nervous system. This is crucial for a socially appropriate response and is done by mirror neurons, which relay the impulses onto the premotor cortex [66]. It is a self-referential emotional cognition, in order to compare and relate the emotional state of others with our own. 'Theory of Mind' allows the awareness of the fact that the mental state of others differs from ours, and to be understood it has to be adopted and evaluated from our own perspective. Atypical neural activation occurred in ASD individuals who were asked to evaluate other people and their own facial emotional response, as compared to control subjects. For example, activation of the prefrontal cortex occurred dorsally in ASD and ventrally in control subjects. This may underlie disturbed empathy in autism [67].

The fMRI findings in autism reflect aberrant function in both white matter axons and gray matter areas. Underconnectivity (distant) and overconnectivity (local) in white matter, in addition to underactivation (frontal) and overactivation (posterior) in gray matter, characterize the array of heterogenous findings in autism.

3. Conclusion

Social and language developments are inseparable domains in human communication. Joint attention as a social cognitive skill, being a core component in both social and language development, has been recognized as deficient in autism-related research. Further research attempts in this domain are warranted due to a few number of participants in research addressing joint attention. There are unraveling fMRI findings implicating several areas as the prefrontal cortex, the posterior superior temporal gyrus, and the functional anterior-posterior cerebral connectivity. There is persistent need to address joint attention more fully and variably in intervention of autism for the sake of better outcomes. Joint attention is a skill that is acquired very early in life and is adherent to typical language development and use among humans. Language use is typically the most pervasively affected linguistic category in autism.

Author details

Marwa Saleh* and Aya Adel

*Address all correspondence to: marwa.saleh7@gmail.com

Unit of Phoniatrics, Department of Otolaryngology, Ain Shams University, Cairo, Egypt

References

[1] Vaughan A, Mundy P, Block J, Delgado C, Gomez Y, Meyer J, et al. Child, caregiver, and temperament contributions to infant joint attention. Infancy. 2003; 4: 603–616. doi: 10.1207/S15327078IN0404_11

[2] Baron-Cohen S, Allen J, Gillberg C. Can autism be detected at 18 months? The needle, the haystack, and the CHAT. British Journal of Psychiatry. 1992; 161: 839–843.

[3] Kasari C, Paparella T, Freeman S, Jahroni LB. Language outcome in autism: Randomized comparison of joint attention and play interventions. Journal of Consulting and Clinical Psychology. 2008; 76: 125–137. doi:10.1037/0022-006X.76.1.125

[4] Adrien JL, Lenoir P, Martineau J, Perrot A, Hameury L, Larmande C, Sauvage D. Blind ratings of early symptoms of autism based upon family home movies. Journal of the American Academy of Child and Adolescent Psychiatry. 1993; 32: 617–626.

[5] Osterling J, Dawson G. Early recognition of children with autism: a study of first birthday home videotapes. Journal of Autism and Developmental Disorders. 1994; 24: 247–257.

[6] Baranek GT. Autism during infancy a retrospective video analysis of sensory-motor and social behaviors at 9-12 months of age. Journal of Autism and Developmental Disorders. 1999; 29: 213–224.

[7] Werner E, Dawson G, Osterling J, Dinno N. Brief report: recognition of autism spectrum disorder before one year of age: a retrospective study based on home videotapes. Journal of Autism and Developmental Disorders. 2000; 30: 157–162.

[8] Tomasello M, Carpenter M, Liszkowski U. A new look at infant pointing. Child Development. 2007 May–June; 78 (30): 705–722.

[9] Barkow JH, Cosmides L, Tooby J, editors. The Adapted Mind: Evolutionary Psychology and the Generation of Culture. 391–428 p. London: Oxford University Press; 1992.

[10] Wetherby AM, Warren SF, Reichle J, editors. Transitions in Prelinguistic Communication. 15–38 p. Baltimore MD: Paul H. Brookes; 1998.

[11] Bakeman R, Adamson L. Coordinating attention to people and objects in mother-infant and peer-infant interaction. Child Development. 2007; 55: 1278–1289.

[12] Mundy P. New perspectives on the role of joint attention in language development. In: Keynote Address Given to the 27th Annual Symposium for Research on Child Language Disorders; 2006; Madison, WI.

[13] Corkum V, Moore C. Origins of joint visual attention in infants. Developmental Psychology. 1998; 34: 28–38.

[14] Mundy P. Joint attention and social-emotional approach behavior in children with autism. Development and Psychopathology. 1995; 7: 63–82.

[15] Adamson LB, Bakeman R, Deckner DF. The development of symbol-infused joint attention. Child Development. 2004; 75: 1171–1187. doi:10.1111/j.1467-8624.2004.00732.xView

[16] Bruner J. Child's talk: Learning to Use Language. New York: Norton & Company; 1985.

[17] Tomasello M, Mannle S, Kruger A. The linguistic environment of one to two-year old twins. Developmental Psychology. 1986; 22: 169–176.

[18] Leslie A. Pretense and representation: the origins of "Theory of mind". Psychological Review. 1987; 94: 412–426.

[19] Whiten A, editor. Natural theories of mind: evolution, development, and simulation of everyday mindreading. 233–251 p. Cambridge, MA: Basil Blackwell; 1991.

[20] Lifter K, Sulzer-Azaroff B, Andersen S, Cowdery GE. Teaching play activities to preschool children with disabilities: the importance of developmental considerations. Journal of Early Intervention. 1993; 17: 139–159.

[21] Baron-Cohen S. Autism and symbolic play. British Journal of Developmental Psychology. 1987; 5: 129–148.

[22] Atlas JA. Play in assessment and intervention in the childhood psychosis. Child psychiatry and Human Development. 1990; 21: 119–133.

[23] Jarrold C, Boucher J, Smith P. Symbolic play in autism: a review. Journal of Autism and Developmental Disorders. 1993; 23: 281–307.

[24] Kasari C, Gulsrud A, Wong C, Kwon S, Locke J. Randomized controlled caregiver mediated joint engagement intervention for toddlers with autism. Journal of Autism and Developmental Disorders. 2010; 40: 1045–1056. doi:10.1007/s10803-010-0955-5

[25] Holmes E, Willoughby T. Play behavior of children with autism spectrum disorders. Journal of Intellectual and Developmental Disability. 2005; 30: 156–164. doi:10.1007/s10803-012-1467-2

[26] Keen D. Verifying teacher perceptions of the potential communicative acts of children with autism. Communication Disorders Quarterly. 2002; 23: 133–142. doi: 10.1177/15257401020230030201

[27] Keen D, Sigafoos J, Woodyatt G. Teacher responses to the communicative attempts of children with autism. Journal of Developmental and Physical Disabilities. 2005; 17: 19–33. doi:10.1007/s10882-005-2198-5

[28] Moore C, Dunham P, editors. Joint Attention: Its Origins and Role in Development. Psychology Press: Routledge Taylor and Francis Books; 2014.

[29] Chiang C, Soong W, Lin T, Rogers S. Nonverbal communication skills in young children with autism. Journal of Autism and Developmental Disorders. 2008; 38: 1898–1906. doi: 10.1007/s10803-008-0586-2

[30] Mundy P, Sigman MD, Ungerer J, Sherman T. Defining the social deficits of autism: the contribution of non-verbal communication measures. Journal of Child Psychiatry and Allied Disciplines. 1986; 27(5): 657–669.

[31] Macdonald R, Andersen J, Dube WV, Geckeler A, Green G, Holcomb W. et al. Behavioral assessment of joint attention: a methodological report. Research in Developmental Disabilities. 2006; 27: 138–150. doi:10.1016/j.ridd.2004.09.006

[32] Gazzaniga MS, Ivry RB, Mangun GR. Cognitive Neuroscience: the Biology of the Mind, 4th ed. New York: Norton; 2002.

[33] Ashwin C, Hietanen JK, Baron-Cohen S. Atypical integration of social cues for orienting to gaze direction in adults with autism. Molecular Autism. 2015; 6: 5. doi:10.1186/2040-2392-6-5

[34] Ristic J, Mottron L, Friesen CK, Iarocci G, Burack JA, Kingstone A. Eyes are special but not for everyone: the case of autism. Cognitive Brain Research. 2005; 24: 715–718. doi: 10.1016/j.cogbrainres.2005.02.007

[35] Posner MI, Snyder CR, Davidson BJ. Attention and detection of signals. Journal of Experimental Psychology. 1980; 109: 160–174.

[36] Greenway R, Plaisted K. Top-down attentional modulation in autistic spectrum disorders is stimulus-specific. Psychological Science. 2005; 16: 987–994. doi:10.1111/j.1467-9280.2005.01648.x

[37] Landry R, Bryson SE. Impaired disengagement of attention in young children with autism. Journal of Child Psychology and Psychiatry. 2004; 45: 1115–1122. doi: 10.1186/2040-2392-6-5

[38] Bayliss AP, di Pelligrino G, Tipper SP. Sex differences in eye gaze and symbolic cueing of attention. Quarterly Journal of Experimental Psychology. 2005; 58A: 631–650.

[39] Pellicano E, Maybery M, Durkin K, Maley A. Multiple cognitive capabilities/deficits in children with an autism spectrum disorder: "Weak" central coherence and its relation-

ship to theory of mind and executive control. Development and Psychopathology. 2006; 18: 77–98.

[40] O'Riordan MA, Plaisted KC, Driver J, Baron-Cohen S. Superior visual search in autism. Journal of Experimental Psychology: Human Perception and Performance. 2001; 27: 719–730.

[41] DeMeyer MK, Alpern GD, Barton S, DeMeyer WE, Churchill DW, Hingtgen JN, Bryson CQ, Pontius W, Kimberlin C. Imitation in autistic, early schizophrenic, and non-psychotic subnormal children. Journal of Autism and Childhood Schizophrenia. 1972; 2(3): 264–287.

[42] Ming X, Brimacombe M, Wagner GC. Prevalence of motor impairment in autism spectrum disorders. Brain and Development. 2007; 29: 565–570. doi:10.1016/j.braindev.2007.03.002

[43] Mundy P, Card J, Fox N. Fourteen-month cortical activity and different infant joint attention skills. Developmental Psychobiology. 2000; 36: 325–338.

[44] Posner M, Rothbart M. Educating the Human Brain. Washington DC: American Psychological Association; 2007.

[45] Jellema T, Baker C, Wicker B, Perrett D. Neural representation for the perception of intentionality of actions. Brain and Cognition. 2000; 44: 280–302.

[46] Mundy P. The neural basis of social impairments in autism: the role of the dorsal medial-frontal cortex and anterior cingulate system. Journal of Child Psychology and Psychiatry. 2003; 44: 793–809.

[47] Mundy P, Newell L. Attention, joint attention, and social cognition. Current Directions in Psychological Science. 2007; 16(5): 269–274. doi:10.1111/j.1467-8721.2007.00518.x

[48] Vissers ME, Cohen MX, Geurts HM. Brain connectivity and high functioning autism: a promising path of research that needs refined models, methodological convergence, and stronger behavioral links. Neuroscience and Biobehavioral Reviews. 2012; 36: 604–625. doi:10.1016/j.neubiorev.2011.09.003

[49] Just MA, Keller TA, Malave VL, Kana RK, Varma S. Autism as a neural systems disorder: a theory of frontal- posterior underconnectivity. Neuroscience and Biobehavioral Reviews. 2012; 36(4): 1292–1313. doi:10.1016/j.neubiorev.2012.02.00730

[50] Just MA, Pelphrey KA, editors. Development and brain systems in autism. 35-63 p. New York: Psychology Press; 2013. doi:10.4324/9780203073353, 1

[51] Just MA, Cherkassky VL, Keller TA, Minshew NA. Cortical activation and synchronization during sentence comprehension in high-functioning autism: evidence of underconnectivity. Brain. 2004; 127: 1811–1821.

[52] McFadden K, Minshew NJ. Evidence for dysregulation of axonal growth and guidance in the etiology of ASD. Frontiers in Human Neuroscience. 2013; 7: 671. doi:10.3389/fnhum.2013.00671

[53] Williams JHG, Waiter GD, Perra O, Perrett DI, Whiten A. An fMRI study of joint attention experience. NeuroImage. 2005; 25(1): 133–140.

[54] Dichter GS. Functional magnetic resonance imaging of autism spectrum disorders. Dialogues in Clinical Neuroscience. 2012; 14(3): 319–351.

[55] Geschwind DH, Levitt P. Autism spectrum disorders: developmental disconnection symptoms. Current Opinion in Neurobiology. 2007; 17: 103–111. doi:10.1016/j.conb.2007.01.009

[56] Johnson MH, Dziurawiec S, Ellis H, Morton J. Newborns' preferential tracking of face-like stimuli and its subsequent decline. Cognition. 1991; 40:1–19.

[57] Klin A, Jones W, Schultz R, Volkmar F, Cohen D. Visual fixation patterns during viewing of naturalistic social situations as predictors of social competence in individuals with autism. Archives of General Psychiatry. 2002; 59: 809–816.

[58] Grill-Spector K, Knouf N, Kanwisher N. The fusiform face subserves face perception, not generic within-category identification. Natural Neuroscience. 2004; 7: 555–562.

[59] Pelphrey KA, Morris JP, McCarthy G, Labar KS. Perception of dynamic changes in facial affect and identity in autism. Social Cognitive and Affective Neuroscience. 2007; 2: 140–149. doi:10.1093/scan/nsm010

[60] Pierce K, Redcay E. Fusiform function in children with an autism spectrum disorder is a matter of "who." Biological Psychiatry. 2008; 64: 552–560. doi:10.1016/j.biopsych.2008.05.013

[61] Hadjikhani N, Joseph RM, Snyder J, et al. Activation of the fusiform gyrus when individuals with autism spectrum disorder view faces. Neuroimage. 2004; 22: 1141–1150. doi:10.1016/j.neuroimage.2004.03.025

[62] Baron-Cohen S, Ring HA, Bullmore ET, Wheelwright S, Ashwin C, Williams SC. The amygdala theory of autism. Neuroscience and Biobehavioral Reviews. 2000; 24: 355–364.

[63] Critchley HD, Daly EM, Bullmore ET, et al. The functional neuroanatomy of social behavior: changes in cerebral blood flow with autistic disorder process facial expressions. Brain. 2000; 123: 2203–2212.

[64] Davis M, Whalen PJ. The amygdala: vigilance and emotion. Molecular Psychiatry. 2001; 6: 13–34.

[65] Bookheimer SY, Wang AT, Scott A, Siqman M, Dapretto M. Frontal contributions to face processing differences in autism: evidence from fMRI of inverted face processing.

Journal of the International Neuropsychological Society. 2008; 14(6): 922–932. doi: 10.1017/S135561770808140X

[66] Leslie KR, Johnson-Frey SH, Grafton ST. Functional imaging of face and hand imitation: towards a motor theory of empathy. Neuroimage. 2004; 21(2): 61–67. doi:10.1016/j.neuroimage.2003.09.038

[67] Schulte-Ruther M, Greimel E, Markowitsch HJ, Kamp-Becker I, Remschmidt H, Fink GR, Piefke M. Dysfunctions in brain networks supporting empathy: an fMRI study in adults with autism spectrum disorders. Society for Neuroscience. 2011; 6(1): 1–21. doi: 10.1080/17470911003708032

Section 6

Interventions and Treatments of Autism

Chapter 12

Mindfulness and Autism Spectrum Disorder

Renee L. Cachia

Additional information is available at the end of the chapter

http://dx.doi.org/10.5772/65394

Abstract

The use of mindfulness interventions for individuals with autism spectrum disorder (ASD) is a relatively new research area, which has followed a more established body of research investigating the efficacy of mindfulness interventions for parents of children with ASD. Given the chronic stress levels experienced by parents and high anxiety and stress levels in individuals with ASD, such research is well justified. The utility of mindfulness in clinical practice for individuals with ASD and their parents will be discussed. This chapter aims to evaluate the research literature, identify important limitations, and propose crucial directions for future research. Acknowledgment of the impact of attitudes, social bias, and a generational shift that may be accelerating the salience of mindfulness is discussed. The author aims to emphasize the importance of high-quality future research with robust methodological designs to clearly identify the potential role for mindfulness in this population. Despite having a solid foundation of *preliminary* findings, it is important that researchers refine current procedures and evaluation of mindfulness interventions for individuals with ASD and their parents while carefully selecting measures that are not solely self-report or parent report.

Keywords: autism, mindfulness, meditation, stress, parenting

1. Introduction

The adverse role of stress, fear, and anxiety in individuals with autism spectrum disorder (ASD) was identified in Kanner's [1] first description of autism in his pioneering paper *Autistic Disturbances of Affective Contact*. The implications of stress and anxiety in individuals with ASD have been investigated over decades, yet we are still analyzing their detrimental impact on the developmental trajectory and mental health of individuals with ASD [2–4]. Psychological stress occurs when an individual perceives that environmental demands tax or exceed his or her adaptive capacity [5]. While stress is a universal human experience, which can be helpful at times, prolonged or chronic elevated stress levels are detrimental to an individual's health and well-being [6]. In contrast, anxiety is an emotion characterized by an unpleasant state of uneasiness and worry, which is often accompanied by nervous behavior, and has the potential to result in a clinical anxiety disorder [7–9]. Chronic stress and anxiety are experienced by many individuals with ASD, however, have also been consistently associated with parenting a child with ASD [10–12]. There is preliminary evidence to suggest that mindfulness training reduces stress and results in a myriad of positive changes in individuals with ASD and their parents. This chapter will review the literature and aim to analyze the participants, methodologies, interventions, and research designs across the body of work in order to determine the robustness of the findings. The implications for the clinical application and directions for the future research on mindfulness interventions for individuals with ASD and their parents will be discussed.

2. Discussion

2.1. Autism, stress and anxiety

The detrimental role of stress and anxiety experienced by individuals with ASD has been investigated over decades. Kanner proposed that "the child's behavior is governed by an anxiously obsessive desire for the maintenance of sameness" ([1], p. 245), and a number of early researchers argued that the core features of behavior of those with ASD, engagement in obsession and stereotypical and repetitive behavior, were a function of managing anxiety and distress [13–15]. Similarly, more recent research has found that the level of anxiety in adults with ASD is three times higher than adults with intellectual disability [16]. This study found that the higher the anxiety and stress levels in the adults with ASD, the less likely they were able to cope with change, sensory stimuli, and what they perceived to be unpleasant events.

A literature review conducted by MacNeil et al. [17] found that adolescents with ASD experience greater levels of anxiety than the general community population. Such levels were similar to those with clinically significant levels of anxiety, however, often presented different patterns of anxiety compared to other clinical groups. Previous research has attributed symptoms of social anxiety in adolescents with ASD to factors including social skill deficits and heightened physiological arousal [18]. Similar to the role of anxiety in adults as described by Kanner [1] and Gillott and Standen [16], Wood and Gadow [19] suggest that anxiety may play three roles for adolescents with ASD: (1) a downstream consequence of ASD symptoms (e.g., via stress generation through social rejection), (2) a moderator of ASD symptom severity, such that certain core autism symptoms like social skill deficits and repetitive behaviors may be exacerbated by anxiety, and (3) a proxy of core ASD symptoms. A noteworthy finding and reoccurring theme across the literature that discusses the prevalence of anxiety in adolescents with ASD is that regardless of how it is measured, anxiety is common in children and adolescents with ASD, despite not always displaying age-typical symptoms [4].

Children with ASD also display high anxiety levels, particularly on measures that identify traits of separation anxiety and obsessive-compulsive disorder [20]. In a study that recorded cortisol levels as a measure of stress in children with ASD, increased cortisol was observed following exposure to a novel, nonsocial stimulus [21]. Thus, the desire for sameness and avoidance of novel stimuli may play a role in symptoms of stress and anxiety in children with ASD, which appears to remain high and potentially increase in adolescence and adulthood. The increase in stress and anxiety from adolescence to adulthood may also be moderated by poor social skills and social rejection. This is detrimental to the development and quality of life for individuals with ASD across the trajectory of their life span. It is essential that interventions successfully target these symptoms in order to maximize the developmental potential and quality of life for individuals with ASD.

2.2. Autism and parent stress

Over time, researchers have consistently shown that parenting a child with ASD is associated with a multitude of challenges and daily stressors. More recently, researchers have also found that parents of children with ASD experience higher stress levels, in addition to symptoms of anxiety and depression when compared to parents of typically developing children and parents of children with other disabilities including Down syndrome, behavioral disorders, and fragile X syndrome [10, 22–25]. Early research reports from the 1970s indicated that parents of children with ASD have a reduced quality of life, high parental burnout, and regular feelings of isolation [12]. In 1984, a book titled *The Effects of Autism on the Family* discussed the issue of parent stress on the family system throughout the manuscript [26]. Marcus [27] proposed that the "unrelieved care" of raising a child with ASD appears foremost among parent stressors. Marcus [27] and Sullivan et al. [12] acknowledged that the severity and long-withstanding nature of ASD, in parallel with the lack of available and appropriate resources, is a key driver of parent stress. Other factors that Marcus [27] proposed that contribute to the physical and emotional exhaustion and parental burnout include difficulties in obtaining a proper diagnosis and appropriate supportive services, pervasive loneliness, and isolation due to raising a child with high needs, inadequate supportive services, and neglect of personal, social, and medical needs of parents. Despite this research being published 32 years ago and the significant advancements in the field of psychological intervention over the last three decades, similar, if not identical, issues potentially still mediate stress levels and burnout in parents of children with ASD today.

The age of receiving an ASD diagnosis is reducing due to increases in early screening and improved diagnostic tools [28–30]. However, parents still report that receiving a diagnosis can be a difficult and stressful experience [31]. Once a child receives a diagnosis of ASD, parents may experience a myriad of negative emotions characterized by guilt, blame, and fear [32]. Many parents also report feelings of grief and loss as they adjust to not having a typically developing child [33]. Such emotions, coupled with high levels of stress, anxiety, and depressive symptoms, result in these parents being psychologically vulnerable. At the same time, parents may be managing conflict and challenging behavior with their child, dealing with problems at childcare centers or schools, caregiving for other children, keeping their household functioning, working, and coping with financial stressors. There is no cure for ASD, and it is considered a lifelong condition; however, parents are likely to seek a treatment to alleviate symptoms in their child. Thus, at this time of heightened stress, parents are exposed to conflicting treatment information and are responsible for selecting the best intervention and treatment approach for their child, which is likely to result in further distress. Due to misleading information, parents often partake in treatments that lack empirical support [34]. To this end, there is often financial strain on parents when they are trialing and maintaining treatment approaches. Due to the multitude of factors described, parents of children with ASD are among the most stressed and at-risk parents in society; however, there are limited evidence-based procedures designed to address such issues.

2.3. What is mindfulness?

Mindfulness can be simply defined as paying attention in a particular way: on purpose, in the present moment, and nonjudgmentally [35]. Known as the "father of mindfulness" in the Western world, Kabat-Zinn [35] proposes that mindfulness aims to cultivate nonjudgmental and nonreactive attention to experiences in the present moment, including our body sensations, cognitions, emotions, and urges. Mindfulness is an ancient Buddhist practice, however, has profound relevance to modern psychology. Hassed and Chambers ([36], p. 6) propose that mindfulness is "a mental discipline aimed at training attention," and they quoted a classic textbook in psychology by William James ([37], p. 5), whereby James proposed that "the faculty of voluntarily bringing back a wandering attention over and over again, is the very root of judgment, character and will." The notion of training attention is not a new phenomenon in psychology.

Mindfulness constitutes formal practice, known as mindfulness meditation, and informal practice, which involves our sensory experiences, moment to moment, in everyday life. Kabat-Zinn [38] outlines that the purposeful control of attention, of that we refer to as mindfulness, can be learned through meditation. Mindfulness meditation is commonly referred to as a state that can become a mental position that facilitates the ability to disengage a given experience from an associated emotion, resulting in a mindful or skillful response to a situation [39, 40]. Seemingly simple, however not necessarily easy to achieve. Further, it requires effort and discipline as it works against our habitual awareness and automaticity [41]. Gunaratana [42] rightfully suggests that mindfulness cannot be entirely captured with words because it is a subtle, nonverbal experience.

The term mindfulness or meditation may provoke attitudes or preexisting assumptions that may be inaccurate. While many individuals may consider mindfulness a spiritual endeavor or a religious practice, it is vital that we are critical and rigorous in evaluating the psychological literature and base our opinions on a foundation of evidence-based research that consists of robust methodologies and accuracy in reporting results. Mindfulness-based stress reduction (MBSR) programs have been found to be effective in resulting in positive change and are being utilized in clinical practice in a wide variety of clinical populations. Keng et al. [43] conducted a comprehensive empirical review of 16 randomized control trials (RCTs) that implemented an MBSR program among both clinical and nonclinical populations. They found a reduction in symptoms of psychological distress, anxiety, depression, anger, rumination, cognitive disorganization, posttraumatic avoidance symptoms and medical symptoms. Keng and colleagues [43] also proposed a myriad of significant positive effects of the MBSR program including an improvement in positive affect, a sense of spirituality, empathy, a sense of cohesion, mindfulness, forgiveness, self-compassion, satisfaction with life, and quality of life. The 16 RCTs included in this review consisted of participants that were students, community adults, professionals, cancer patients, fibromyalgia patients, generalized social anxiety disorder patients, adults with high stress, and patients with multiple sclerosis, which highlights the versatility of mindfulness-based interventions [43].

The feasibility of utilizing mindfulness training as a sustainable, time-effective, and cost-effective tool for individuals caring with others with disabilities is gaining increased academic attention. A leading research team in the field of mindfulness and developmental disabilities recently conducted a benefit-cost analysis of implementing a mindfulness-based positive behavior support (MBPBS) training program to staff of community group homes for individuals with developmental disabilities [44]. Outcome measures included the frequency of verbal redirection and physical restraint, staff stress levels, and turnover, in addition to staff and peer injuries. They found significant reductions in the use of verbal redirection, complete disuse of physical restraints within a few weeks of MBPBS training, and cessation of staff and peer injuries. In addition to substantial financial savings due to staff participation in the program, results showed a significant reduction in staff stress, and there was no staff turnover during this program. Such findings are important to replicate in parents of children with ASD which may be further extended to caring staff and teachers, in terms of conducting a cost-benefit analysis.

2.4. What is mindful parenting?

Mindful parenting brings the elements of mindfulness to parenting, first described by Kabat-Zinn and Kabat-Zinn ([45], p. 71) as paying attention to your child and your parenting in a particular way: intentionally, here and now, and nonjudgmentally which "calls to wake up to the possibilities, the benefits, and the challenges of parenting with a new awareness and intentionality." A more recent definition by the pioneer of mindful parenting refers to "the awareness that emerges through paying attention, on purpose, in the present moment, and nonjudgmentally to the unfolding of experience moment by moment" ([46], p. 145). Experts have long argued that mindful parenting is a fundamental parenting skill [45, 47]. When compared with traditional forms of mindfulness, mindful parenting is a relatively new phenomenon which has demonstrated an increase in both research and awareness recently regarding its efficacy in clinical and nonclinical populations.

Mindful parenting programs were developed to reduce parenting stress; however, recent research has found a myriad of positive outcomes in parents that utilize mindfulness in interactions with their children [48, 49]. A literature review by Bögels et al. [48] proposed that mindful parenting improved parent-child interactions in mental health settings which was characterized by changes in parents including increased attention, reduced stress and preoccupation, improved executive functioning, breaking the cycle of repeating dysfunctional schemes from their own upbringing, and increasing self-nourishing attention. Research conducted by the same research team found that mindful parenting training resulted in an improvement in parenting, parental stress and reactivity to stressors, parental experiential avoidance, parent and child behavior and emotional problems, and general mindfulness in parents, in addition to improvements in the process of co-parenting and marital functioning [48, 50, 51]. Furthermore, mindful parenting may be essential in promoting positive relationships and psychological well-being in parents and their children.

2.5. Mindful parenting and autism

Based on the research of Sameroff [52, 53], Singh and colleagues [54] outlined that transactional analysis indicates that parents and children are active participants in the development of the children, including their problem behaviors. Therefore, utilizing tools to teach parents to reduce their stress levels in order to alter parent-child transactions that may impact the development or maintenance of problem behaviors in their children is warranted [54]. Given parenting a child with ASD has been consistently correlated with high levels of stress, depression, anxiety, and reduced quality of life due to the ongoing nature of care [10, 22, 55], researchers such as Singh and colleagues [54] have investigated the efficacy of mindful parenting in this population.

A recent systematic review conducted by the current author and her colleagues investigated the impact of mindfulness interventions in parents of children with ASD across ten studies [56]. All 10 included studies contributed at least one self-report finding supporting the effectiveness of mindfulness interventions in reducing stress and increasing psychological well-being in parents. Seven studies that measured parental stress as a primary variable found decreased levels on self-report measures in parents of children with ASD associated with mindfulness training [44, 57–62]. Three studies reported that their physiological findings, which included measures of cortisol levels and galvanic skin response, signified reduced stress levels and emotional responses [62–64]. In addition, four studies found decreased self-reported depression post-mindfulness training [58, 59, 63, 64]. Across the 10 included studies, many improvements related to broad psychological well-being were noted, including reductions in overall health complaints, mood disturbances, and self-reported somatic symptoms. An increase in self-perceived general health, greater satisfaction with their parenting skills, and increased mindfulness and quality of life in parents were also reported.

In the same systematic review [56], two longitudinal studies presented alluring findings that extend the potential of mindful parenting programs, reporting a positive indirect ripple effect of parental mindfulness training in reducing aggressive behavior and increasing compliance in their children with ASD, with effects lasting up to 12 months [44, 54]. The authors reported that following mindfulness training, these children were engaging in very little, if any, aggressive behavior. This review provides preliminary evidence that mindful parenting interventions may be effective in enhancing positive outcomes in parents of children with ASD, and in turn, these results have the potential to trigger a positive ripple effect to their children and promote healthy behavior.

Surprisingly, eight studies utilized broad mindfulness programs, and only two studies, de Bruin and colleagues [57] and Singh and colleagues [54], utilized specific mindful parenting programs. The mindfulness interventions resulted in positive changes in parents; however, the development of a mindful parenting program specific to parenting ASD or further evaluating the effectiveness and efficacy of current programs may be essential.

2.6. Mindfulness in individuals with autism

Research evaluating the effectiveness of mindfulness interventions in individuals with ASD is very new and is significantly behind the mindfulness research literature in other populations. This may be surprising among clinicians who provide counseling and cognitive therapy to individuals with ASD. The most recent systematic review conducted by the current author and her colleagues identified only six studies and investigated the efficacy of mindfulness interventions in reducing stress, anxiety, depression, rumination, aggression, and increasing positive affect and psychological well-being in individuals with ASD [65]. The participants ranged in the studies from children and adolescents to high-functioning adults. A quality assessment rated three studies as weak, one as adequate and two as strong in research design strength. One study measured the effects of mindfulness in children and their parents. In contrast, three studies investigated outcomes in adolescents and two in adults with high-functioning ASD. The findings of this review will be examined in further detail.

Results of one study indicated that an 8-week mindfulness program, followed by 12 months of mindfulness training, led to an increase in the quality of family life, a reduction in stress in parents, and a reduction in anxiety and thought problems in children with ASD [66]. The effects were cumulative throughout the 12 months of practice. While this result is positive, it is largely based on self-report measures of child behavior and parent stress. A good preliminary finding, however, replication and refinement of direct observational data collection in future research, is essential. Similarly, de Bruin and colleagues [57] conducted a mindfulness program designed specifically to help adolescents cope with common stressors associated with ASD in parallel to the mindful parenting program. This study found a significant increase in quality of life which remained at follow-up and a significant decrease in rumination from pretest to follow-up [57]. Parents also reported that their children's social responsiveness significantly improved at follow-up, in addition to social cognition, social communication, and reduced preoccupations at posttest. The authors proposed that these results may represent improvements in the adolescents' theory of mind, central coherence, and executive functioning. While these findings are an important step forward in investigating the impact of mindfulness in developing social awareness and cognition in adolescents with ASD, this study is also reliant on self-report measures of such variables. In order to validate the proposed positive impacts of mindfulness training as reported by Hwang and colleagues [66] and de Bruin and colleagues [57], future research must move away from solely utilizing self-report or parent-report measures of behavior and develop superior methodological designs that potentially include mixed methods such as structured measures of direct behavioral observation and physiological changes that may be complimented by self-report measures. In consideration of parent-report measures, utilizing either parents or siblings to calculate interobserver agreement (IOA) may be beneficial.

A research team based in the United States led by Singh published several studies that found mindfulness to be effective in reducing aggression, resulting in positive changes in individuals with a range of conditions including intellectual disability, conduct disorder, mental illness, and Prader-Willi syndrome [67–70]. More recently, this research team turned their attention to investigating the effectiveness of Singh's "Soles of the Feet Program" for adolescents with ASD [71, 72]. One parent recorded incidents of aggression, whereby another family member also recorded incidents 30% of the time in order to determine IOA. In one study, the adolescents' incidents of aggression reduced significantly, with no instances observed during the last 3 weeks of mindfulness practice and with no episodes of physical aggression occurring within a 4-year follow-up [71]. The other study also found that incidents of aggression reduced significantly, whereby aggression occurred at a rate of about once per year during a 3-year follow-up period [72].

Two recent studies investigated the psychological effects of a mindfulness intervention in adults with ASD with an average to high intellectual quotient (IQ) and verbal ability (VA) [73, 74]. Kiep and colleagues [73] adopted a within-group pre- and post-comparison design, whereby they reported improvements in symptoms of anxiety, depression, agoraphobia, somatization, inadequacy in thinking and eating, distrust and interpersonal sensitivity, sleeping problems, general psychological and physical well-being, and rumination during the intervention phase. The decline in rumination was related to the effect of the intervention on symptoms of depression both during and after the intervention and to symptoms of anxiety post intervention. They also proposed that participants displayed an increase in positive affect while hostility did not change. Although no differences were found between self-reported symptoms from baseline to 9 weeks after treatment, the authors suggested that this represented stable treatment results over time. In contrast, Spek and colleagues [74] conducted an RCT, and despite being considered the gold standard research design, this was a unique design among this research literature. The authors proposed that there was a reduction in symptoms of anxiety, depression, and rumination in the intervention group that was not present in the control group of adults. In addition, positive affect increased in the intervention group as opposed to the control group. These studies are pivotal in promoting future research in using mindfulness in adults with ASD. When interpreting such results, it is important to consider that these two studies were conducted by the same research team. In summary, they reported a reduction of symptoms based on self-report measures which are, however, only representative of adults with an average or high IQ and VA, otherwise often referred to as high-functioning ASD.

2.7. Future research and directions

The rapid propagation of the awareness and use of mindfulness in clinical and nonclinical practice, in addition to the research literature, may be indicative of a socially accepted phenomenon that is potentially influenced at a generational level. Due to the wide acceptance and increasingly prevalent discussion around mindfulness meditation in academic and nonacademic literature, the language is becoming more salient. This is potentially influenced by the expeditious development of websites, resources, mobile applications, and awareness on social media platforms, which may be creating a social bias. While a common saying is that "the research is finally catching up to the practice," we must carefully communicate the robust empirical support, particularly when we are working with high-risk, clinical populations. As previously mentioned, parents of children with ASD already face difficult decisions relating to optimal treatment choice for their child and family; therefore, it is important that researchers and practitioners commit to scientific integrity and evidence-based practice.

At this point in time, there are solid *preliminary* findings to suggest that mindfulness-based interventions may result in effective positive change in individuals with ASD. As discussed throughout this chapter, the body of research is currently inconclusive, despite having a general positive trend in results across studies. A major limitation is that there is an overrepresentation and reliance on self-report and parent-report questionnaires as a measure of stress, anxiety, parent-child interactions, quality of life, social responsiveness, and behavior. While this validates the need for future research to take superior precision in choice of measures, it does not constitute empirical support to conclude that mindfulness is effective in creating such change in individuals with ASD. Secondly, the research is scarce when investigating each age group individually, from children to adolescence and adulthood. Future research should investigate each stage of the life span to clarify the impact of mindfulness practice on each age group specifically. There is also minimal evidence on using mindfulness for individuals that are considered have low-functioning or nonverbal ASD. Such contrasts are important to make for the future application of mindfulness in this population. The evidence base for using mindfulness as an intervention to *parents* of children with ASD is more developed. This research has consistently shown reduced stressed, anxiety, depressive symptoms, and a range of improvements in broad psychological well-being. However, this body of research consists of studies that utilize mostly self-report measures of psychological stress, symptoms, and well-being. Likewise, future research should aim to design more robust designs by including a variety of measures including structured observations and physiological findings, in addition to parent report. As four studies in our review [65] utilized an acceptance and commitment therapy (ACT) intervention which is based on the principles of mindfulness, future research should contrast if ACT is superior to sole mindfulness interventions.

In summary, it is essential that future research refines current methodological issues, adopts high-quality measures of treatment fidelity, and includes a range of valid data collection measures across participants of different ages and levels of functioning to add meaningful research to the current evidence base. It will be beneficial to include an economic evaluation of implementing mindfulness interventions for individuals with ASD and their parents in order to determine the cost-effectiveness. Future research should investigate how mindfulness may compliment and advance current evidence-based treatments in reducing symptoms for individuals with ASD, such as applied behavior analysis (ABA)-based early intervention and cognitive behavior therapy (CBT) [75, 76]. As mindfulness generally does not teach explicit developmental skills, it may be most effective in reducing stress and increasing psychological well-being in individuals with ASD and therefore indirectly increase their skill acquisition and ability to develop cognition while engaging in other interventions. The role of mindfulness in individuals with ASD may be pivotal; however, further clarification of the clinical utility of mindfulness in best practice is required.

3. Conclusions

The use of mindfulness interventions in individuals with ASD is a relatively recent research area, which has followed the more established body of research investigating the efficacy of mindfulness interventions for parents of children with ASD. Given the chronic stress endured in parents, in addition to high anxiety and stress levels in individuals with ASD, such research is well justified. The two systematic reviews discussed in this chapter encapsulate the existing body of research evaluating the efficacy of mindfulness interventions in individuals with ASD and their parents [56, 65]. It can be concluded that mindfulness interventions may be considered an evidence-based intervention in parents of children with ASD; however, additional research is required in order to be considered as evidence-based practice in individuals with ASD. That point notwithstanding the positive and promising results that have been presented. As proposed in our review [65], it is essential that researchers continue to refine mindfulness-based intervention procedures and their evaluation, aimed at maximizing the efficacy of current interventions available for individuals with ASD and their parents.

Acknowledgements

I would like to acknowledge the support and contribution of my PhD supervisors at Monash University, Professor Dennis Moore and Dr. Angelika Anderson.

Author details

Renee L. Cachia

Address all correspondence to: renee.cachia@monash.edu

Faculty of Education Monash University, Clayton, Australia

References

[1] Kanner, L. Autistic disturbances of affective contact. Nervous Child. 1943;2:217–250. DOI: 10.1097/00005053-197105000-00012

[2] Groden, J., Cautela, J., Prince, S., & Berryman, J. The impact of stress and anxiety on individuals with autism and developmental disabilities. In: Schopler, E. & Mesibov, G. B., editors. Behavioral Issues in Autism. US: Springer; 1994. p. 177–194. DOI: 10.1007/978-1-4757-9400-7_9

[3] Turner, L. B. & Romanczyk, R. G. Assessment of fear in children with an autism spectrum disorder. Research in Autism Spectrum Disorders. 2012;6(3):1203–1210. DOI: 10.1016/j.rasd.2012.03.010

[4] White, S. W., Oswald, D., Ollendick, T., & Scahill, L. Anxiety in children and adolescents with autism spectrum disorders. Clinical Psychology Review. 2009;29(3):216–299. DOI: 10.1016/j.cpr.2009.01.003

[5] Cohen, S., Kessler, R. C. & Gordon, U. L. Strategies for measuring stress in studies of psychiatric and physical disorder. In: Cohen, S., Kessler, R. C. & Gordon, U. L, editors. Measuring Stress: A Guide for Health and Social Scientists. New York: Oxford University Press; 1995. p. 3–26.

[6] McEwen, B. S. Protective and damaging effects of stress mediators. New England Journal of Medicine. 1998;338(3):171–179. DOI: 10.1056/NEJM199801153380307

[7] Seligman, M. E. P., Walker, E. F., Rosenhan, D. L. Abnormal Psychology. 4th ed. New York: W.W. Norton & Company; 2000.

[8] Bouras, N., Holt, G. Psychiatric and Behavioral Disorders in Intellectual and Developmental Disabilities. 2nd ed. US: Cambridge University Press; 2007.

[9] American Psychiatric Association. Diagnostic and Statistical Manual of Mental Disorders. 5th ed. VA: American Psychiatric Publishing; 2013. 189 p.

[10] Bitsika, V., & Sharpley, C. F. Stress, anxiety and depression among parents of children with autism spectrum disorder. Australian Journal of Guidance and Counselling. 2004;14(2):151–161. DOI: 10.1017/S1037291100002466

[11] Holroyd, J., & McArthur, D. Mental retardation and stress on the parents: A contrast between Down's syndrome and childhood autism. American Journal of Mental Deficiency. 1976;80(4):431–436

[12] Sullivan, R. C., Ward, D., Faragoh, E., Hagamen, M. B., Foster, R. E., & LaVigna, G. W. The burn-out syndrome. Journal of Autism and Developmental Disorders. 1979;9(1): 111–126. DOI: 10.1007/BF01531298

[13] Despert, J. L. The Emotionally Disturbed Child: Then and Now. New York: Robert Brunner; 1965.

[14] Howlin, P. Prognosis in autism: do specialist treatments affect long-term outcome? European Child & Adolescent Psychiatry. 1997;6(2):55–72. DOI: 10.1007/BF00566668

[15] Howlin, P. Psychological and educational treatments for autism. Journal of Child Psychology and Psychiatry. 1998;39(3):307–322. DOI: 10.1111/1469-7610.00327

[16] Gillott, A., & Standen, P. J. Levels of anxiety and sources of stress in adults with autism. Journal of Intellectual Disabilities. 2007;11(4):359–370. DOI: 10.1177/1744629507083585

[17] MacNeil, B. M., Lopes, V. A., & Minnes, P. M. Anxiety in children and adolescents with autism spectrum disorders. Research in Autism Spectrum Disorders. 2009;3(1):1–21. DOI: 10.1016/j.rasd.2008.06.001

[18] Bellini, S. The development of social anxiety in adolescents with autism spectrum disorders. Focus on Autism and Other Developmental Disabilities. 2006;21(3):138–145. DOI: 10.1177/10883576060210030201

[19] Wood, J. J., & Gadow, K. D. Exploring the nature and function of anxiety in youth with autism spectrum disorders. Clinical Psychology: Science and Practice. 2010;17(4):281–292. DOI: 10.1111/j.1468-2850.2010.01220.x

[20] Gillott, A., Furniss, F., & Walter, A. Theory of mind ability in children with specific language impairment. Child Language Teaching and Therapy. 2004;20(1):1–11. DOI: 10.1191/0265659004ct260oa

[21] Corbett, B. A., Mendoza, S., Abdullah, M., Wegelin, J. A., & Levine, S. Cortisol circadian rhythms and response to stress in children with autism. Psychoneuroendocrinology. 2006;31(1):59–68. DOI: 10.1016/j.psyneuen.2005.05.011

[22] Dumas, J. E., Wolf, L. C., Fisman, S. N., & Culligan, A. Parenting stress, child behavior problems, and dysphoria in parents of children with autism, Down syndrome, behavior disorders, and normal development. Exceptionality: A Special Education Journal. 1991;2(2):97–110. DOI: 10.1080/09362839109524770

[23] Abbeduto, L., Seltzer, M. M., Shattuck, P., Krauss, M. W., Orsmond, G., & Murphy, M. M. Psychological well-being and coping in mothers of youths with autism, down syndrome, or fragile X syndrome. American Journal on Mental Retardation. 2004;109(3):237–254. DOI: 10.1352/0895-8017

[24] Dabrowska, A., & Pisula, E. Parenting stress and coping styles in mothers and fathers of pre-school children with autism and Down syndrome. Journal of Intellectual Disability Research. 2010;54(3):266–280. DOI: 10.1111/j.1365-2788.2010.01258.x

[25] Griffith, G. M., Hastings, R. P., Nash, S., & Hill, C. Using matched groups to explore child behavior problems and maternal well-being in children with Down syndrome and autism. Journal of Autism and Developmental Disorders. 2010;40(5):610–619. DOI: 10.1007/s10803-009-0906-1

[26] Schopler, E., & Mesibov, G. B., editors. The effects of autism on the family. 1st ed. US: Springer Science & Business Media; 2013.

[27] Marcus, L. M. Coping with burnout. In: Schopler, E., & Mesibov, G. B., editors. The effects of autism on the family. 1st ed. US: Springer; 1984. p. 311–326.

[28] Barbaro, J., & Dissanayake, C. Early markers of autism spectrum disorders in infants and toddlers prospectively identified in the Social Attention and Communication Study. Autism. 2013;17(1):64–86. DOI: 10.1177/1362361312442597

[29] Johnson, C. P., & Myers, S. M. Identification and evaluation of children with autism spectrum disorders. Pediatrics. 2007;120(5):1183–1215. DOI: 10.1542/peds.2007-2361

[30] Kleinman, J. M., Ventola, P. E., Pandey, J., Verbalis, A. D., Barton, M., Hodgson, S., et al. Diagnostic stability in very young children with autism spectrum disorders. Journal of Autism and Development Disorders. 2008;38(4):606–615. DOI: 10.1007/s10803-0 07-0427-8

[31] Siklos, S., & Kerns, K. A. Assessing the diagnostic experiences of a small sample of parents of children with autism spectrum disorders. Research in Developmental Disabilities. 2007;28(1):9–22. DOI: 10.1016/j.ridd.2005.09.003

[32] Navot, N., Jorgenson, A. G., Vander Stoep, A., Toth, K., & Webb, S. J. Family planning and family vision in mothers after diagnosis of a child with autism spectrum disorder. Autism. 2016;20(5):605–615. DOI: 10.1177/1362361315602134

[33] Myers, B. J., Mackintosh, V. H., & Goin-Kochel, R. P. "My greatest joy and my greatest heart ache:" Parents' own words on how having a child in the autism spectrum has affected their lives and their families' lives. Research in Autism Spectrum Disorders. 2009;3(3):670–684. DOI: 10.1016/j.rasd.2009.01.004

[34] Green, V. A., Pituch, K. A., Itchon, J., Choi, A., O'Reilly, M., & Sigafoos, J. Internet survey of treatments used by parents of children with autism. Research in Developmental Disabilities. 2006;27(1):70–84. DOI: 10.1016/j.ridd.2004.12.002

[35] Kabat-Zinn, J. Full Catastrophe Living: Using the Wisdom of Your Mind and Body to Face Stress, Pain, and Illness. New York: Delacorte; 1990.

[36] Hassed, C., & Chambers, R. Mindful Learning: Reduce Stress and Improve Brain Performance for Effective Learning. NSW: Exisle Publishing; 2014.

[37] James, W. The Principles of Psychology. MA: Harvard University Press; 1890.

[38] Kabat-Zinn, J. An outpatient program in behavioral medicine for chronic pain patients based on the practice of mindfulness meditation: theoretical considerations and preliminary results. General Hospital Psychiatry. 1982;4(1):33–47. DOI: 10.1016/0163-83 43(82)90026-3

[39] Kutz, I., Borysenko, J. Z., & Benson, H. Meditation and psychotherapy: a rationale for the integration of dynamic psychotherapy, the relaxation response, and mindfulness meditation. The American Journal of Psychiatry. 1985;142(1):1–8.

[40] Breslin, F. C., Zack, M., & McMain, S. An information-processing analysis of mindfulness: Implications for relapse prevention in the treatment of substance abuse. Clinical Psychology: Science and Practice. 2002;9(3):275–299. DOI: 10.1093/clipsy.9.3.275

[41] Kabat-Zinn, J. Wherever You Go, There You are: Mindfulness Meditation in Everyday Life. New York: Hyperion; 1994.

[42] Gunaratana, B. H. Mindfulness in Plain English. MA: Wisdom Publications; 2002.

[43] Keng, S. L., Smoski, M. J., & Robins, C. J. Effects of mindfulness on psychological health: A review of empirical studies. Clinical Psychology Review. 2011;31(6):1041–1056. DOI: 10.1016/j.cpr.2011.04.006

[44] Singh, N.N., Lancioni, G. E., Winton, A. S., Karazsia, B. T., Myers, R. E., Latham, L. L., & Singh, J. Mindfulness-based positive behavior support (MBPBS) for mothers of adolescents with autism spectrum disorder: effects on adolescents' behavior and parental stress. Mindfulness. 2014;5(6):646–657. DOI: 10.1007/s12671-014-0321-3

[45] Kabat-Zinn, M., & Kabat-Zinn, J. Everyday Blessings: the Inner Work of Mindful Parenting. New York: Hyperion; 1997.

[46] Kabat-Zinn, J. Mindfulness-based interventions in context: past, present, and future. Clinical Psychology: Science and Practice. 2003;10(2):144–156. DOI: 10.1093/clipsy.bpg016

[47] Steinberg, L. The 10 basic principles of good parenting. New York: Simon & Schuster; 2004.

[48] Bögels, S. M., Lehtonen, A., & Restifo, K. Mindful parenting in mental health care. Mindfulness. 2010;1(2):107–120. DOI: 10.1007/s12671-010-0014-5

[49] Bögels, S., & Restifo, K. Mindful Parenting: A Guide for Mental Health Practitioners. New York: Springer; 2014.

[50] Bögels, S. M., Hellemans, J., van Deursen, S., Römer, M., & van der Meulen, R. Mindful parenting in mental health care: effects on parental and child psychopathology, parental stress, parenting, coparenting, and marital functioning. Mindfulness. 2014;5(5):536–551. DOI: 10.1007/s12671-013-0209-7

[51] Bögels, S. M., Hoogstad, B., van Dun, L., de Schutter, S., & Restifo, K. Mindfulness training for adolescents with behaviour disorders and their parents. Behavioral and Cognitive Psychotherapy. 2008;36(2):193–209. DOI: 10.1017/S1352465808004190

[52] Sameroff, A. J. General systems theories and developmental psychopathology. In: Cicchetti, D. & Cohen, D. J., editors. Developmental Psychopathology: Vol. 1. Theory and Methods. New York: John Wiley; 1995. p. 659–695.

[53] Sameroff, A. J. Ports of entry and the dynamics of mother-infant interventions. In: Sameroff, A. J., McDonough, S. C. & Rosenblum, K. L., editors. Treating Parent-Infant Relationship Problems: Strategies for Intervention. New York: Guilford Press; 2004. p. 3–8.

[54] Singh, N. N., Lancioni, G. E., Winton, A. S., Fisher, B. C., Wahler, R. G., Mcaleavey, K., Singh J., Sabaawi, M. Mindful parenting decreases aggression, noncompliance, and self-injury in children with autism. Journal of Emotional and Behavioral Disorders. 2006;14(3):169–177. DOI: 10.1177/10634266060140030401

[55] Estes, A., Munson, J., Dawson, G., Koehler, E., Zhou, X.H., & Abbott, R. Parenting stress and psychological functioning among mothers of preschool children with autism and developmental delay. Autism. 2009;13(4):375–387. DOI: 10.1177/1362361309105658

[56] Cachia, R. L., Anderson, A., & Moore, D. W. Mindfulness, stress and well-being in parents of children with autism spectrum disorder: a systematic review. Journal of Child and Family Studies. 2016;25(1):1–14. DOI: 10.1007/s10826-015-0193-8

[57] de Bruin, E. I., Blom, R., Smit, F. M., van Steensel, F. J., & Bögels, S. M. MYmind: Mindfulness training for Youngsters with autism spectrum disorders and their parents. Autism. 2015;19(8):906–914. DOI: 10.1177/1362361314553279

[58] Benn, R., Akiva, T., Arel, S., & Roeser, R. W. Mindfulness training effects for parents and educators of children with special needs. Developmental Psychology. 2012;48(5): 1476–1487. DOI: 10.1037/a0027537

[59] Blackledge, J. T., & Hayes, S. C. Using acceptance and commitment training in the support of parents of children diagnosed with autism. Child & Family Behavior Therapy. 2006;28(1):1–18. DOI: 10.1300/J019v28n01_01

[60] Ferraioli, S. J., & Harris, S. L. Comparative effects of mindfulness and skills-based parent training programs for parents of children with autism: feasibility and preliminary outcome data. Mindfulness. 2013;4(2):89–101. DOI: 10.1007/s12671-012-0099-0

[61] Kowalkowski, J. D. The impact of a group-based acceptance and commitment therapy intervention on parents of children diagnosed with an autism spectrum disorder [dissertation]. US: Master's Theses and Doctoral Dissertations; 2012. 1–120 p.

[62] Ruiz-Robledillo, N., Sarinana-Gonzalez, P., Perez-Blasco, J., Gonzalez-Bono, E., & Moya-Albiol, L. A mindfulness-based program improves health in caregivers of people with autism spectrum disorder: A pilot study. Mindfulness. 2015;6(4):767–777. DOI: 10.1007/s12671-014-0316-0

[63] Hahs, A. D. A Comparative Analysis of Acceptance and Commitment Therapy and a Mindfulness-based Therapy with Parents of Individuals Diagnosis: Experiment 1 [dissertation]. US: ProQuest Dissertations and Theses; 2013a. 46–71 p.

[64] Hahs, A. D. A Comparative Analysis of Acceptance and Commitment Therapy and a Mindfulness-based Therapy with Parents of Individuals Diagnosed with Autism Spectrum Disorder: Experiment 2 [dissertation]. US: ProQuest Dissertations and Theses; 2013b. 66–79 p.

[65] Cachia, R. L., Anderson, A., & Moore, D. W. Mindfulness in Individuals with Autism Spectrum Disorder: a Systematic Review and Narrative Analysis. Review Journal of Autism and Developmental Disorders. 2016;3(2):1–14. DOI: 10.1007/s40489-016-0074-0

[66] Hwang, Y. S., Kearney, P., Klieve, H., Lang, W., & Roberts, J. Cultivating mind: mindfulness interventions for children with autism spectrum disorder and problem behav-

iours, and their mothers. Journal of Child and Family Studies. 2015;24(10):3093–3106. DOI: 10.1007/s10826-015-0114-x

[67] Singh, N. N., Lancioni, G. E., Winton, A. S., Singh, J., Curtis, W. J., Wahler, R. G., & McAleavey, K. M. Mindful parenting decreases aggression and increases social behavior in children with developmental disabilities. Behavior Modification. 2007;31(6):749–771. DOI: 10.1177/0145445507300924

[68] Singh, N. N., Lancioni, G. E., Singh, A. N., Winton, A. S., Singh, J., McAleavey, K. M., & Adkins, A. D. A mindfulness-based health wellness program for an adolescent with Prader-Willi syndrome. Behavior Modification. 2008;32(2):167–181. DOI: 10.1177/0145 4455807308582

[69] Singh, N. N., Lancioni, G. E., Winton, A. S., Singh, A. N., Adkins, A. D., & Singh, J. Clinical and benefit–cost outcomes of teaching a mindfulness-based procedure to adult offenders with intellectual disabilities. Behavior Modification. 2008;32(5):622–637. DOI: 10.1177/0145445508315854

[70] Singh, N. N., Wahler, R. G., Adkins, A. D., Myers, R. E., & Mindfulness Research Group. Soles of the feet: A mindfulness-based self-control intervention for aggression by an individual with mild mental retardation and mental illness. Research in Developmental Disabilities. 2003;24(3):158–169. DOI: 10.1016/S0891-4222(03)00026-X

[71] Singh, N. N., Lancioni, G. E., Singh, A. D., Winton, A. S., Singh, A. N., & Singh, J. Adolescents with Asperger syndrome can use a mindfulness-based strategy to control their aggressive behavior. Research in Autism Spectrum Disorders. 2011;5(3):1103–1109. DOI: 10.1016/j.rasd.2010.12.006

[72] Singh, N. N., Lancioni, G. E., Manikam, R., Winton, A. S., Singh, A. N., Singh, J., & Singh, A. D. A mindfulness-based strategy for self-management of aggressive behavior in adolescents with autism. Research in Autism Spectrum Disorders. 2011;5(3):1153–1158. DOI: 10.1016/j.rasd.2010.12.012

[73] Kiep, M., Spek, A. A., & Hoeben, L. Mindfulness-based therapy in adults with an autism spectrum disorder: do treatment effects last? Mindfulness. 2015;6(3):637–644. DOI: 10.1007/s12671-014-0299-x

[74] Spek, A. A., van Ham, N. C., & Nyklíček, I. Mindfulness-based therapy in adults with an autism spectrum disorder: a randomized controlled trial. Research in Developmental Disabilities. 2013;34(1):246–253. DOI: 10.1016/j.ridd.2012.08.009

[75] Lang, R., Regester, A., Lauderdale, S., Ashbaugh, K., & Haring, A. Treatment of anxiety in autism spectrum disorders using cognitive behaviour therapy: A systematic review. Developmental Neurorehabilitation. 2010;13(1):53–63. DOI: 10.3109/17518420903 236288

[76] Peters-Scheffer, N., Didden, R., Korzilius, H., & Sturmey, P. A meta-analytic study on the effectiveness of comprehensive ABA-based early intervention programs for children with autism spectrum disorders. Research in Autism Spectrum Disorders. 2011;5(1):60–69. DOI: 10.1016/j.rasd.2010.03.011

Chapter 13

Constructing Healthy Experiences through Human-Animal Interactions for Autistic Children and Their Families: Implications for Research and Education

Alina S. Rusu

Additional information is available at the end of the chapter

http://dx.doi.org/10.5772/65395

Abstract

A significant body of research in the field of animal assistance in autism spectrum disorder (ASD) therapy indicates that positive human-animal interactions (HAIs), such as playing with therapy dogs or dogs presence while reading Social Stories, improve the social interactions and the level of the behavioral indicators of positive moods (smiling, laughing) in autistic children. In this chapter, we aim to present a series of evidence-based modalities of including animal-assisted activities in standard therapeutic settings but also in the home environment (e.g., interactions with family animals), targeting the socio-emotional development of autistic children and their optimal communication with the family members, including the companion animals. The studies presented here are discussed from the perspective of potential mechanisms, such as oxytocin system, and several attachment-related views. Our studies point toward the valorization of companion animals in the process of development and optimizing the interpersonal communication abilities of ASD children in a positive and engaging manner for both humans and animals.

Keywords: human-animal interactions, animal-assisted enhanced therapy, autistic children, socio-emotional skills

1. Introduction

A significant body of research in the field of animal assistance in the therapy of autism spectrum disorders (ASD) indicates that positive human-animal interactions (HAI), such as playing with therapy dogs or dogs presence while reading Social Stories (SS), have the potential to improve the social interactions at level of displaying behavioral indicators of positive moods (smiling, laughing) in autistic children [1, 2]. It appears that the direct contact with life forms other than humans, especially companion animals, has a modulatory effect on the psychophysiological parameters associated to social interactions [3, 4]. In this light, oxytocin, which is a hormone produces in the hypothalamus, has been considered an optimal candidate for the investigation of the beneficial psycho-physiological effects of friendly interactions with animals in general population and in ASD children [3]. It is hypothesized that the interaction between the hypothalamic-pituitary-adrenal (HPA) axis and the oxytocin system might be the central neurobiological mechanism behind the beneficial psychophysiological effects of the positive HAI, such as stress reduction and facilitation of social extroversion. Physical contact is considered a classical marker of secure attachment and caregiving relationship, and it is often assumed that oxytocin system might be activated in situations that involve direct physical contact, such as play with peers or positive human-animal interactions [3, 5]. Also, the effect of a friendly animal on the perception of the human in its company and on the facilitation of interpersonal interactions is known in the literature as *the social catalyst effect* [3].

Experts in the area of HAI management indicate a large and growing number of companion animals within EU countries, including Romania, i.e., there are an estimated number of 64 million cats and 60 million dogs in EU countries [6]. While it is well known that companion animals can make crucial contributions to human societies as working animals, a growing scientific body of evidence supports the benefits of animals in human healthcare, especially in the case of socially impaired children (ASD children). Recent statistics indicate a prevalence of autistic children and adolescents in Romania of around 15,000 [7]. Also, there is a growing interest of autism-oriented associations toward the inter-professional educational and therapeutic methods, such as animal-assisted therapy (AAT) and activities. Based on this growing interest of professionals in the field of autism toward the benefits of positive human-animal interactions, in this chapter, we aim to present a series of evidence-based studies that have investigated several modalities of including positive animal-assisted activities in standard therapeutic settings targeting the socio-emotional development of ASD children. The modalities presented here can be easily designed and implemented in the home environment of ASD children (i.e., interactions with other family members and resident companion animals).

2. Social Story in the presence of dogs: an animal-assisted enhanced method

The first study to be described in this chapter combines an already validated method addressing the social skills of ASD children, i.e., Social Story (SS) method [8], with the presence of therapy animals (dogs). The method of designing and incorporation of the dog presence in the Social Story procedure will be presented, as well as the ways of assessing significant outcome variables at behavioral level. Animal-assisted interventions (AAI) have started to be approached by specialists designing therapeutic programs for children with social impairments, such as ASD children, which appear to perceive and comprehend animal communication better than the human communication [9, 10]. It is generally acknowledged that one of the most important deficits that ASD individuals experience across their life span is the impairment in social abilities [11]. Recently, several authors in the ASD field suggested that the use of all the possible elements of social environment, including companion animals, should be considered when planning therapeutic interventions for ASD children [10]. Our study [1] describes for the first time in the ASD literature the effects and the procedure of implementing the dog presence in the Social Story method [12], under the form of a low-cost and short-term intervention (3 months), with significant results on the social ability development of ASD children.

It is generally acknowledged that humans and animals (especially companion animals) tend to naturally establish connections based on attachment, empathy, and affection [5]. The human-animal bond is considered to be an authentic one if the following criteria are met: (1) it involves a continuous relationship, not a temporary one and (2) it brings reciprocal benefits on humans and animals [5, 13]. There is evidence that ASD individuals appear to better perceive and comprehend animal nonverbal communication than the verbal and nonverbal human communication [10], which might indicate that dogs communicate their intentions on a level that ASD children find easier to understand [9].

When directed toward a specific objective and delivered in a structured and documented manner, animal-assisted activities become components of animal-assisted therapy [5]. According to Delta Society [14], which is one of the most active organizations in the field of therapeutic HAI, animal-assisted therapies (AATs) are goal-directed interventions, which are delivered by a health/human service professional with specialized expertise and within the scope of practice of his/her profession. AATs include animal-assisted activities aiming to improve the physical, social, emotional, and cognitive functioning of several categories of persons [5, 13], and it can be incorporated in a large variety of standard procedures for physiological recovery, attention-related problems, speech-related problems, depression treatments, successful aging programs for institutionalized elderly persons, etc. [15, 16].

In the case of ASD children, specialists agree that social impairment does not necessarily imply a lack of desire or interest of children to socially interact, but rather a lack of necessary social skills to successfully carry out social interactions [11]. In this direction, several types of interventions are focusing on improving the social skills of ASD children, and among them, Social Story [8] is one of the most popular methods used in special education in general and in the treatment of autism, in particular. Social Story (SS) method aims at providing ASD individuals with the social information and procedural knowledge they lack and thus helping them develop appropriate behaviors in social interactions and interpersonal relationships [8, 17]. It is assumed that SS provides a learning environment that might help the children to better understand and internalize appropriate social behavioral elements [18]. Over the last decade, several authors have evaluated and validated the effectiveness of the SS method in decreasing the frequency and the intensity of several problematic behaviors, such as aggression, screaming, grabbing toys, and crying [17], and in increasing the frequency and intensity of desirable behaviors, such as greeting and sharing things, playful behavior, etc. [11]. In many of these studies, SS has been used either as a sole intervention [11] or combined with other interventions, such as verbal and pictorial prompts, reinforcement of appropriate responses, robot-assisted programs [19], and various priming strategies [20].

In line with the trend depicted in the ASD literature of developing enhanced therapy plans, we performed an exploratory investigation entitled *Interaction with a therapy dog enhances the effects of Social Story method in autistic children* [1], aiming to combine the Social Story method [12] with naturally occurring elements that are supposed to be socially relevant to autistic individuals, such as therapy dogs. The main hypothesis was that a social environment heterospecifically enriched by the presence of a therapy dog while reading a Social Story might improve the effectiveness of the method at level of increasing the social abilities of ASD children. Two social skills were targeted: (1) the ability to greet a social partner and (2) the ability to introduce oneself to a social partner, following a standard *single-subject research design*. This exploratory investigation took place at a Romanian therapy center for ASD children (Transylvania Autism Association). Each participant had one 15-min intervention session per day (i.e., Social Story or Social Story plus dog presence), twice per week, for a period of three month (March–June 2012). An individualized Social Story was designed for each participant by the child's therapist together with the experimenter, by using Gray's construction guidelines [12]. A Labrador retriever dog, Arwan (male, 2 years), and his handler were involved in the study (the team was certified in AAT). Prior to the study, the AAT team had several visits to the Autism Day Center.

The dependent variables were the following: (1) frequency of appropriate social interactions relevant to the target social skill, (2) level of prompt needed to provide the expected social response, and (3) frequency of initiations of the social interactions relevant to the target social skill. Hypotheses were constructed for each of the variable, assuming that, compared to the sessions in which the Social Story was solely administrated, the enhanced version of the SS (SS plus dog presence) will be associated with a higher frequency of the appropriate social interactions, a lower level of prompt provided by the therapist (Note: A total level of prompt was considered here, comprising the sum of verbal prompt, gestural prompt, and the combination of the two; the lack of prompt was also recorded; for a detailed description of the coding system of the prompt, see Ref. [1].) and a higher level of initiations of appropriate social interactions. The following events were considered as appropriate social interactions: (a) any verbal, physical, or gestural appropriate response to the presence of a social partner; (b) any comment or a relevant question addressed to a social partner; (c) any appropriate response to questions or comments of a social partner; and (d) any direct eye contact or at least a look toward a social partner [11].

The exploratory study included three single case experiments, each one consisting of a succession of three phases (phases A, B and C). In the phase A (i.e. the baseline phase), each child was observed for 15 minutes of social interactions that required the usage of a specific social skill, which was aimed to be improved by the phase B (i.e. the Social Story method) or by the phase C (i.e. SS plus dog presence). For each participant, the Social Story was introduced prior the observation period. After six sessions, the intervention was withdrawn to the baseline condition. All the sessions were video-recorded and analyzed frame by frame for the extraction of behavioral data.

The analysis of the *frequency of the appropriate social interactions* relevant to the target social skills revealed that, for the first participant, the frequency did significantly improve from a mean value of 0.33 (SD = 0.51) in the baseline to a value of 5.16 (SD = 0.75) in the first phase of the SS plus dog presence intervention ($U = 0.00$, $p < 0.05$). The withdrawal of the SS plus dog presence intervention was associated with a decrease in the frequency to a mean value of 3.33 (SD = 0.51), followed by a nonsignificant increase when the SS intervention was introduced in the phase C. The size effect when comparing the two interventions had a high value (Cohen's d = 0.83, $p < 0.05$). For the other two participants, no significant increase in the frequency of the appropriate social interactions neither after the introduction of the SS intervention nor after the introduction of the SS plus dog presence intervention was registered.

The results on the *level of prompt needed to provide the expected social response* indicated that, for the first participant, as soon as the SS plus dog presence intervention was introduced, there was a significant decrease in the total level of prompt, from a mean value of 5.00 (SD = 0.00) to a value of 0.66 (SD = 0.81) after the first intervention (phase C; $U = 0.00$, $p < 0.02$). When the SS plus dog presence intervention was withdrawn, the level of prompt did increase (mean value = 2.50, SD = 0.51), yet it remained lower than the baseline values (Cohen's d = 0.47; $p < 0.05$). For the second participant, the data showed a decreasing trend during the initial baseline, but not significant. When the SS intervention was introduced (phase B), the decrease in the level of prompt was observed (mean value = 1.50, SD = 0.83). At the subsequent withdrawal of the SS intervention, the value of the level of prompt did not change, indicating no treatment reversal. When SS plus dog presence was introduced in phase C, the level of prompt decreased to a mean value of 0.66 (SD = 0.51), but with no significance. For the third participant, the SS plus dog presence intervention was associated with a significant decrease in the level of prompt. The value of the prompt level continued to significantly decrease throughout the SS plus dog presence intervention, compared to the baseline phase (*U* Mann-Whitney = 4.5, $p < 0.05$).

The results on the *frequency of the initiations of social interactions* indicate that, for all the three participants, no initiations were registered in the baseline phase. In the case of the first participant, the SS plus dog presence intervention was associated with a significant increase in the frequency of the initiations (mean = 2.33, SD = 0.11; *U* Mann-Whitney = 0.00, $p < 0.05$). After the introduction of the SS intervention, a small but nonsignificant increase in the frequency of the social initiations was observed compared to the baseline level. For the second participant, there was no significant difference in the level of the social initiations between the baseline and the SS intervention (phase B). The introduction of the SS plus dog presence intervention was a marked by an increase in the frequency (mean value for phase A = 0.16, SD = 0.40; mean value for phase B = 0.16, SD = 0.40; mean value for phase C = 2.0, SD = 0.89). In the case of the third participant, SS intervention was associated with a slight, but not significant increase in the frequency of social initiations, whereas the introduction of the SS plus dog presence intervention was associated with a sudden and significant increase in the frequency (mean = 2.33, SD = 0.81). The frequency of the social initiations was significantly higher in the Social Story plus dog presence intervention than the second baseline phase (*U* Mann-Whitney = 1.5, $p < 0.05$). The comparison of the SS and SS plus dog presence interventions indicated a high-effect size for all the three participants (Cohen's d = 0.83 for the first participant, $d = 0.92$ for the second one, and $d = 0.79$ for the third participant, $p < 0.05$).

In conclusions, the findings of this exploratory investigation of the effects of the combined methods SS plus dog presence indicate that the presence of the therapy dog was associated with a statistically significant increase in the frequency of the social initiations for all the participants and a significant decrease in the level of prompt needed to perform the specific social tasks in two of the participants in the study. The frequency of the appropriate social interactions appeared to significantly increase in the dog presence only in one out of the three participants in the study. It is important to mention that, in this study, the aim was to explore the minimal elements (i.e., the presence of the animal) needed for inclusion of a trained dog in the therapeutic context, without any other exercises, such as active playing on specific commands. In summary, our findings suggest that the presence of a dog while reading a SS is a low-cost method that can bring significant improvements to the Social Story therapy method, by increasing the frequency of social initiations and by decreasing the level of prompt that ASD children usually need from their therapists to perform appropriate social interactions. The findings presented here come in line with the results of previous studies on the effectiveness of animal-assisted therapy in enhancing the social motivation and communication of autistic children [21, 22].

3. Active participation of dogs in therapy of ASD children: dog-assisted functional play

The next study refers to the investigation of the effects of *active participation* of therapy dogs in the functional play of autistic children, targeting the development of their imitation skills, task performance, and communication with others. ASD children are often characterized by deficits in social abilities, narrowed or lack of motivation for different activities, and the presence of repetitive behavioral patterns [23]. Also, compared to their typically developed peers, ASD children are often described as having limited playing abilities, and when engaged in leisure activities, they often tend to rely on the help of others [24].

Playing behavior is often considered in the literature as providing opportunities to practice already acquired abilities or to acquire new ones in a safe and encouraging environment [25]. Functional play (which is related to the cognitive development) is defined as the specific use of an object or conventional association of several objects in the context of everyday life activities in the direction of developing functional individual autonomy [26]. In ASD children, the deficits in the capacity to pretend are related to a series of difficulties in the following abilities: (1) realize the need for reciprocity, (2) recognize different interpretations of actions, and (3) use imagination [24]. Another deficit of the ASD children, often placed within the category of theory of mind that might impair their ability to play and to properly interact within the play context, is their impaired ability to recognize that other persons make different interpretations of the events, according to their own knowledge and experiences [27, 28].

Play is considered to offer an optimal context to learn about social aspects, such as trust, negotiation, and compromises, as well as to explore the environment and to perceive its physical and social safety [29, 30]. During the symbolic play, typically developed children tend to explore social roles and rules in order to build a common understanding language with their play partner [30]. Because ASD children are generally known to have a low motivation level to share experiences, their imagination capabilities and the symbolic communication do not always appear to be reflected in their playing activities [24]. Hence, compared to the playing behavior of typically developed children, the play of ASD children is short in duration, and it has fewer functional and symbolic play sequences [27]. Also, the ASD children show lower levels of appropriate use of objects [31], less variety in play, and fewer functional and age-appropriate activities [32], as well as the tendency to use repetitive and precise verbal and/or gesture elements, which are rarely spontaneous [33, 34]. Although they may engage in symbolic play, ASD children often appear not to realize the need to motivate their social partners to play with them, and even in the case of verbally functional ASD children, they tend to display a passive participation in the play [34]. The term motivation refers here to the child's observable behavioral reactions to external stimuli, so that increased motivation is reflected by an increased responsiveness to social and environmental stimuli, as well as by a short latency of response to elements of the social interaction repertoire, such as instructions and questions [35].

The passive participation in play of ASD children, along with their low level of motivation to get involved in the social interactions that are normally expected to take place during play [35], is often interpreted as indifference to ambient stimuli [36]. Compared to typically developed children, ASD children appear to assess social stimuli in an atypical manner and tend to pay more attention to objects than to people [37]. Also, common indicators of joint attention, such as eye contact with other humans during social interactions, as well as spontaneous initiations of activities, are less frequent or less visible in the case of ASD children [38]. These deficits are being associated in the literature with a low level of general social motivation, i.e., *the social motivation model*, which can be observed from early childhood, and it might have consequences on the development of other aspects of their social life later on [39–41].

In order to develop social skills that are typical for a certain chronological age, especially in relation to the play behavior, which represents one of the most positive and basic ways of social interactions in humans and it has a significant moderating value of the family cohesion and of the individual quality of life, early therapeutic interventions are seriously considered in the case of ASD children. There is a consensus in the literature regarding the importance and benefits of early therapeutic interventions targeting the development and improvement of social skills in autistic children, including their playing abilities [42]. In this regard, literature analysis reveals a wide variety of therapeutic approaches, such as applied behavior analysis (ABA), peer-mediated intervention [43], robot-assisted therapy [19], video modeling, and Social Stories [12]. These methods can be efficient by themselves, or they can be administered in an enhanced form of combinations of elements and procedures. For example, the efficiency of Social Story method (originally developed by Gray [12]) can be enhanced at level of efficiency by the assistance of the therapist by a social robot who tells the Social Story while automatically expressing emotions [19] or by the presence of a therapy dog while reading the Social Story and asking the ASD children several comprehensive questions [1].

Literature in the field of ASD treatment supports more and more the positive effects of including therapy dogs in the therapeutic plans of ASD children aiming to improve their socio-emotional skills, especially because the interaction with animals is usually constructed on the species-specific playful and exploratory behavioral tendencies of the dogs, as well as on their evolved abilities to understand human emotions, which are expressed at verbal and nonverbal levels [44, 45]. In a play context (ball game, playing with a stuffed animal, and playing with a real dog), ASD children manifested an increased frequency of social initiations with the therapist in the condition of playing with the dog [46]. In another study that incorporated playing activities with dogs in a 15-week program of standard occupational therapy [47], data indicated a higher frequency of social initiations in the case of ASD children in the experimental group than those from the control group (occupational therapy). However, most of the studies cited above do not refer to the possibility of including the positive interactions with companion and/or therapy animals in the functional plays which children tend to naturally display during childhood and which are commonly incorporated in the educational curricula of children with special needs in the direction of improving their functional autonomy in everyday life situations.

The aim of the present study was to investigate the efficiency of actively including a therapy dog in the functional play of ASD children, by using a *randomized clinical trial* type of design. Based on the positive results regarding the efficiency of dog presence in Social Story method [1], the functional play of *bathing a doll* was incorporated in a SS scenario, in which the instructions and questions were specially adapted to the context of bathing (the SS was identical for the experimental and control groups). The bathing theme, which is an important component of nurturing behavior and human quality of life, was chosen based on autonomy-related needs identified by the therapists of the ASD children. Functional play consisted in "bathing the doll" game, in which the object of bathing was a medium-size doll and a real dog (experimental group), respectively, a doll, and a toy dog, similar in size to the real dog (control group).

The hypotheses were the following: (1) the play-related task performance of ASD children in the experimental group (functional play with a real dog) will be higher than the task play-related performance of ASD children in the control group (functional play with a toy dog). The play-related task performance was assessed by the frequency of imitations of the therapist's movements and the frequency of physical and verbal answers to the instructions and questions included in the adapted SS scenario; (2) the level of motivation to participate in the play of the children from the experimental group will be higher than the children from the control group (response latency to instructions and questions and frequency of the joint attention events).

The study included 20 children from the Day Center of Transylvania Autism Association (Romania). Participation of each child was based on informal consent signed by the parents. The study was conducted by two master students, under the supervision of the author, in collaboration with the psychologist of the Day Center. The ASD children (age between 3 and 9 years) had no allergies to animals or history of aggression with dogs. The playing session took place in the occupational therapy room of the Day Center, which was a carpeted room with a surface of 12 m^2. The therapy dog (Loki) was a male cocker spaniel, 8 years old, certified for animal-assisted therapy. The handler, who was also a psychologist, participated in all the play sessions. Loki was specially included in this study due to his high level of willingness to positively interact with children (playing with toys, retrieving the ball, playing football, etc.).

The experimental procedure consisted in eight functional play sessions for each ASD child (two sessions/week) and three follow-up sessions (two months after the post-intervention phase), with the length duration of 15 min (in average)/session, with slight variations depending on the behavioral particularities of each child. The first two sessions allowed us to establish a basal level for each of the dependent variables and to distribute the children in a randomized manner in the experimental ($N = 10$) and control ($N = 10$) groups. The children from the control group were then individually administered the functional bathing game (bathing the doll and a toy dog) and a Social Story adapted to the bathing situation, several comprehensive questions on the utility and components of bathing, while the experimental group was administered the functional game (bathing the doll) and bathing-related activities with a real dog. The social scenario was similar for both groups of ASD children.

The structure of the functional play consisted in a set of specific items, such as a toy bath tube, a comb, a brush, a towel, and a toy bottle of shampoo, which were introduced to the child alongside a protocol of 28 steps, embedded in a bathing-related Social Story. The protocol included 10 instructions (e.g., *open the shampoo bottle; let's brush the hair of the doll; let's brush the fur of the dog.*), five contextual questions (e.g., *what do you need to wash the hair of the doll? How do you brush your hair?*), and four imitation tasks (e.g., *look, can you do like I do?*). For each task, the child was expected to offer a verbal and/or physical response in a maximum of 5 s; After 5 s, in the absence of an answer, the therapist was allowed to prompt the child toward the optimal answer (i.e., prompt was offered either verbal, gestural, or in a combined version). The dependent variables related to the efficiency of the functional play in the two conditions (functional play with a toy dog and functional play with a real dog) were *play task performance* and *motivation to participate in the play.*

Play task performance was assessed by (1) the frequency of physical answers to the instructions, (2) frequency of imitations of the therapist's movements (after the instruction to imitate was given), and (3) frequency of verbal answers to the questions included in the protocol. *Frequency of physical answers to the instructions* refers to the numbers/sessions of the proper physical responses of the ASD children to the instructions given by the therapists, in accordance to the intervention protocol. *Imitation* refers here to the voluntary copying of the therapist's movement by the child, following the therapist's instruction, regardless of the level of familiarity with the movement [48]. In the case of children with motor disabilities, successful imitation is also counted for the partial copying of the movement, not only for the complete copying. *Frequency of verbal answers to the questions* refers to the numbers/sessions of the proper verbal responses of the ASD children to the instructions given by the therapists, in accordance to the intervention protocol. A latency period of 5 s was assigned for the answer to appear. After 5 s, the therapist was allowed to offer a prompt to the child in the direction of the proper answer.

Motivation to participate in the functional play was assessed by (1) response latency to verbal questions (latency lower or equal to 5 s, i.e., verbal answers without any prompt from the therapist) and (2) the frequency of joint attention events. Motivation to participate in the play refers to the child's enthusiasm and tendency to direct his/her playing-related interests to others, in order to develop the social interaction context needed for the play to take place [49]. *Response latency* was assessed by the time in seconds of the verbal and/or physical response of the child from the moment the therapist was giving a verbal instruction, a question, or an imitation task. After 5 s of waiting for an answer to occur, a prompt was offered by the therapist in the direction of the proper answer. The frequency of responses with latency lower than 5 s was counted for each session. *Joint attention* was measured by the frequency of voluntary eye contact of the child with the therapist during each play session. All the play sessions were recorded based on the informal consent signed by the parents. The first two play sessions were considered the pre-intervention phase, followed by six sessions. Among these six sessions, the last two were considered the post-intervention phase. After 2 months, another two sessions were conducted, which are considered the follow-up phase. Statistical analysis was conducted in order to reveal the differences between the control and the experimental groups on each of the dependent variables.

3.1. Effects of playing with real dog on the play task performance

The results on the *frequency of physical answers to the instructions* indicated that the two groups of ASD children started from similar frequencies of physical answers of children to the instructions of the therapist (Mann-Whitney test, $U = 43$, $Z = -0.53$, $p = 0.56$), while in the post-intervention phase, a significant difference between groups was recorded ($U = 14$, $Z = -2.78$, $p < 0.05$), in the favor of the experimental group. The effect of the interactions with the real dog was statistically significant (Cohen's $d = 1.44$). In the follow-up phase, the difference between groups was also significant ($U = 7.5$, $Z = -2.82$, $p < 0.05$, Cohen's $d = 1.73$). For the experimental group, we recorded a statistical difference between pre- and post-intervention phases at level of the frequency of physical answers to the instructions ($\chi^2 = 13.24$, $p < 0.05$), while no statistical difference was recorded for the control group between the phases. For the experimental group, the effect of the interaction with the real dog on the physical answers to the instructions was preserved from the post-intervention phase to the follow-up phase ($Z = -0.37$, $p = 0.7$).

The analysis of *frequency of imitations* in the pre-intervention phases indicated that the two groups started from similar levels of frequency ($U = 43.50$, $Z = -0.51$, $p = 0.6$), while in the post-intervention phase, the experimental group manifested a significantly higher frequency of imitations than the control group ($U = 1$, $Z = -2.75$, $p < 0.05$, Cohen's $d = 1.41$). In the follow-up, the difference between groups remained in the same direction and significant ($U = 6.5$, $Z = -3.09$, $p < 0.05$, Cohen's $d = 1.58$). While no significant evolution was recorded for the control group, the post hoc analysis for the experimental group revealed a significant improvement at level of frequency of imitations from pre-intervention to post-intervention ($Z = -2.04$, $p < 0.05$) but without statistical significance from post-intervention to the follow-up phase ($Z = -0.99$, $p = 0.31$).

Data collected on the *frequency of verbal answers to questions* in the pre-intervention phase indicated no differences between the two groups ($U = 39.50$, $Z = -0.81$, $p = 0.639$). Also, in the post-intervention phase, no significant difference between groups was registered ($U = 25.50$,

$Z = -1.38$, $p = 0.166$), as well as in the follow-up phase ($U = 22$, $Z = -1.38$, $p = 0.168$). No statistical differences were registered for the two groups from the pre- to post-interventions and for the post-intervention to the follow-up phase.

3.2. Effects of playing with real dog on the motivation of ASD children to participate in the play

The analysis of the *response latency to verbal questions* revealed that the two groups started from similar levels of response latency to verbal questions in the pre-intervention phase (Mann-Whitney test, $U = 46$, $Z = -0.3$, $p = 0.57$), while in the post-intervention phase, a significant difference between groups was recorded, with the experimental group having lower values of the response latency to verbal questions ($U = 10.5$, $Z = -2.98$, $p = 0.003$, Cohen's $d = 1.78$). The difference between groups in the post-intervention phase was also statistically significant ($U = 2$, $Z = -3.28$, $p < 0.05$, Cohen's $d = 2.61$). Statistically significant differences were registered for the experimental group of ASD children between the pre- to post-intervention phases ($\chi^2 = 12.40$, $p < 0.05$) and between the post-intervention phase and the follow-up. No significant differences were registered for the control group between the phases.

The two groups (control and experimental) started from similar levels of *frequency of joint attention episodes* (eye contacts with the therapist in the context of the functional play) in the pre-intervention phase ($U = 34$, $Z = -0.93$, $p = 0.34$). Significant differences were registered in post-intervention ($U = 23$, $Z = -2.06$, $p < 0.05$), indicating that the ASD children from the experimental group had a higher frequency of joint attention episode than those from the control group (Cohen's $d = 0.87$). While for the control group there were no significant differences between phases, for the experimental group, there was a significant difference between the post-intervention and the follow-up ($Z = -2.53$, $p = 0.01$), but not between the pre- and post-interventions.

The aim of the present study was to investigate the efficiency of actively including a therapy dog in the functional play of ASD children, by using a randomized clinical trial type of design. The theme of bathing process, which is an important component of nurturing behavior and human quality of life, was chosen based on autonomy-related needs identified by the therapists of the ASD children. Functional play consisted in "bathing the doll" game, in which the object of bathing was a medium-size doll and a real dog (experimental group), respectively, a doll, and a toy dog, similar in size to the real dog (control group). Our results indicated a significant positive effect of playing with the therapy dogs (comparisons between the experimental and control groups) at level of the following variables: frequency of physical answers to the instructions offered by the therapist in the context of the adapted social scenario to the bathing game, frequency of imitations (playing with the real dog was associated with a higher frequency of imitations than the condition of playing with a toy dog), response latency to the verbal instructions (ASD children from the experimental group, even though did not differ significantly in the frequency of verbal responses from the control group, had a shorter latency to respond to the verbal instructions), and frequency of joint attention episodes (ASD children that played with a real dog had significantly higher frequency of joint attention episodes in the post-intervention phase than the children in the control group). To summarize, the active interaction with the real dog in the context of functional play was associated with a significant improvement of the indicators of motivation of ASD children to participate in the play and to maintain the social interactions with the therapist during this activity. Because the active interaction with the dog involved direct contact with the animal, we can conclude that our data support the hypothesis of social catalyst effect of positive human-animal interactions [3].

Besides the quantitative data presented above, several qualitative data provided by the parents of ASD children indicated that some of the children expressed willingness to participate to the therapy sessions where the real dog was present and, in one case of a child with motor disability, his ability to stand up (gross motor skills) has improved due to his motivation to move closer to the dog during the interactions. Some of the ASD children were also reported to show a higher interest toward their family pets (dogs and cats), and they were more willing to participate in games and other activities involving the animal and their siblings or other family members, such as fetching the ball games or brushing and feeding the dogs. To summarize, functional play for ASD children can be significantly enhanced in terms of efficacy by the active inclusion of therapy animals (in therapy or educational settings) or of resident companion.

While in this study, the interaction with the dog took place indoor (the occupational therapy room) and it was included in the specific steps of the adapted Social Story scenario, in the next study, we aimed to investigate the association of active playing with behavioral indicators of positive moods in ASD children of two types of outdoor positive human-animal interactions, such as (1) active playing with dogs in a structured manner (i.e., agility type of exercises, in an organized spatial environment) or (2) in a free style (playing fetch the ball, football, running around, and walking the dog). Also, in this study, we aimed to investigate not only the behavioral indicators of positive affects in humans but also in dogs, by using methods from ethology (the scientific study of animal behavior), such as focal animal sampling and sequential analysis.

4. Agility exercises for ASD children and their families: free-style play or structured activities?

While most of the families with children, including children with special needs, tend to adopt companion animals, not all of them are aware of the importance of spending quality time with their pets in activities involving direct contact (play, agility), which is an important prerequisite of the benefits of social catalyst effect of animals in human life to occur [50]. Positive interactions between humans and dogs, such as play, petting, talking to the dog [51], or even prolonged eye contact [52], are known to be associated with health benefits for both species. It is generally acknowledged that animal assistance can provide opportunities for motivational, educational, recreational, and/or therapeutic benefits to enhance the quality of life of humans, especially in the socio-emotional skills' development of children with autism.

There are studies indicating that in the case of ASD children, "there is low baseline cardiac parasympathetic activity with evidence of elevated sympathetic tone" [53, 54], which might predispose them to express high levels of stress and anxiety. However, there is a growing scientific evidence of the positive outcomes of interactions with animals in many dimensions of the social life of ASD children, such as increase in frequency of imitations during functional play; increase in initiations of social interactions; decrease in the number, duration, and intensity of stereotypic behaviors [1, 55]; as well as decreased social anxiety [21]. Hence, a possible explanation of the positive effects of human-animal interactions in the case of autistic children is that the parasympathetic nervous system (PNS) becomes activated through the positive interactions with the animals, which are known to be more tolerated by ASD children (as a presence and as object of active interactions) than human individuals [54]. Although dogs are known for their evolved abilities for understanding human facial and vocal emotions [44, 45], they may encounter difficulties when interacting with human individuals with deficits at level of expressing emotions, such as ASD children. Such difficulties might be associated with signs of stress in animals that might impair not only the efficiency of the therapy interventions but also the well-being of the therapy animals and their motivation to further participate in assistance activities.

The aspect of well-being of dogs involved in animal-assisted interventions has become of great concern for specialists designing this type of interventions, which are more and more aware that interactions with sentient beings involve responsibilities for their biological needs [56]. In this regard, assessment techniques (behavioral, physiological, or combinations) to assess the well-being of therapy animals are highly recommended. Several authors investigating the stress indicators concluded that working long hours with no breaks was associated with high level of cortisol (stress hormone) in therapy dogs [57, 58]. Familiarity with the therapy environment was associated with a decrease in the cortisol level in therapy dogs [58].

In the present study, we aimed to investigate the effect at level behavioral indicators of positive affects in ASD children and dogs of two types of outdoor activities with dogs, which can be easily organized in the open spaces of any institution or in the home courtyards. The first type of activity was a structured one, inspired from the agility sport, in which a handler directs a dog through an obstacle course, without touching or leading the dog in a leash. In the case of autistic children, the structure activity was adapted to their special needs, so that a double leash was provided, one for the handler and one for the child. Hence, the structured activities are placed within the category of para-agility (i.e., the dog is directed not only by the handler but also by a person with special needs). The structured activities were implemented in collaboration with a local dog training school (Cluj-Napoca, Romania), within a research grant on the improvement of socio-emotional abilities of ASD children. The second type of activity consisted in free-style interactions, such as walking the dog (by using a double leash) and playing fetch the ball and football with the dog, in an *ad hoc* succession of playing and walking. During playing, the leash of the dog was removed by the handler, who was present during the whole session. The two types of activities were compared in terms of frequency of behavioral indicators of positive affects (e.g., smile and laughing for the child, tail wagging and petting acceptance for the dog).

Having in mind that interactions with animals offer continuous possibilities for positive design and behavioral engineering of healthy human and animal life experiences, this is an exploratory investigation of two types of dog-children outdoor interactions, aiming to identify the optimal associations of activity sequences and behavioral indicators of positive affects in human and animals in order to offer further guidelines for constructing optimal human-animal interactions in both institutional (therapy and educational) settings and in home environment.

Eleven children diagnosed with autism (ages between 4 and 12 years, enrolled at the Day Center of Transylvania Autism Association (Cluj-Napoca, Romania) participated in the program, based on informal consent signed by their parents. Prescreening for their inclusion in the animal-assisted activities indicated no allergies and no history of aggression with animals. All the families of the children had animals at home (dogs and/or cats). Each child was able to communicate using verbalization and each of them was able to walk. The program took place outdoor, in the courtyard of the Day Center, from April to July 2015. Six certified therapy dogs of different breeds (three Australian shepherd, one male and two females; one female beagle; one male cocker Spaniel; and one male former stray dog) together with their handlers participated in the program. All the dogs belonged to the Pet Joy Dog Training School (Cluj-Napoca, Romania). The handlers were certified in AAT, with previous experience on working with ASD children.

Before the beginning of the program, two visits of the dogs were organized at the Center, so the children had the chance to familiarize with the presence of the animal-assisted therapy teams. Each session had duration of 20 min, with slight variations. In the structured interaction sessions (SIS), after a demonstration offered by the handler and the dog, the dog was individually led by the children through an agility arena, consisting of a line of five obstacles and a play tunnel (3 m length). The handler was always present next to the child, as well as the therapist (the last one intervenes only when the child did not understand the guidance offered by the handler or when the child specifically asked for help). The structured sessions were designed in a way that encouraged positive human-animal interactions, so that the children were instructed to verbally praise the dog after each segment of the agility course and to offer small items of food reward (after a short previous training on how to properly offer dry food to the dogs). Also, depending on their time availability, parents were invited to assist the sessions and qualitative feedback was collected from them (perception of the utility of exercises, perception of signs of joy and motivation to play expressed by their children compared to other activities, etc.). In the unstructured interaction sessions (UIS), the dog and child were allowed to walk and play freely (fetch the ball, football, or other types of play-related activities), being closely supervised by the handler and the therapist from the Day Center. Dog walking was done with the help of a double leash system, which was gradually removed, and only one leash remained attached to the dog's collar. The succession of SS and SS was randomly established for each child, but they were always delivered within the same time interval of 2 h/day.

The behavioral indicators of the positive affects in children and of the lack of distress in dogs were selected from previous studies found in the literature, in which significant associations were found between several behavioral elements and physiological markers of stress, such as gazing into dog's eyes was associated with the activation of parasympathetic nervous system [52]; petting and playing with the dog were associated with oxytocin release and decrease in

http://dx.doi.org/10.5772/65395

cortisol [51, 59]; laughter and smile were associated with dog presence [1]. The behavioral indicators (activity, gestures, and postures) of positive affects in children toward the dogs were coded as it follows [54]: petting the dog, reaching for the dog, touching the dog, playing with the dog (usually the play involved activities such as throwing the ball by hand or hitting the ball by foot, in order for the dog to fetch it or to push the ball with the nose), gazing into the dog's eyes, smiling while interacting with the dog, and laughing while interacting with the dog. The behavioral indicators of positive affects of dogs toward children were considered the following: playing with the child, gazing into the child's eyes, acceptance of being touched, acceptance of being petted, and tail wagging while interacting with the child.

Each session was video-recorded, based on the informal consent signed by the parents of the ASD children [54]. The recorded materials were analyzed frame by frame using continuous sampling and focal individual observations. Among the recorded sessions, those that allowed the extraction of data (high-quality records) were 28 structured interaction sessions (SIS) and 13 unstructured interaction sessions (UIS) for the extraction of behavioral indicators of children toward the dogs and 27 SS and 7 US for the extraction of behavioral indicators of the positive affects of dogs toward children. For each session, the behavioral indicators were registered as sequences (one sequence followed by another), and chains of sequences were generated for each session. Transition matrices between behavioral sequences were generated for each session, allowing for the calculation of relative frequencies of occurrence of each behavioral indicator per time unit, i.e., 60 s. The relative frequencies of behavioral indicators of positive affects in children and dogs were then compared between structured and unstructured sessions.

The analysis of the results is presented in summary (for details on the results, see [54]). Even though the one-way ANOVA analysis revealed no statistically significant differences between the behavioral indicators of positive affects of dogs toward children (SIS, N = 22 = 22, m = 1.42, SD = 0.41), in the unstructured sessions (walking, playing fetch and football), dogs expressed more behavioral indicators of positive affects toward children (UIS, N = 7, m = 1.66, SD = 0.42) than in the structured sessions (SIS, N = 28 = 22, m = 1.42, SD = 0.41). Data on the behavioral indicators of positive affects of children toward dogs, although with no statistical significance (one-way ANOVA, F = 0.60, p = 0.44), indicated that the mean value in the structured sessions (SS, N = 28, m = 1.78, SD = 0.45) was higher than in the unstructured ones (UIS, N = 13, m = 1.66, SD = 0.72).

Our findings indicated that the structured human-animal positive interactions (para-agility exercises) were associated with higher mean values of the behavioral indicators of positive affects displayed by the ASD children toward the dog, whereas the free play style (unstructured interactions) was associated with a higher mean value of the positive behaviors displayed by dogs toward the children. It is important to mention that para-agility exercises involved more guidance from the handler compared to the free-style interactions with the dogs. The guidance from the handler might have functioned as gestural and verbal prompts for the children, who, as a consequence, might tended to pay more attention to the handlers than to the dogs. This aspect might be considered of important educational and therapeutic value in terms of mediating the development of interpersonal interactions (child handler) in a playful environment, in which the main action agent is the animal.

Another important aspect revealed by our data in terms of considering it for designing future positive ASD children-animal interactions is that each type of session had specific predominant behavioral indicators of the positive affects [54]. For example, in the structured sessions (SS), the predominant behavior of children toward the dog was petting the dog (i.e., direct contact with the dog), while in the unstructured sessions, the predominant one was playing with the dog by using the toys provided. Hence, in the case of ASD children, we can conclude that a structured environment of HAI is associated with higher opportunities of direct contact with the animals. As pointed out in the literature, the direct contact with animals is an important prerequisite for psychophysiological positive effects of animal assistance to occur, i.e., release of oxytocin and decrease in stress hormones. Also, in the case of structured sessions, the dogs accepted more petting behavior from ASD children than in the case of unstructured sessions, in which they responded to the play invitations and/or initiated the play, but they received a lower level of petting and touching. Also, in the unstructured sessions, dogs had more eye contacts with the handlers than with the children, as they were looking for a security base during the interactions.

Further studies are necessary to assess the physiological indicators of positive affects in children and animals in order to compare the similarities and differences in terms of facilitating the positive affects in children and animals. This preliminary study [54] indicates that both types of interactions (structured and unstructured activities) were associated with behavioral indicators of positive affects of humans toward animals (smiling, laughing, petting) and of animals toward humans (acceptance of petting, initiations of play, eye contact). Even though the sample size was a small one, the results of this investigation indicated that one should consider a *combination of both types of exercises* when designing outdoor animal-assisted activities for ASD children in institutions or at home, in the direction of creating the chance for healthy experiences to occur for both humans and animals. Agility routes can be easily set up in any type of environment, by using low-cost elements to build up mazes and/or simple barriers to be crossed by dogs. Besides the therapeutic value that animal assistance is known to have upon the socio-emotional development of ASD children, the animal-assisted structured activities such as para-agility have the potential to increase the motivation of ASD children for physical activity.

In line with the existing literature, the studies presented in this chapter indicate positive results of the incorporation of animal assistance in standard therapeutic methods for ASD children and also in play-type interactions, which can be easily organized at institutional level or at home, together with their family members, including the resident companion animals. Recent surveys indicate that dogs are the most common pets in Romania [60] and that they are affordable companion animals to families with children with special needs, such as autistic children. In this light, the findings of the studies presented in this chapter represent valuable guidelines of designing low-cost and efficient animal-assisted interactions, taking into considerations the well-being of both humans and animals. Our studies point toward the valorization of companion animals in the process of developing and optimizing the interper-

http://dx.doi.org/10.5772/65395

sonal communication abilities of ASD children in a positive and engaging manner for both humans and animals. Also, it is important to consider that, in order to optimally implement animal-assisted activities by professionals and parents of ASD children, appropriate theoretical and practical knowledge of the principles of human-animal interactions and zoonotic risk management are mandatory. These healthy principles addressing the quality of life of both humans and animals are often found under the umbrella of *One Health concept*, which implies a multidimensional and inter-professional partnership between specialists and beneficiaries of human-animal interactions, in the direction of promoting human and animal well-being [61].

Acknowledgements

The first and the second studies were supported by the research grant PN-II-RU-TE-3-2011-3-0080 (director: Alina S. Rusu). The third study was supported by the research grant PN-II-PT-PCCA-2013-4-0781 (director: Alina S. Rusu). The author would like to thank all the research team members (master students, PhD students, and research assistants) that have contributed to the data collection, analysis, and elaboration of the papers cited in this chapter. A special thank goes to the personnel of Transylvania Autism Association for facilitating the access to the ASD children and their families, as well as to the teams (handlers and dogs) of Pet Joy Dog Training School, Cluj-Napoca, Romania.

Author details

Alina S. Rusu

Address all correspondence to: alina.rusu@ubbcluj.ro

Faculty of Psychology and Sciences of Education, Babeș-Bolyai University, Cluj-Napoca, Romania

References

[1] Grigore AA, Rusu AS. Interaction with a therapy dog enhances the effects of social story method in autistic children. Society & Animals. 2014 Apr 22;22(3):241–61.

[2] Prothmann A, Bienert M, Ettrich C. Dogs in child psychotherapy: Effects on state of mind. Anthrozoos: A Multidisciplinary Journal of the Interactions of People & Animals. 2006 Sep 1;19(3):265–77.

[3] Beetz A, Uvnäs-Moberg K, Julius H, Kotrschal K. Psychosocial and Psychophysiological effects of human-animal interactions: The possible role of Oxytocin. Frontiers in Psychology. 2012;3:1–15.

[4] Wilson EOO. Biophilia. Cambridge, MA: Harvard University Press; 1984.

[5] Chandler CK. Animal Assisted Therapy in Counseling. London, United Kingdom: Routledge; 2011.

[6] Home. Home [Internet]. 2015 [cited 2016 Aug 17]. Available from: http://www.callistoproject.eu/joomla/

[7] Europe A. Latest news [Internet]. 2016 [cited 2016 Aug 17]. Available from: http://www.autismeurope.org/

[8] Gray CA, Garand JD. Social stories: Improving responses of students with autism with accurate social information. Focus on Autism and Other Developmental Disabilities. 1993 Apr 1;8(1):1–10.

[9] Hirschfeld LA, Gelman SA. Mapping the Mind: Domain Specificity in Cognition and Culture. Cambridge: Cambridge University Press; 1994.

[10] Prothmann A, Ettrich C, Prothmann S. Preference for, and responsiveness to, people, dogs and objects in children with autism. Anthrozoos: A Multidisciplinary Journal of the Interactions of People & Animals. 2009 Jun 1;22(2):161–71.

[11] Scattone D. Social skills interventions for children with autism. Psychology in the Schools. 2007;44(7):717–26.

[12] Gray C. Carol Gray – social stories; [Internet]. 2016 [cited 2016 Aug 17]. Available from: http://carolgraysocialstories.com/about-2/carol-gray/

[13] Fine AH. Handbook on Animal-Assisted Therapy: Theoretical Foundations and Guidelines for Practice. 2nd ed. Amsterdam: Elsevier/Academic Press; 2006.

[14] Fredrickson M, Howie AR, Burch M, Shay E, Albert T. The pet partners team training course: A Delta Society program for animal-assisted activities and therapy. 5th ed. Renton, WA: The Society; 2000.

[15] Nimer J, Lundahl B. Animal-assisted therapy: A meta-analysis. Anthrozoos: A Multidisciplinary Journal of the Interactions of People & Animals. 2007 Sep 1;20(3): 225–38.

[16] Chitic V, Rusu AS, Szamoskozi S. The effects of animal assisted therapy on communication and social skills: A meta-analysis. Transylvanian Journal of Psychology [Internet]. 2016 Mar 2 [cited 2016 Aug 17];13. Available from: http://connection.ebscohost.com/c/articles/79980461/effects-animal-assisted-therapy-communication-social-skills-meta-analysis

[17] Kuoch H, Mirenda P. Social story interventions for young children with autism spectrum disorders. Focus on Autism and Other Developmental Disabilities. 2003 Jan 1;18(4):219–27.

[18] Sansosti FJ, Powell-Smith KA, Kincaid D. A research synthesis of social story interventions for children with autism spectrum disorders. Focus on Autism and Other Developmental Disabilities. 2004 Jan 1;19(4):194–204.

[19] Vanderborght B, Simut R, Saldien J, Pop C, Rusu AS, Pintea S, et al. Using the social robot probo as a social story telling agent for children with ASD. Interaction Studies Social Behaviour and Communication in Biological and Artificial Systems. 2012;13(3): 348–72.

[20] Crozier S, Tincani MJ. Using a modified social story to decrease disruptive behavior of a child with autism. Focus on Autism and Other Developmental Disabilities. 2005 Jan 1;20(3):150–7.

[21] O'Haire ME. Animal-assisted intervention for autism spectrum disorder: A systematic literature review. Journal of Autism and Developmental Disorders. 2012 Nov 5;43(7): 1606–22.

[22] Solomon O. What a dog can do: Children with autism and therapy dogs in social interaction. Ethos; 2010 Mar;38(1):143–66.

[23] Association the AP, Association AP. Diagnostic and statistical manual of mental disorders, text revision (DSM-IV-TR). 4th ed. Arlington, VA: American Psychiatric Association; 2000.

[24] Hobson RP. Understanding self and other. Behavioral and Brain Sciences. 2004 Feb; 27(01):109–110.

[25] Naber FBA, Bakermans-Kranenburg MJ, van Ijzendoorn MH, Swinkels SHN, Buitelaar JK, Dietz C, et al. Play behavior and attachment in toddlers with autism. Journal of Autism and Developmental Disorders. 2007 Sep 26;38(5):857–66.

[26] Ungerer JA, Sigman M. Symbolic play and language comprehension in autistic children. Journal of the American Academy of Child Psychiatry. 1981 Mar;20(2):318–37.

[27] Baron-Cohen S, Leslie AM, Frith U. Does the autistic child have a "theory of mind"? Cognition. 1985 Oct;21(1):37–46.

[28] Yirmiya N, Solomonica-Levi D, Shulman C, Pilowsky T. Theory of mind abilities in individuals with autism, down syndrome, and mental retardation of unknown Etiology: The role of age and intelligence. Journal of Child Psychology and Psychiatry. 1996 Nov;37(8):1003–14.

[29] Ainsworth MDS. The Bowlby-Ainsworth attachment theory. Behavioral and Brain Sciences. 1978 Sep;1(03):436.

[30] Casby MW. The development of play in infants, toddlers, and young children. Communication Disorders Quarterly. 2003 Jan 1;24(4):163–74.

[31] Freeman BJ, Ritvo ER, Schroth PC. Behavior assessment of the syndrome of autism: Behavior observation system. Journal of the American Academy of Child Psychiatry. 1984 Sep;23(5):588–94.

[32] Mundy P, Sigman M, Kasari C. A longitudinal study of joint attention and language development in autistic children. Journal of Autism and Developmental Disorders. 1990 Mar;20(1):115–28.

[33] Jordan R. Social play and autistic spectrum disorders: A perspective on theory, implications and educational approaches. Autism. 2003 Dec 1;7(4):347–60.

[34] Sherratt D, Peter M. Developing Play and Drama in Children with Autistic Spectrum Disorders. London: David Fulton Publishers; 2001.

[35] Koegel RL, Bradshaw JL, Ashbaugh K, Koegel LK. Improving question-asking Initiations in young children with autism using pivotal response treatment. Journal of Autism and Developmental Disorders. 2013 Sep 7;44(4):816–27.

[36] Sigman M, Dijamco A, Gratier M, Rozga A. Early detection of core deficits in autism. Mental Retardation and Developmental Disabilities Research Reviews. 2004 Nov;10(4): 221–33.

[37] Sasson NJ, Turner-Brown LM, Holtzclaw TN, Lam KSL, Bodfish JW. Children with autism demonstrate circumscribed attention during passive viewing of complex social and nonsocial picture arrays. Autism Research. 2008;1(1):31–42.

[38] Petrina N, Carter M, Stephenson J. The nature of friendship in children with autism spectrum disorders: A systematic review. Research in Autism Spectrum Disorders. 2014 Feb;8(2):111–26.

[39] Dawson G, Toth K, Abbott R, Osterling J, Munson J, Estes A, et al. Early social attention impairments in autism: Social orienting, joint attention, and attention to distress. Developmental Psychology. 2004;40(2):271–83.

[40] Schultz RT, Grelotti DJ, Klin A, Kleinman J, Van der Gaag C, Marois R, et al. The role of the fusiform face area in social cognition: Implications for the pathobiology of autism. Philosophical Transactions of the Royal Society B: Biological Sciences. 2003 Feb 28;358(1430):415–27.

[41] Chevallier C, Kohls G, Troiani V, Brodkin ES, Schultz RT. The social motivation theory of autism. Trends in Cognitive Sciences. 2012 Apr;16(4):231–9.

[42] Howlin P. Practitioner review: Psychological and educational treatments for autism. Journal of Child Psychology and Psychiatry. 1998 Mar;39(3):307–22.

[43] Hundert J, Rowe S, Harrison E. The combined effects of social script training and peer buddies on generalized peer interaction of children with ASD in inclusive classrooms. Focus on Autism and Other Developmental Disabilities. 2014 Feb 27;29(4):206–15.

[44] Andics A, Gácsi M, Faragó T, Kis A, Miklósi Á. Voice-sensitive regions in the dog and human brain are revealed by comparative fMRI. Current Biology. 2014 Mar;24(5):574–8.

[45] Albuquerque N, Guo K, Wilkinson A, Savalli C, Otta E, Mills D. Dogs recognize dog and human emotions. Biology Letters. 2016 Jan;12(1):20150883.

[46] Martin F, Farnum J. Animal-assisted therapy for children with pervasive developmental disorders. Western Journal of Nursing Research. 2002 Oct 1;24(6):657–70.

[47] Sams MJ, Fortney EV, Willenbring S. Occupational therapy incorporating animals for children with autism: A pilot investigation. American Journal of Occupational Therapy. 2006 May 1;60(3):268–74.

[48] Volkmar FR, Cohen DJ. Handbook of Autism and Pervasive Developmental Disorders, Diagnosis, Development, Neurobiology, and Behavior, volume 1, 3rd ed. Volkmar MFR, Paul R, Klin A, editors. New York: John Wiley & Sons; 2005.

[49] Landreth GL, Homeyer LE, Glover GJ, L GL, Sweeney DS. Play Therapy Interventions with Children's Problems: Case Studies with DSM-IV Diagnoses. reth LH, editor. New York, NY, United States: Jason Aronson Inc. Publishers; 1996.

[50] Beetz A, Julius H, Turner D, Kotrschal K. Effects of social support by a dog on stress modulation in male children with insecure attachment. Frontiers in Psychology, 2012;3:1–9.

[51] Odendaal JS., Meintjes R. Neurophysiological correlates of affiliative behaviour between humans and dogs. The Veterinary Journal. 2003 May;165(3):296–301.

[52] Nagasawa M, Mitsui S, En S, Ohtani N, Ohta M, Sakuma Y, et al. Oxytocin-gaze positive loop and the coevolution of human-dog bonds. Science. 2015 Apr 16;348(6232):333–6.

[53] Ming X, Julu POO, Brimacombe M, Connor S, Daniels ML. Reduced cardiac parasympathetic activity in children with autism. Brain and Development. 2005 Oct;27(7):509–16.

[54] Pop D, Rusu AS, Miresan V. The development of a canine Para-Agility program: Positive affects in children with autism and in therapy dogs. Bulletin of University of Agricultural Sciences and Veterinary Medicine Cluj-Napoca Animal Sciences and Biotechnologies. 2016 Feb;73(1):1–6.

[55] Redefer LA, Goodman JF. Brief report: Pet-facilitated therapy with autistic children. Journal of Autism and Developmental Disorders. 1989 Sep;19(3):461–7.

[56] Podberscek AL. Positive and negative aspects of our relationship with companion animals. Veterinary Research Communications. 2006 Aug;30(S1):21–7.

[57] Haubenhofer DK, Kirchengast S. Physiological arousal for companion dogs working with their owners in animal-assisted activities and animal-assisted therapy. Journal of Applied Animal Welfare Science. 2006 Apr;9(2):165–72.

[58] Glenk L, Kothgassner O, Stetina B, Palme R, Kepplinger B, Baran H. Therapy dogs' salivary cortisol levels vary during animal-assisted interventions. Animal Welfare. 2013 Aug 1;22(3):369–78.

[59] Handlin L, Hydbring-Sandberg E, Nilsson A, Ejdebäck M, Jansson A, Uvnäs-Moberg K. Short-term interaction between dogs and their owners: Effects on oxytocin, cortisol, insulin and heart rate—An exploratory study. Anthrozoos: A Multidisciplinary Journal of the Interactions of People & Animals. 2011 Sep 1;24(3):301–15.

[60] Cocia RI, Rusu AS. Attitudes of Romanian pet caretakers towards sterilization of their animals: Gender conflict over male, but not female, companion animals. Anthrozoos: A Multidisciplinary Journal of the Interactions of People & Animals. 2010 Jun 1;23(2): 185–91.

[61] Evans BR, Leighton FA. A history of one health. Revue Scientifique et Technique de l'OIE. 2014 Aug 1;33(2):413–20.

Chapter 14

Sociocultural Perspective on Autism Intervention

Elizabeth Hughes Fong and Helen Lee

Additional information is available at the end of the chapter

http://dx.doi.org/10.5772/65965

Abstract

The landscape of the population in the United States is diversifying, as are the individuals who have a diagnosis of autism spectrum disorder. Autism spectrum disorder now affects one of out every 68 children. Although the diagnostic criteria do not differ, there are differences in time of diagnosis, treatment and acceptability of the diagnosis in various cultures, which is important for clinicians to understand. One approach to autism intervention is applied behavior analysis (ABA), which seeks to intervene on socially significant behavior. In addition, to using an approach such as ABA, which emphasis social significance, individuals may also use a cultural broker. The cultural broker can help to bridge the gap between parties and promote more effective treatment experience and thus help to ensure a more culturally sensitive approach to intervention.

Keywords: autism spectrum disorder, cultural competence, applied behavior analysis, cultural broker, social validity, culture

1. Introduction

According to the *Diagnostic and Statistical Manual of Mental Disorders* [1], autism spectrum disorder (ASD) is a neurodevelopmental disorder which can be broadly characterized by deficits in social communication and restricted interests and repetitive behaviors. Autism spectrum disorder has implications in the individual's ability to develop and maintain social relationships and function in society, and its symptoms can be recognized and diagnosed by 3 years of age.

Autism is considered a global health issue affecting individuals across diverse cultures [2, 3]. The prevalence of ASD in the United States is high, affecting roughly 1 in 68 children. However, this rate may be even higher considering that the ethnic and racial minority children are currently believed to be underdiagnosed due to barriers with accessibility to evaluation, diagnosis, and services [4]. Together with greater awareness across the world, there has been increasing interests both nationally and internationally to develop effective autism intervention treatment.

Among the number of intervention approaches that are currently available to treat autism, the literature suggests that behavior-focused interventions are arguably the most widely used and accepted in the field [5, 6]. Based on the science of applied behavior analysis (ABA), behavior analytic intervention programs are primarily designed to teach new skills and modify problem behavior by manipulating some aspects of the environment [7]. In particular, behavior therapists are taught to develop the intervention goals, methods, and implementations in line with clients' needs and the norms of social community [8, 9].

With the greater recognition of cultural diversity of individuals with ASD and their families across the world and in the United States, there is also a growing need to develop culturally sensitive ASD intervention programs. A culturally sensitive intervention program recognizes that clients from diverse cultural backgrounds can be best served when their needs are addressed with respect to the sociocultural contexts of their past developmental histories and current adaptive environment [4]. Such a program integrates an appropriate cultural view in assessing, designing, and implementing the program, and in approaching clinician-client relationship. Moreover, culturally sensitive intervention programs are embedded within a larger social cultural context of support, especially within a community of professionals who work as cultural mediators between the mainstream culture and the autism community. Such mediations between the mainstream and autism communities create a crucial social space or buffer for exchanges of ideas and conversations and adaptive interaction to take place, and it strengthen the long-term intervention effect.

We first discuss the cultural role in conceptualization and treatment of autism and disability in general, and then the importance of considering culture in developing behavior analysis interventions. We also discuss the role of greater professional community as cultural mediators between the mainstream and the autism spectrum community, highlighting the importance of cumulative efforts from the ABA perspective and professional community support in intervention outcome. Ultimately, we point out that in order for an intervention to be successful, it needs to be sustainable over time not only in the individual and family levels, but also in the social cultural community level as well.

2. Disability, autism and culture

The discovery of autism as well as the development of its intervention treatment have been largely originated in Western cultures and thinking. The significant early work by American doctor Leo Kanner and German doctor Hans Asperger in the 1940s have significantly contributed in establishing autism as a disorder that is currently known in the modern world. Similarly, ABA interventions are based primarily on the scholarly work of behaviorism, particularly by Skinner's [10] radical behaviorism, which highlighted the importance of deciphering particularities of environmental condition on organism's behavior.

http://dx.doi.org/10.5772/65965

Understandably, beyond Western cultures, there is significant variance regarding the meaning of disability and autism, and different ways individuals and families cope with the impact of the conditions. Some cultures may perceive the symptoms of a disability as a part of individuals' personality traits such as "stubbornness" or "laziness," and avoid seeking a necessary treatment. A mismatch on the cultural perceptions about behavior between ethnic and racial minority families and health professionals from the mainstream culture can also influence how families cope and seek help for treatment. For example, studies suggested that European American parents may be more likely to agree with the assessment of their child's behavior by a teacher than Asian/Pacific Islander and African American parents [11]. As a result, such culture-specific responses can potentially impact the interventions recommended by a treatment team, with European American children more likely to participate in intervention programs and receiving treatment via parent support more immediately than Asian children. On the other hand, the cultural differences in perceiving behavior have also contributed to over-diagnoses of behavior problems of minority students due to the cultural biases of educational and mental health administrators [12, 13].

Culture may also impact the diagnosis of autism, the time of diagnosis, as well as the access to services. For example, in the US, European Americans are diagnosed on average 1.5 years before their ethnic minority counterparts [14], allowing European American children for more immediate access to interventions for autism, in comparison to their minority counterparts. Across the world, in Egypt, autism has been often considered analogous to mental retardation or even a curse by folk belief, and children have been sometimes caged as a result [15]. In China, autism has been conceptualized as a disease of the 'rich and lazy' and its treatments included walking long distances in heavy clothing and weight training [16]. In Ethiopia, many individuals believed that children who have autism were possessed by the devil due to their parent's sins and attribute largely to supernatural explanations as the cause of autism, and the families live with high levels of stigma [17]. However, nowadays, there are growing global health initiatives to enhance understanding for autism and its symptoms and to stimulate greater acceptance of those who are diagnosed with ASD by their community [18].

Consequently, the treatment of autism in some parts of the world has included the use of folk healers and religious rituals, or forced isolation from the community. For ABA therapists, when treating families whose cultural beliefs and practices related to autism may be differ from the therapists, it may be important for the therapists to not only educate themselves about their client's culture but also educate their clients about the evidence-based literature findings which is guiding the therapists' intervention practice [4]. Furthermore, the clients who are disconnected from the community may need to be educated about the process and best ways to navigate some of the challenges to obtaining care from their state and federal level systems (e.g., health care and educational systems).

In sum, differences in cultural notions about typical human development and disability can influence different ways in which individuals perceive autism and seek treatment [4]. When there is perceived cultural difference between the therapists and clients, it is more critical for the therapists to understand their clients' cultural views and strategy the best way to create common treatment goals, procedures, and outcome assessments together with their clients and families.

3. Culture and behavior analysis

In discussing various intervention programs to teach individuals with ASD socially appropriate behaviors and communication skills, it is often ignored that there is social cultural diversity in human behavior across communities. Culture refers to the historical patterns of meanings embodied in various forms of symbols that pervade in a community and which are transmitted to the next generation of offspring [19]. It shapes individuals' values, beliefs, and behaviors including different ways they display emotion, communicate needs and wants to others, and approach inter-personal relationships. Skinner [10, 20] has also noted that culture represents the collection of operants or contingencies unique to a social community.

Applied behavior analysis is one of the most common interventions used with individuals who have autism and has been used to develop a number of popular behavior-focused intervention programs used today, including pivotal response training, early intensive behavioral intervention, and positive behavior interventions [21]. Behavior analysis focuses on teaching and shaping-specific behavior by manipulating the behavior's functional relationship with the environment [7]. Environmental variables such as conditions which precede (antecedents) and follow (consequence) the behavior and motivational factors like individuals' state of deprivation and satiation are analyzed in order to identify reasons for the prevalence of the behavior, i.e., increasing or decreasing manner in the given context.

Considering that defining characteristics of autism are concern with difficulties in social interaction and verbal and nonverbal communication [1], the key goals of ASD intervention have traditionally focused on addressing these deficits. However, the traditional methods of teaching communicative skills and other living skills have largely occurred in restricted learning environment with limited considerations for social cultural norms and values.

There are a number of ways cultural knowledge can help develop effective behavior analytic programs, especially for naturalistic setting-based intervention. Cultural knowledge can guide behavior analysts to design more contextually appropriate intervention programs by helping them to recognize variations of different forms of antecedent and reinforcers and understand their functional relationships. The different forms include verbal and nonverbal behaviors of individuals and agencies or structures at the institutional level that control contingencies. For example, all verbal relations are considered operants with different verbal forms controlled by consequences, all of which are unique to different cultural communities [10, 20, 22]. A verbal community shapes speaker and listener behavior by teaching specific and shared verbal forms and their consequent behavior through group practices [10, 20]. At a basic level, when an English speaker says, "give me an apple," the linguistic 'form' or meaning for the request can only elicit proper action from the same linguistic community (English), not from other linguistic communities. Moreover, when an individual with autism from an English-speaking North American community hands an apple to the speaker in response, s/he may be considered to have mastered fluency skill level. However, a child from a culture that emphasize social hierarchy and respect toward authority figures and elders may need to be further trained on how to properly hand the apple to an authority figure or elder with two hands and a posture for respect to be considered mastered the fluency. As Vargas [22] has noted, language does not exist in static symbolic forms but rather in dynamic action forms including utterances, writings, and bodily gestures which carry with them implicit meanings that are not directly communicated. Skinner [20] also emphasized that verbal behavior is not restricted to any particular mode of behavior but any behavior reinforced through mediation of other people (speaker) and can include any movement capable of affecting another organism.

When programs are culturally sensitive, they integrate culturally appropriate forms of antecedents and reinforcements from the natural environment. Individuals' perception of what is desired or aversive of symbolic systems of objects, events, and behaviors is often heavily influenced by the prior experience in the social environment. For example, children may respond better with a type of tangible reinforcement (e.g., food or toy) when it is more familiar and desirable to them. Children in northern Europe may respond more favorably to liquorish candy than sesame snacks which are more popular in Asia. When providing social praise for positive reinforcement, behavior analysts can consider different ways cultures express emotion and praise or disappointment. Studies have shown that Western cultures encourage their children to value autonomy and independence while Asian cultures encourage their children to value collective needs and group harmony and emotional control in public [23, 24]. An individual who grew up in a culture that values emotional control and avoids high intensity social expression of affect may be unfamiliar and uncomfortable by loud and highly energetic praise which individuals who grew up in Western cultures may prefer. In such settings, more toned down subtle forms of praise may work better as positive social reinforcement, while the high intensity expression of praise may serve an aversive function. Therefore, a culturally sensitive program considers not only different types of reinforcement but also different potential functions, they may serve related to their environmental history. In addition, a culturally sensitive program can help individuals to generalize better across contexts by minimizing the gap between the teaching session and everyday interaction.

In interpersonal communication, cultural knowledge can enhance the ABA therapists' ability to communicate with their clients about the intervention more effectively. When therapists understand ones' own cultural biases and cultural differences in their clients' values, beliefs, and communication styles, therapists can develop ways to build rapport and quality relationships with clients and communicate more effectively [25].

In order to ensure social relevance of intervention, ABA frequently employs various social validity assessments [26]. When working with culturally diverse clients, utilizing social validity measures frequently to ensure the goals, methods, and outcomes of intervention are accepted by the clients would be particularly critical. Although more work is needed to modify currently existing validity forms in culturally sensitive ways, it would be important to be aware of them. They include Lennox and Milternberger's [27] 12 factors for treatment acceptability, Winett et al.'s [28] epidemiological conceptualization of social validity, Gresham and Lopez's [29] conceptualization of social validity as the accumulation of multiple sources of information from culturally relevant key stake holders, Kennedy's [30, 31] maintenance model of social validity, or Carter's [32] distributive model of treatment acceptability. Examples of format treatment acceptability measurement instruments include the:

Treatment Evaluation Inventory, Treatment Evaluation Inventory-Short Form, Treatment Acceptability Rating Form, Treatment Acceptability Form Revised, Intervention Rating Profile, Intervention Rating Profile 1.5 m, Children's Intervention Rating Profile, Behavior Intervention Rating Scale, Intervention-Process Rating Scale (IPRS), and Abbreviated Acceptability Rating Profile [33].

4. Cultural brokers of autism intervention

A comprehensive treatment intervention for autism often involves a number of service professionals with diverse areas of expertise from the community. The role of the professionals as essential cultural mediators is often shadowed by the social interest for the effectiveness of the intervention service as a product they deliver to the clients [34]. However, it should be acknowledged that various professionals in the community such as those working in education, health, and social service systems also serve a critical role as social mediators. As a collective, they help to bridge the gap in knowledge between the broader cultural community and the autism community. Through their cultural mediation, the cultural broker helps to create an important inclusive social environment or space, one that which disabled individuals can practice, make progress and connect with the general population [34, 35].

In the field of education, cultural brokers may be teachers, instructional aides, school counselors, community members, after school program staff, students, siblings, school liaisons, and parent liaisons [34]. On the behalf of the student and family, within the educational setting, brokering activities may include, translation, assistance with navigating, interpreting the educational system, development of advocating skills, assistance with social skills, and potential employment opportunities for the student and their family. In addition, cultural brokers might inform the school staff about the cultural practices of the student and their family, as well as how to successfully work within any differences [34]. Ultimately, use of a cultural broker in the educational process can help address barriers between the student, family and school, which is important as the previous literature outcomes emphasize the importance of a school home collaboration for student success.

Professionals serving as cultural brokers or intermediary can help to translate information between the autism community which include individuals with ASD and their families and the mainstream social cultural communities which they are part of. According to Lo [36], professionals can serve as cultural brokers who help to bridge, link, or mediate between groups or persons from different cultures. Cultural brokers work to reduce conflict, or bring about change by bridging or linking groups of culturally different individuals together [37]. This often involves rapport, trust, long-term relationships, building of networks, and cultural labor, which can take considerable times and effort on the part of the clinician.

According to Jezewski and Sotnik [37], there are three stages of brokering process. The first stage involves identifying problem of a breakdown or conflict in the communication between the parties. Second, the intervening condition stage involves integrating culturally relevant factors in analyzing the problem, devising appropriate strategies, and evaluating outcomes.

http://dx.doi.org/10.5772/65965

During this stage, the intervention strategies are examined critically with respect to the potential explanations for the success or failure interventions. Here, cultural brokers might advocate for particular strategies, mediate between groups for greater understanding, help professionals and clients network to broader community, and help negotiate different views different parties may have. In the process, much work is devoted for professionals' ability to establish trust and rapport and bonds with their clients. In the final stage, the intervention outcomes are evaluated and deemed to be successful or unsuccessful. An intervention is deemed successful when bonds are established between individuals from different cultures but unsuccessful when intervention continues to involve a breakdown in services.

5. Conclusion and future direction

Autism has become a global health concern, affecting individuals across diverse cultural populations. The effective treatment of autism, especially involving teaching of socially adaptive skills, needs to consider appropriate sociocultural contexts of their clients' living environment [4]. Cultural values, beliefs, and practices which play key roles individuals' conceptualization and choice for treatment of autism are not consistent across cultures, and it behooves therapists to be informed about cultural perspectives that are different than their own.

To develop culturally sensitive intervention programs for individuals with autism, it would be important for therapists to be aware of their own biases, as these biases related to treatment, cause, and diagnostic views may not be in agreement with how a family or their culture conceptualizes the process [25]. Thus, it is recommended that regular validity checks are performed with the family and other stakeholders to ensure the proper representation of the family culture during intervention team meetings.

By taking the time to understand the needs of the clients and families in the context of their social cultural environment, therapists motivate greater family engagement in treatment services, compliance with treatment planning and recommendations, all of which contribute to better treatment outcomes. Together with the supports from cultural brokers from diverse fields of expertise in the community, socioculturally grounded intervention programs for individuals with autism can offer valuable opportunities to acquire skills that are more functionally adaptive to their cultural environment.

Author details

Elizabeth Hughes Fong[1]* and Helen Lee[2]

*Address all correspondence to: efong@sju.edu

1 Saint Joseph's University, Philadelphia, United States of America

2 University Boston, Boston, United States of America

References

[1] Diagnostic and statistical manual of mental disorders DSM-5 (2013). Arlington, V.A.: American Psychiatric Association.

[2] Baxter, A. J., Brugha, T. S., Erskine, H. E., Scheurer, R. W., Vos, T., & Scott, J. G. (2015). The epidemiology and global burden of autism spectrum disorder. Psychological Medicine, *45*, 601–613.

[3] Tomlinson, M., Yasamy, M. T., Emerson, E., Officer, A., Richler, D., & Saxena, S. (2014). Setting global research priorities for developmental disabilities, including intellectual disabilities and autism. Journal of Intellectual Disability Research, *58*, 1121–1130.

[4] Tek, S., & Landa, R. J. (2012). Differences in autism symptoms between minority and non-minority toddlers. Journal of Autism and Developmental Disorders, *42*(9), 1967–1973.

[5] Green, V. A., Pituch, K. A., Itchon, J., Choi, A., O'Reilly, M., & Sigafoos, J. (2006). Internet survey of treatments used by parents of children with autism. Research in Developmental Disabilities, *27*, 70–84.

[6] Sallows, G. O., & Graupner, T. D. (2005). Intensive behavioral treatment for children with autism: four-year outcome and predictors. American Journal on Mental Retardation, *110*(6), 417–438.

[7] Cooper, J. O., Heron, T. E., & Heward, W. L. (2007). Applied behavior analysis, 2nd ed. Upper Saddle River, N.J.: Pearson Prentice Hall.

[8] Turner, L. B., Fischer, A. J., & Luiselli, J. K. (2016). Towards a competency-based, ethical, and socially valid approach to the supervision of applied behavior analytic trainees. Behavior Analysis in Practice, 1–12.

[9] Wolf, M. M. (1978). Social validity: the case for subjective measurement or how applied behavior analysis is finding its heart1. Journal of Applied Behavior Analysis, *11*(2), 203–214.

[10] Skinner, B. F. (1972). Beyond freedom and dignity. New York: Bantam Books.

[11] Mandell, D. S., & Novak, M. (2005). The role of culture in families' treatment decisions for children with autism spectrum disorders. Mental Retardation and Developmental Disabilities Research Reviews, *11*(2), 110–115.

[12] Fletcher, T. V., & Navarrete, L. A. (2011). Learning disabilities or difference: a critical look at issues associated with the misidentification and placement of hispanic students in special education programs. Rural Special Education Quarterly, *30*, 30.

[13] Irvine, J. J. (2012). Complex relationships between multicultural education and special education an African American perspective. Journal of Teacher Education, *63*, 268–274.

[14] Ennis-Cole, D., Durodoye, B. A., & Harris, H. L. (2013). The impact of culture on autism diagnosis and treatment: considerations for counselors and other professionals. The Family Journal, *21*, 279–287.

[15] Gharib, M. (2016). She turned the pyramids blue – and got Egyptians to talk about autism. Retrieved from: http://www.npr.org/sections/goatsandsoda/2016/06/20/478548029/she-turned-the-pyramids-blue-and-got-egyptians-to-talk-about-autism

[16] Connor, N. (2016). Autistic boy, 3, dies after punishing exercise at China centre. The Telegraph. Retrieved from: http://www.telegraph.co.uk/news/2016/05/07/autistic-boy-3-dies-after-punishing-exercise-at-china-centre/

[17] Tilahun, D., Hanlon, C., Fekadu, A., Tekola, B., Baheretibeb, Y., & Hoekstra, R. A. (2016). Stigma, explanatory models and unmet needs of caregivers of children with developmental disorders in a low-income African country: a cross-sectional facility-based survey. BMC Health Services Research, *16*, 152.

[18] Tekola, B., Baheretibeb, Y., Roth, I., Tilahun, D., Fekadu, A., Hanlon, C., & Hoekstra, R. A. (2016). Challenges and opportunities to improve autism services in low-income countries: lessons from a situational analysis in Ethiopia. Global Mental Health, *3*, e21.

[19] Geertz, C. (1973). The interpretation of cultures: Selected essays (Vol. 5019). New York, N.Y: Basic books.

[20] Skinner, B. F. (2014). Verbal behavior. Cambridge, M.A.: B.F. Skinner Foundation Reprint Series

[21] Lord, C., & McGee, J. P. (2001). Educating children with autism. Washington DC: National Academic Press.

[22] Vargas, E. A. (2013). The Importance of form in Skinner's analysis of verbal behavior and a further step. The Analysis of Verbal Behavior, *29*(1), 167.

[23] Tsai, J. L., & Levenson, R. W. (1997). Cultural influences on emotional responding Chinese American and European American dating couples during interpersonal conflict. Journal of Cross-Cultural Psychology, *28*(5), 600–625.

[24] Tsai, J. L., Levenson, R. W., & Carstensen, L. L. (2000). Autonomic, subjective, and expressive responses to emotional films in older and younger Chinese Americans and European Americans. Psychology and Aging, *15*(4), 684.

[25] Fong, E. H., Catagnus, R. M., Brodhead, M. T., Quigley, S., & Field, S. (2016). Developing the cultural awareness skills of behavior analysts. Behavior Analysis in Practice, *9*, 84–94.

[26] Finn, C. A., & Sladeczek, I. E. (2001). Assessing the social validity of behavioral interventions: a review of treatment acceptability measures. School Psychology Quarterly, *16*(2), 176.

[27] Lennox, D. B., & Milternberger, R. G. (1990). On the conceptualization of treatment acceptability. Education and Training in Mental Retardation, *25*, 211–224.

[28] Winett, R. A., Moore, J. F., & Anderson, E. S. (1991). Extending the concept of social validity: behavior analysis for disease prevention and health promotion. Journal of Applied Behavior Analysis, *24*, 215–230.

[29] Gresham, F. M., & Lopez, M. F. (1996). Social validation: a unifying concept for school-based consultation research and practice. School Psychology Quarterly, *11*(3), 204.

[30] Kennedy, C. H. (2002). The maintenance of behavior change as an indicator of social validity. Behavior Modification, *26*, 594–606.

[31] Kennedy, C. H. (2002b). Toward a socially valid understanding of problem behavior. Education and Treatment of Children, 25, 142–153.

[32] Carter, S. L. (2008). A distributive model of treatment acceptability. Education and Training in Developmental Disabilities, *43*, 411–420.

[33] Carter, S. L. (2009). The social validity manual: A guide to subjective evaluation of behavior interventions. Burlington, M.A.: Academic Press.

[34] Yohani, S. (2013). Educational cultural brokers and the school adaptation of refugee children and families: challenges and opportunities. Journal of International Migration and Integration, *14*(1), 61–79.

[35] National Center for Cultural Competence, Georgetown University Center for Child and Human Development, Georgetown University Medical Center (2004). What Is the Role of Cultural Brokers in Health Care Delivery? Rockville, M.D.: National Health Service Corps, Bureau of Health Professions Health Resources and Services Administration, U.S. Department of Health and Human Services.

[36] Lo, M. C. M. (2010). Cultural brokerage: creating linkages between voices of lifeworld and medicine in cross-cultural clinical settings. Health, *14*(5), 484–504.

[37] Jezewski, M. A., & Sotnik, P. (2001). Culture brokering: providing culturally competent rehabilitation services to foreign-born persons. Buffalo, N.Y.: CIRRIE Monograph Series, Center for International Rehabilitation Research Information and Exchange.

Chapter 15

Physical Activity in Individuals with Autism Spectrum Disorders (ASD): A Review

Sara M. Scharoun, Kristen T. Wright,
Jennifer E. Robertson-Wilson, Paula C. Fletcher and
Pamela J. Bryden

Additional information is available at the end of the chapter

http://dx.doi.org/10.5772/66680

Abstract

Current recommendations indicate that children and youth ages 5–17 should participate in 60 min and adults in 150 min of moderate-to-vigorous physical activity daily. Research suggests that physical activity levels of individuals with autism spectrum disorder (ASD) are lower than typically developing and developed peers. Despite evidence for PA decreasing negative behaviors and promoting positive behaviors, individuals with ASD may be less motivated and less likely to participate. Individuals with ASD may be more likely to be overweight or obese than their typically developing counterparts as a result of decreased activity levels. Conflicting findings regarding PA levels in individuals with ASD have been reported. Given mixed evidence, further inquiry is warranted. The present chapter provides a review of literature pertaining to PA in individuals with ASD. Four databases were searched. Predetermined search terms and inclusion/exclusion criteria were clearly outlined to identify relevant articles which were then critically appraised. This research provides a greater understanding of the status of PA participation of individuals with ASD.

Keywords: physical activity, autism spectrum disorder, exercise, recreation, leisure

1. Introduction

Numerous physical and mental health benefits have been attributed to regular participation in physical activity (PA) and limited sedentary behavior [1–3]. Nevertheless, global levels of insufficient PA are reported, and physical inactivity levels are rising [4, 5]. The World Health Organization (WHO) [5] recommends that children and youth ages 5–17 should participate in 60 min and adults ages 18–64 should participate in 150 min of moderate-to-vigorous PA (MVPA) daily. For individuals with autism spectrum disorder (ASD), recent reports indicate that the levels of PA are significantly lower than typically developing and developed peers [6].

The WHO estimates one person in 160 has an autism spectrum disorder [7]. A group of neurodevelopmental disorders diagnosed in childhood and persisting throughout life, ASD is characterized by varying challenges with communication, social interaction, and repetitive behaviors and movements [8]. Although not recognized as a formal diagnostic feature, sensorimotor impairments have also been identified as a cardinal feature of ASD [9, 10]. Furthermore, comorbid conditions typically manifest in individuals with ASD, including attention-deficit hyperactivity disorder (ADHD), anxiety disorders, and chronic sleeping problems [11–13].

The aforementioned difficulties and comorbid conditions combined have been shown to significantly impact the quality of life for individuals with ASD [14]. Despite evidence for PA decreasing negative behaviors and promoting positive behaviors [15], individuals with ASD may be less motivated and less likely to participate in PA [16]. As a result of decreased activity levels, individuals with ASD are more likely to be overweight or obese than their typically developing counterparts [6], thus leading to further health-related challenges. Notwithstanding the previous literature, conflicting findings regarding physical activity in individuals with ASD have also been reported. In one recent example, Corvey et al. [17] identified no relationships between ASD and overweight or physical activity after controlling for comorbidities and medications. Tyler et al. [18] found that, despite being less active than their typically developing peers, children with ASD did meet physical activity guidelines set out by the US Department of Health and Human Services (i.e., 60 min of moderate-to-vigorous PA/day). Clearly, further inquiry is warranted.

The present chapter provides a review of literature pertaining to physical activity in individuals with ASD. Four research questions were assessed as follows: (1) What is the status of PA participation; (2) Does PA decrease negative behaviors and/or promote positive behaviors; (3) What facilitators and barriers exist; and (4) What PA intervention programs have demonstrated effectiveness?

2. Methods

In July of 2016, a computerized search of four electronic databases (PubMed, PSYCHINFO, Web of Science, and EBSCOhost) was conducted. Two sets of key words were used in the search strategy to identify articles that included participants with ASD (Autism Spectrum Disorder, ASD, Autism, Autistic disorder, Pervasive Developmental Disorder Not Otherwise

Specified, Asperger's syndrome) and that included PA (physical activity, exercise, recreation, leisure, fitness, athletics, sport, and playing). Search terms were entered based on specific format requirements of each database.

Inclusion and exclusion criteria were as follows: Articles must have been available in English and published within the last decade (i.e., 2006–2016). Only studies with quantitative designs were included. In the case of mixed designs, qualitative data are not presented in results. Participants (no age restrictions) must have been diagnosed with an ASD according to current or previous iterations of diagnostic criteria. Due to the difference in classification, each article discussed in this review will utilize the terminology from each respective publication. Studies that included individuals with other disabilities and/or disorders were included only if individuals with ASD were separated as a subgroup for analyses and interpretation of results. Finally, a specific PA intervention, outcome, or predictor must have been present. Studies were excluded if PA was not separated from generally defined "play," "leisure," or "recreational activities."

PA was defined in accordance with the WHO [5], Centers for Disease Control and Prevention (CDC) [19], and Compendium of Physical Activities [20]. The WHO [5] defines PA as "any bodily movement produced by skeletal muscles that requires energy expenditure" (p. 53). Similarly, the CDC [19] Glossary of Terms describes PA as "any bodily movement produced by the contraction of skeletal muscle that increases energy expenditure above a basal level" (p. 1). After consulting the Compendium of Physical Activities [20], the definition of PA was narrowed for the purpose of the current review. As such, the definition of PA was concurrent with the CDC [19] and the definition of health-enhancing PA described as "activity that, when added to baseline activity, produces health benefits. Brisk walking, jumping rope, dancing, playing tennis or soccer, lifting weights, climbing on playground equipment at recess, and doing yoga are all examples of health-enhancing physical activity" (p. 1). Studies were excluded if the PA did not fit this definition.

Figure 1 depicts a summary of the phases of the review process. The initial search produced 1823 articles. Titles were screened to remove irrelevant articles and duplicates. The first two authors subsequently appraised abstracts. Finally, full texts were assessed based on the specific inclusion and exclusion criteria outlined previously. A total of 69 articles were included in the final review. Articles were sorted into five categories: (1) levels of PA (n = 10); (2) predictors related to PA (n = 4); (3) PA related to other outcome variables (n = 4): (4) PA interventions leading to changes in other outcome variables (n = 30); and (5) interventions that lead to changes in PA (n = 5). Categories 1 (levels of PA) and 2 (predictors related to PA) were combined in consideration of articles that assessed both variables (n = 16 for a total n = 30). Each article was critically analyzed based on the following components: descriptive information, research methodology, participant characteristics, physical activity measures and/or intervention, outcome measures, and overall findings. Findings were then synthesized.

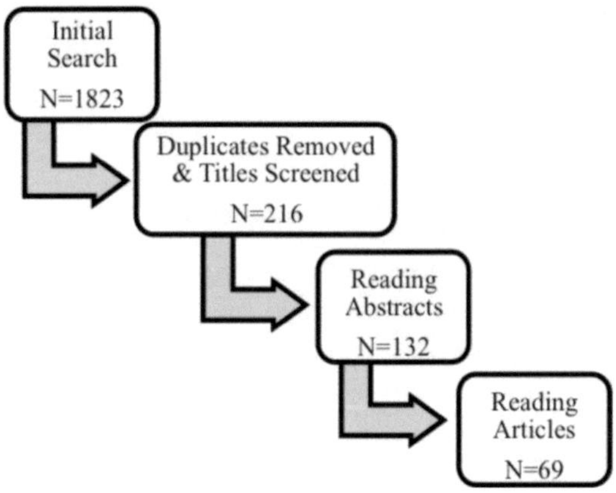

Figure 1. Summary of the different phases of the review.

3. Results

3.1. Levels of PA and predictors related to PA

Thirty cross-sectional studies (see **Table 1**) that assessed levels of PA (n = 10) [18, 21–28], predictors related to PA, (n = 4) [6, 30–32], or both (n = 16) [16, 17, 33–46] were obtained. Accelerometers were implemented as a primary measure in 59% of studies [16, 18, 21, 24–29, 33, 34, 37, 40, 42–44] and greater than half of studies were published in the USA (n = 15) [6, 17, 18, 21, 23, 24, 27, 31–33, 35, 39–41, 54] or Taiwan (n = 8) [16, 25, 26, 28, 29, 42–44]. Twenty-one articles included more male than female participants [6, 17, 18, 21–27, 30–35, 37–41, 45, 46], and seven studies included only male participants [16, 28, 29, 30 42–44]. Participants ranged in age from 3 to 21 years of age. Taken together, findings revealed lower levels of PA in individuals with ASD when compared directly to their typically developing peers [16, 18, 22, 23, 26, 28, 33, 36, 43, 44, 46], previous reports of typically developing children and/or CDC requirements [21, 27, 29, 38]; however, other studies reported no difference. More specifically, Boddy et al. [34] identified similar PA levels, albeit few children were active enough to meet recommended guidelines. Macdonald et al. [24] identified no difference when controlling for intelligence quotient, severity, and gender. Similarly, Corvey et al. [17] found no association between ASD and PA, although children with more severe symptoms were more sedentary. Pan et al. [43] revealed no difference in PA levels; however, children with ASD accumulated fewer steps per minute. Predictors related to PA included age, sex, family structure, SES, and the number and types of barriers and facilitators. For example, PA was greater in males than females [7] and decreased as a function of increasing age [21, 24, 27, 29, 33, 37, 38, 41].

3.2. PA related to other outcome variables

Four studies [47–49] were included (see **Table 2**), 75% of which were conducted in the USA [47, 48, 59]. Three studies included more male participants than females [47, 49, 50]. One study included participants between the ages of 4 and 6 years of age [49], whereas the remaining studies assessed 9- to 17-year-olds [47, 48, 50]. Studies were cross-sectional in nature,

Author(s)	Year/ Country	Purpose	Participants	Method	Primary measures	Main findings
Ayvazoglu et al. [21]	2015 USA	Assess MVPA	ASD: N = 6 (ages 4–13, 4 male; 1 A, 2 HFA, 1 PDD-NOS, 2 AS), 6 mothers (ages 30–51)	Cross-sectional	RT3 accelerometer—7d—MVPA	- Low levels of MVPA—2/6 children close to CDC recommendations - Decrease in PA with age
Borremans et al. [22]	2010 Finland	Assess physical fitness and PA levels	AS: n = 30 (ages 15–21, 21 male), TD: n = 30 (ages 16–19, 21 male)	Cross-sectional	Eurofit, PARQ	- ASD: Lower physical fitness scores and levels of PA; Less intense PA; Prefer solitary activities
Breslin et al. [23]	2015 USA	Determine HR response and PA levels in response to free play PE experience	ASD: n = 3, all male, TD: n = 4 (2 male) (ages 4.33–6.83)	Single-subject design	Actiheart HR monitor — PAHR—Tues/Thurs every other week for 6 weeks—morning free play	- ASD and TD: Similar HR response before, during, and after play session - ASD: % Time above PAHR-50 greater for TD - ASD: Less MVPA vs. TD
Macdonald et al. [24]	2011 USA	Describe sedentary and MVPA patterns with age	ASD: N = 72 (ages 9–18, 55 male)	Cross-sectional	Actical® accelerometer—7d prior to adapted PA intervention—4 days included: sedentary activity, MVA, VPA; WASI; SRS; BMI	- No difference in PA based on IQ, severity or gender - Differences in sedentary/MVPA time (total, in school, after school and evening): older children more sedentary and less active
Pan [25]	2008b Taiwan	Compare PA (ASD, WD) during inclusive recess settings	ASD: n = 24 (ages 7–12, 23 male;12 mild/HFA, 9 7moderate A, 3 AS), WD: n = 24 (ages 7–12, 23 male)	Cross-sectional	GT1M ActiGraph accelerometer—5d PA: % time MVPA (daily overall recess, AM/PM1,2,3, lunchtime	- Activity levels during overall recess: WD greater than ASD - No pattern in MVPA according to specific recess time period (WD+ASD)
Pan [26]	2008a Taiwan	Compare PA (PE + recess), assess contribution to health-related guidelines, assess MVPA	ASD: n = 24 (ages 7–12, 23 male, 20 A, 3 AS, WD: n = 24 (ages 7–12, all male)	Cross-sectional	GT1M ActiGraph accelerometer—5d: %MVPA (PE and recess)	- ASD: Greater %MVPA during PE vs. recess relative to time spent in settings - ASD and WD: Activity levels similar during PE but ASD less active during recess vs. WD
Pan and Frey [27]	2006 USA	Examine weekday/ weekend PA and within day-time period to determine patterns	ASD: N = 30 (ages 10–19, 27 male; 14 A, 12 AS, 4 PDD-NOS)	Cross-sectional	MTI 7164 uniaxial accelerometer—4d: CPM, MVPA (total, 5-/10/20-min bouts; CAAL	- Participants less active vs. previous reports on TD peers - Decline in PA with age - Some meet recommended amount – varies with age - No patterns in overall PA/MVPA

Author(s)	Year/ Country	Purpose	Participants	Method	Primary measures	Main findings
Pan et al. [28]	2015 Taiwan	Assess PA (school day), compliance with guidelines for MVPA, and if compliance differs (ASD vs. TD)	ASD: n = 30,TD: n = 30 (ages 12–17, all male)	Cross-sectional	GT1M ActiGraph accelerometer—5d: daily average PA: CPM, %MPA, %VPA, %MVPA; total during periods	- Daily PA (CPM, %MPA, %MVPA) higher among TD - All more active in PE vs. recess, lunchtime, and after-school - ASD: lower time in MVPA vs. TD (PE, recess and lunchtime) - ASD: lower compliance with MVPA guidelines during each period of day
Pan et al. [29]	2011 Taiwan	Examine differences in patterns PA among weekdays/weekend days and among different time periods	ASD: N = 35 (ages 7–12, lower gr. 1–2: n = 13; middle gr. 3–4: n = 13; upper gr. 5–6: n = 9; all male, 13AS, 22 A)	Cross-sectional	MTI Actigraph 7164 accelerometer—% total PA, CPM, %MPA, %VPA, %MVPA	- No differences in MVPA for each time period to daily total MVPA, but differences in periods - Lower grade more active overall - Upper grade more active on weekdays - Lower/middle grade more active on weekend
Tyler et al. [18]	2014 USA	Determine physical fitness and PA levels	ASD: N = 17, (ages 9–17, 9 male), TD: N = 12 (ages 9–14, 6 male)	Cross-sectional	ActiGraph GTX3+ accelerometer: 7d 20-meter multistage shuttle run, sit-and-reach test, handgrip, BMI	- ASD more sedentary, less physically active (less time in LPA, MPA and MVPA) and fit (strength) compared to TD, but flexibility, aerobic fitness and BMI similar
Kuo et al. [30]	2013 Canada	Investigate perceptions, and potential factors linked with friendships; Explore activities engaged in with friends, gender differences, and types of friends	ASD: N = 91 (ages 12–18, 74 male), parents: (M_{age} = 47.2% fathers)	Cross-sectional	2 activity reports; questionnaire about relationship with best friend; parent-report family background/friend; SCQ	- ASD: 37% engage in PA with friends (33% of males, 57% of females)
McCoy et al. [6]	2016 USA	Determine relationship between sedentary behaviors, daily PA and BMI	ASD: N = 915 (ages 10–17, 81% male) TD: N = 41,879 (ages 10–17, 52% male)	Secondary analysis	NSCH: Severity/ classification, BMI, PA, screen time, computer usage, electronic media in bedroom, sport/club participation Covariates: age, sex, school setting, household income, highest level of education in household, comorbid ADHD	- ASD more likely to be overweight/obese vs. TD - ASD less likely to engage in regular PA, sports and clubs vs. TD

Author(s)	Year/ Country	Purpose	Participants	Method	Primary measures	Main findings
Obrusnikova and Miccinello [31]	2012 USA	Investigate parent perceptions of factors that influence afterschool PA participation	ASD: n = 104 (ages 5–21; 42% A, 41% AS, 18% PDD-NOS) Parents: n = 103 (ages 29–57, 85 male)	Cross-sectional	Online questionnaire: demographics, ASD diagnosis, relationship to child, advantages/disadvantages, barriers/facilitators to PA	- 69% advantages and 31% disadvantages of afterschool PA participation reported - Physical most frequently cited, followed by psychosocial and cognitive - Disadvantages either psychosocial or physical
Stanish et al. [32]	2015 USA	Assess PA enjoyment, perceived barriers, beliefs, and self-efficacy	ASD: n = 35 (ages 13–21, 29 male); TD: n = 60 (ages 13–18, 36 males)	Cross-sectional (*Test-retest reliability assessed for subset: n = 15 with ASD, n = 20 TD)	26-item closed ended questionnaire—7-items targeted PA enjoyment and preferences for where and with whom youth participate	- Enjoyment of walking/individual sports did not differ (ASD vs. TD), ASD do not like gym glass/team sports; prefer "something else" to sports or exercise in free time; reported sports/exercise a lot of fun, but less than TD - Beliefs: ASD less likely to report sports/exercise as a way to make friends, make them feel good vs. TD; positive response about doing more sports/exercise but less than TD - Barriers: ASD—getting hurt (would stop participation), too hard to learn (low n but greater than TD)
Bandini et al. [33]	2013 USA	Assess PA levels and relationship with BMI	ASD: N = 53 (ages 3–11, 44 male) TD: N = 58 (ages 3–11, 45 male)	Cross-sectional	Actical® accelerometer—7d, min and %time in LPA, MPA, VPA, MVPA; activity count, total daily activity, Checklist: frequencies/types of PA	- No differences overall (ASD/TD) - Control for sex/age: total activity counts/time spent MPA greater in TD - Parental report of time spent in/variety of PAs correlated for both ASD and TD, but ASD: less time/activities, younger greater than older
Boddy et al. [34]	2015 UK	Investigate levels of habitual PA/recess play behaviors, differences by sex, age group, and ID group	N = 70 (ages 5–15, M = 9.97, 57 male)—ASD/non-ASD group—n differed for each measure	Cross-sectional	BMI; ActiGraph accelerometer—3/7d—sedentary time, LPA, MPA, VPA, MVPA; SOCARP	- PA: No difference between groups—few active enough to benefit health - No difference boys/girls - ASD: less time standing, more time engaged in very active PA vs non-ASD

Author(s)	Year/ Country	Purpose	Participants	Method	Primary measures	Main findings
Corvey et al. [17]	2016 USA	Examine obesity/ overweight, sedentary behaviors, and PA levels	N = 65,680 (weighted = 49,586,134)—ASD (ages 12–17, n = 986,352, 816,263 male)	Cross-sectional	NSCH: Obesity, overweight, PA, sedentary behavior	- ASD: Obesity higher - No differences: PA rates/sedentary behavior vs. TD but severe ASD more sedentary
Getchell et al. [35]	2012 USA	Compare EE during walking/running and compare EE/MVPA during Nintendo Wii with walking/ running	HFA: N = 15 (M = 17.50, SD = 2.4, 12 male) TD: N = 15 (M = 17.23, SD = 4.1, 6 male)	Cross-sectional	Actical accelerometer —2 or 3 activities in 2 weeks in PE: EE and MVPA	- Similar EE as TD, but HFA greater in Wii Fit - HFA: Nearly met daily recommended MVPA in DDR
Mangerud et al. [36]	2014 Norway	Assess frequency of PA and participation in individual/team sports, associations across psychiatric disorders, and if PA related to use of psychotropic medication, BMI, and chronic pain.	Clinical: n = 566—ASD: n = 39 (82% AS), TD: n = 8173 (ages 13–18)	Cross-sectional	Questions: Frequency/time spent in PA outside school, chronic pain, BMI, SES	- Threefold increased risk of lower levels of PA overall for ASD - Low levels of PA, and of all groups, lowest participation in team sports - ASD and mood disorders most inactive vs. other disorders
Memari et al. [37]	2013 Iran	Address demographics/ other factors affecting PA and examine time-activity patterns	ASD: N = 90 (ages 7–14, 55 male)	Cross-sectional	GT3X Actigraph™ accelerometer—7d: time sheet/activity log—overall PA, time in PA (weekdays, weekends, in/after-school), survey: health status	- Lowest PA levels in 13-to 14-year-olds, girls (weekdays, after-school, overall), single-parent children, obesity group, with comorbidity - Less active in vs. after-school
Memari et al. [38]	2015 Iran	Assess participation in physical and daily activities and examine individual/social factors contributing to the level of participation in leisure PAs.	HFASD: N = 83 (ages 6–15, 53 male)	Cross-sectional	Checklist adapted from Godin-Shephard Leisure Time Questionnaire, parent-report barriers,	- Few children met minimum PA criteria—only 12% physically active - Low due to finances, lack of resources/ opportunities - Low social/high solitary play during typical day - Male greater than female - Negative effect of age

http://dx.doi.org/10.5772/66680

Author(s)	Year/ Country	Purpose	Participants	Method	Primary measures	Main findings
Must et al. [39]	2015 USA	Compare prevalence of parent-reported child/ family, social, and community barriers and assess association of barriers to PA with parent-reported levels of PA and total screen time	ASD: n = 53 (ages 3–11, 44 male), TD: n = 58 (ages 3–11, 45 male,)	Cross-sectional	17-item questionnaire (perceived child/family, social, community barriers to PA; Questionnaire—types + frequency of PA in 12 months (17 activities total); Question about hours of screen time in past week	- Greater number of child/family, social and community barriers to PA (ASD) for nearly every barrier question; greater than half (ASD) reported 6+ barriers to PA; most common: poor motor skills, behavior and learning problems, need supervision - Similar barriers (ASD/TD): time constraints, lack of transportation, neighborhood safety - ASD: Positive relationship between age and total number of barriers, and social barriers - Total number of barriers: Inversely correlated with number of PA hours and types of activities per year; directly related to total screen time
Obrusnikova and Cavalier [40]	2011 USA	Assess barriers/ facilitators of after-school MVPA and determine if PA patterns exist in relation to barriers	ASD: N = 14 (ages 8–14, M = 10.64, SD = 1.65, 12 male; 1A, 10 AS, 3 PDD-NOS)	Cross-sectional	SRS; Actical accelerometer—7d in 14-d period, Photovoice (barriers/ facilitators of after-school MVPA	- All: More time LPA vs. MVPA - 3 met minimum MVPA on all days, 5 did not meet minimum MVPA on any days - Barriers: time in sedentary activities, lack of partner - Facilitators: good equipment, community programs
Orsmond and Kuo [41]	2011 USA	Describe activities, who engaged with, factors associated with time spent in, and if had effect on symptoms	ASD: N = 103 (ages 12.7–21.8, 75.7% male)	Cross-sectional — From longitudinal	Mother-report 24-h time diaries—activity participation (weekday + weekend day)	- PA third most frequency discretionary activity (47% of participants, total mean = 0.56 h), behind watching TV and computer use - Discretionary time spent along or with mothers, little time with peers - Time use associated with: age, gender, presence of ID, family income, marital status, maternal education

Author(s)	Year/ Country	Purpose	Participants	Method	Primary measures	Main findings
Pan [42]	2009 Taiwan	Examine associations of age, social engagement and PA in structured (PE) and unstructured (recess) play opportunities	ASD N = 25 (ages 7–12, all male, all A)	Cross-sectional	BMI, GTIM ActiGraph—5d, PA—1 PE class + 1 recess: SPM, CPM, MVPA, VPA; Engagement Check	- More active physically/socially during PE vs. recess - Age positively correlated with CPM, SPM in recess, 5-min MVPA in PE, peer-interactive and total social engagement during PE - Non-interactive engagement with adults during PE positively correlated with VPA and SPM
Pan et al. [43]	2011 Taiwan	Assess PA, environment/ personal correlates that influence PA during PE	ASD: n = 19 (M = 14.19, SD = 0.82, all male); TD (n = 76, M = 14.10, SD = 0.80, all male)	Cross-sectional	GTIM ActiGraph—2 PE lessons in 1 week: CPM, SPM, %MPA, %VPA, %MVPA; Social interaction/initiation frequency	- No differences in PA, but ASD lower SPM than TD - Social initiations in ASD positively correlated with CPM, SPM, %MVPA - Social interactions in ASD positively correlated with CPM, %MPA, %VPA, %MVPA - Fitness/free-play: higher MVPA vs. team/ individual activities, more active with female teachers, non-certified teachers, outdoor, in combined spaces (all)
Pan et al. [16]	2011 Taiwan	Examine differences in PA, motivational processes in PE, associations between PA/ patterns of motivational processes	ASD: n = 25 (M = 14.26, SD = 0.89, all male), WD: n = 75 (M = 14.08, SD = 0.80), all male	Cross-sectional	ActiGraph GTM1 accelerometer during 2 PE lessons—%MPA, %VPA, %MVPA, SPM; modified MPES	- ASD: less active (less walking, %MPA, %VPA, %MVPA), variable and externally regulated - ASD: less perceived competence/ relatedness, lower intrinsic motivation, identified regulation and introjected regulation, motivation higher, SDI lower, effort, enjoyment in PE and intention to be active lower - Similar motivational processes for ASD and WD
Pan et al. [44]	2016 Taiwan	Compare physical fitness/PA levels, assess relationships between PA/physical fitness (weekday vs. weekend)	ASD: n = 35; 10 AS, 25 mild AD, without ASD: n = 13 (ages 12–17, all male)	Cross-sectional	BMI; GT1M accelerometer—7d: min/d, MVPA min/d, CPM, %MVPA; BPFT (pre- / post-PA assessment)	- ASD: less active and less MVPA—37% ASD/60% without ASD met daily 60min+ MVPA standard - ASD: lower physical fitness measures, except body composition

http://dx.doi.org/10.5772/66680

Author(s)	Year/ Country	Purpose	Participants	Method	Primary measures	Main findings
Soden et al. [45]	2012 USA	Assess nutritional intake (diet logs and laboratory testing), determine if low BMD is detectable, and quantify/assess clinical/ medical history data correlates, and parental perceptions of lifestyle with BMD	ASD (N = 26, ages 10–18, 21 male; 6 AS, 9 AD, 11 PDD-NOS)	Cross-sectional	- 5-point likert scale (dietary pickiness, PA, sunlight, electronic media use; Fan beam DXA—BMD of lumbar spine); parent-report food, beverage, supplement intake, minutes of sunlight PE and electronic media use over 72 h	- Mean PA less than 1/3 mean electronic media use - Parent rating: 13 extremely/somewhat picky, 13 little to no exercise or less than average amount of exercise, 8 average media greater than 3 h per day - Parents perceptions of PA, electronic media use, sunlight exposure correlated with 3-d activity diaries - High screen time to PA ratio
Taheri et al. [46]	2016 Canada	Compare social participation, quantity and quality of friendships	ASD: n = 232, 79.7% male); TD: n = 210, 69% male); ID: n = 186, 56.8% male); ages 3–19	Cross-sectional	GO4KIDDS questionnaire: child/parent demographics, activities questionnaire, # friends	- ID and ID+ASD less than TD: fewer social activities, participate less often - ID+ASD less than ID in special occasions with friends and in taking lessons

Note: See Appendix A for list of abbreviations used in this table.

Table 1. Articles that assessed levels of PA (light gray), predictors related to PA (dark gray), or both (no shading).

Author(s)	Year/Country	Purpose	Participants	Method	Primary measures	Main findings
Dreyer Gillette et al. [47]	2015 USA	Examine prevalence of overweight/obesity and how health behaviors relate to weight status	N = 45,000 responses (ages 10–17; non-ASD: 50.3% male; ASD: n = 900, 84% male)	Cross-sectional	NSCH: ASD diagnosis, weight/height, sleep, VPA, family meals, time spent watching TV/videos/playing games, with electronic devices, screen in bedroom	- ASD: more likely to have 0 days/week with 20-min VPA; less likely to get 4–6 days of VPA/week - Groups did not differ on likelihood of engaging in VPA 1–3 days/week - ASD: less PA, no differences (sleep, most measures screen time, mealtimes), overweight/obese did not differ from normal weight peers with ASD on days of engaging in VPA
McManus et al. [48]	2012 USA	Examine relationship between parent-child function and adolescent PA/TV viewing, and whether parent-child function is important	N = 86,777, ages 10–17, 1.5(0.1)%A	Cross-sectional	NSCH: Frequency of PA/TV viewing in week; age, race, ethnicity, presence of SHCN, BMI; primary caregiver education, physical health, exercise; family structure, function and income	- Low parent-child function linked to less PA and more TV viewing - Higher parent-child function influential: At mean parent-child function score, adolescents with A 43% less likely to meet PA recommendations; Unit increase in score associated with 39% lower likelihood of engaging in recommended PA
Tatsumi et al. [49]	2014 Japan	Investigate association between daytime PA and sleep quantity/quality	ASD: N = 31 (ages 51–70 months, 25 male); TD: N = 16 (ages 61–68 months, 10 male)	Cross-sectional	Actiwatch 2 accelerometer, 7 days: sleep onset, sleep-end time, total sleep duration, snooze time, sleep %, PA (CPM); CBCL ages 4–18	- 8 CBCL items (withdrawal, anxiety/depression, social problems, thought problems, attention problems, delinquent, and aggressive behaviors) higher in ASD - Sleep % higher, snooze time longer, % poor sleepers greater, TD vs. ASD - PA not different on weekdays (ASD vs. TD) but longer on weekend mornings (ASD) - Sleep % not modulated by PA but sleep onset earlier on active day - PA can advance sleep phase in ASD
Wachob and Lorenzi [50]	2015 USA	Determine relationship that engagement in MVPA has on healthy sleep patterns	ASD: N = 10 (ages 9–16, 9 male)	Cross-sectional	CSHQ; Actigraph GT3X+ (ActiSleep) accelerometer, 7 days: sedentary time, MVPA (weekday, weekend, in school after-school), sleep efficiency, WASO; BMI	- Age contributed to PA - Less active in vs. afterschool - Older participants more sedentary and more disturbed sleep patterns - No relationship: sleep and CSHQ, BMI and test variables - Negative relationship: MVPA and WASO time - more PA children had overall higher sleep quality

Note: See Appendix A for list of abbreviations used in this table.

Table 2. Articles that assessed the relationship between PA and other outcome variables.

assessing the relationship between PA and sleep (n = 2), [49, 50] parent-child functioning (n = 1) [48], TV viewing frequency (n = 1 [48], weight status (n = 1) [47], and child behavior (n = 1) [49]. Findings revealed that: (1) PA is related to sleep [49, 50]; (2) with an increase in parent-child functioning, there is an increase in PA [48]; and (3) overweight/obesity is not related to days of engaging in vigorous PA for children with ASD [47].

3.3. PA interventions leading to change in other outcome variables

Thirty studies [51–80] (see **Table 3**) were included, where over half (n = 16) were published in the USA. Only five articles included individuals over the age of 18 [51, 61, 62, 66, 74]. Eighty percent of the studies were comprised of over half, or all male participants [51, 53, 54, 56–62, 64, 65, 67, 69–75, 77–80]. Nineteen studies used repeated measures designs observing effects pre- and post-intervention [52–56, 58, 60, 61, 64–68, 71–74, 78, 79]. PA interventions most commonly included swimming/aquatic exercise (n = 5) [57, 71–72, 77, 80] and general exercise programs (n = 8, for example, aerobic and weight-bearing exercise, physical education, and recreational programs) [55, 58–59, 61–62, 65–66, 78]. Examples of outcomes included as follows: autistic behaviors and stereotypy [e.g., 53, 65], executive function [51, 73], motor skills [55, 73, 80], sleep [55], anxiety [61, 79] communication/social skills [e.g., 54, 67], exercise specific skills [e.g., 57, 63], and physical fitness [65, 71], where 53.3% of the articles assessed multiple outcomes [51, 55–58, 61, 64, 65, 68, 71–74, 76, 79, 80]. Of the fifty total outcome measures, improvement (n = 41; indicated by ⁺⁺ in **Table 3**), or null effects (n = 9; indicated by ⁺ in **Table 3**) following the PA interventions were reported. Taken together, there is no evidence to suggest that PA interventions have negative effects, nor is there evidence to show one PA intervention is superior to others, likely attributed in part to the multiple outcome measures.

3.4. Interventions that lead to changes in PA

Five studies [81–85] were included (see **Table 4**), of which varying interventions influenced PA. Repeated measures (n = 3) [81, 82, 84] and multiple-baseline (n = 2) [83, 85] designs were used to investigate outcomes pre- and post-intervention. Of these studies, 80% were published in North America (Canada, n = 2; [84, 85] USA, n = 2; [82, 83]). Interventions were mainly PA based (n = 4) [81, 83–85] and included walking, jogging, snowshoeing, and cycling. One study investigated a motor skills intervention. All participant groups included over 50% males, and only two articles included participants over the age of 18 [83, 84]. Four studies [81, 83–85] found an increase in participation and overall levels of PA, whereas one study, focusing on a motor skills intervention, found no difference in PA levels [82]. Together, findings revealed PA and/or health interventions can influence sustained PA levels post-intervention; however, there is insufficient evidence to conclude whether interventions that are not PA-based influence PA levels.

4. Discussion

Taken together, findings revealed lower levels of PA in individuals with ASD [16, 18, 22–23, 26–28, 33, 36, 38, 43, 44, 46]; especially in male children [37, 38] and with increasing age [21,

Authors	Year/ country	Purpose	Participants	Method	Intervention	Outcome measure(s)/number	Main findings
Anderson-Hanley et al. [51]	2011 USA	Assess effects of exergaming on repetitive behaviors and cognitive performance	ASD: N = 22 (ages 8–21, 18 male)	Within-subjects experimental design	DDR or Cybercycling for 20 min	Behavioral assessment: video-taped and coded using GARS-2 Executive function: Digit Span Forward and Backward, The Color Trails Test, and The Stroop task **2 outcomes**	- Behavioral†† and cognitive†† performances increased after exergaming compared to the control condition
Arzoglou et al. [52]	2013 Greece	Investigate effect of a traditional dance program on neuromuscular coordination	ASD: N = 10 (M = 16.8)	Pre-post	Traditional Greek dance: 3x/week, 35-45min	Neuromuscular coordination: KTK Physical characteristics also measured **1 outcome**	- Dance improved the aspects of motor skills and fitness (lateral jumps right to left, lateral movement and repositioning, and total score of test) and neuromuscular coordination††
Bahrami et al. [53]	2012 Iran	Determine if Kata techniques reduce stereotypic behaviors	ASD: N = 30 (ages 5–16, 26 male)	Pre-post	Kata: 14 weeks, 4x/week 30-90 min/session	Stereotypy severity: GARS-2 **1 outcome**	- Kata intervention reduced stereotypic behaviors††
Bahrami et al. [54]	2016 Iran	Determine if karate techniques reduce communication deficits	ASD: N = 30 (ages 5–16, 26 male)	Pre-post	Kata: 14 weeks, 4x/r week, 30–90 min/session	Communication deficits: GARS-2 **1 outcome**	- Karate training improved the communication deficits of children with ASD††
Brand et al. [55]	2015 Switzerland	Explore if aerobic and motor skills training intervention lead to positive changes in sleep and motor skills	ASD: N = 10 (ages 7–13, 5 male; 6A, 3AS, 1 HFASD)	Pre-post	Aerobic exercise and motor skills training: 3x/week for 3 weeks, 30 min biking, 30-min coordination and balance training	Sleep: EEG device, Insomnia Severity Index, Pittsburgh Sleep Quality Index Motor skills: recorded each session, ball skills and balancing **2 outcomes**	- Intervention improved specific motor skills†† (catching, throwing, and balancing) - Improved objectively assessed sleep on nights following PA††

http://dx.doi.org/10.5772/66680

Authors	Year/ country	Purpose	Participants	Method	Intervention	Outcome measure(s)/number	Main findings
Casey et al. [56]	2015 Canada	Evaluate effects of a 12-week therapeutic skating intervention	ASD: N = 2 (ages 7 and 10, both male)	Repeated measures: baseline, weeks 4 and 8	Skating: 1 h 3x/ week, 12 weeks	Dynamic balance: Pediatric Balance Scale and Flamingo Test Functional mobility: 6MWT, Floor to Stand, Timed Up and Go, Timed Up and Down Stairs Test Personal goals: Participant Goal Attainment Scaling **3 outcomes**	- Improvements in balance††, motor behavior, and functional capacity†† following the 12 week skating program - Participant and parental goals were met††
Fragala-Pinkham et al. [57]	2011 USA	Examine effectiveness of a group aquatic exercise program on fitness and swimming skills	ASD: N = 12 (ages 6–12, 11 male; 6AS, 6 PDD-NOS, 1 HFASD)	Randomized control trial; pre- and post-testing	Swimming: 2x/ week for 14 weeks, 40- min sessions	Swimming skills: Swimming Classification Scale, YMCA Water Skills Checklist Cardiorespiratory endurance: half mile walk/run Muscle endurance: curl-up and isometric push-ups Mobility skills: Multidimentional Pediatric Evaluation of Disability Inventory Mobility Scale **4 outcomes**	- Significant improvement in swimming skills†† - No statistically significant results for muscular endurance†, cardiorespiratory endurance†, or mobility†
Fukasawa and Takeda [58]	2012 Japan	Clarify validity of sAA as an index of sympathetic nervous system activity	ASD: N = 7 (ages 107 ± 8 months, all male)	Pre-post	Morning activities: 30 min daily	sAA: sAA monitor Heart rate: pulse oximeter **2 outcomes**	- Post-learning values of sAA and HR significantly higher†† - Total exercise not correlated with change in sAA or HR† - sAA = indicator that can reflect changes in sympathetic nervous system over extended period of time

Authors	Year/ country	Purpose	Participants	Method	Intervention	Outcome measure(s)/number	Main findings
Goodarzi and Hemayattalab [59]	2012 Iran	Assess effects of weight bearing exercise and Ca supplement BMD	ASD: N = 60 (ages 8–10, all male)	Randomized control trial; pre- and post-measurements	Weight bearing exercises: 6 months, 3x/week, 50 min/session Ca: 250 mg/d	BMD: X-ray Absorptiometry **1 outcome**	- Weight bearing exercise and CA affected BMD - Exercise in combination with Ca most effective††
Gruber and Poulson [60]	2016 USA	Assess effects of a parent-implemented graduated guidance and reinforcement to teach yoga poses	ASD: N = 3 (ages 3–4, 2 male)	Multiple baseline design across subjects; pre- and post-testing	Yoga: DVD with a parent, 3x/week, 92 days	Independent responses: If child did same poses as video model Customer satisfaction survey **1 outcome**	- Systematic increase of independent responses across all participants with the introduction of the intervention††
Hillier et al. [61]	2010 USA	Examine reductions in stress and anxiety in response to a low-intensity physical exercise and relaxation intervention	ASD: N = 18 (ages13–27, 16 males; 3A, 5 PDD-NOS, 10 AS	Repeated measures; Pre-post 3 sessions	PA program: 8 weeks, 75-min session 1x/week	Cortisol measured Anxiety: Self-report questionnaire **2 outcomes**	- Significant reduction in levels of cortisol at the end of the exercise sessions†† - Short-term within-session decrease in anxiety††
Judge [62]	2015 USA	Examine the effectiveness of a CBFS for students during PE class	ASD: N = 1 (age 19, male)	Single subject A-B-A-B design	CBFS sessions: 15 sessions, 15 min each	Independent transitioning: observational data **1 outcome**	- Functional relationship between use of a CBFS and number of independent transitions†
Kaplan-Reimer et al. [63]	2011 USA	Evaluate use of an intervention package for teaching indoor rock climbing	ASD: N = 2 (ages 11 and 6, both female)	Non-concurrent multiple baseline design across participants	Rock climbing: 45-min sessions, 3x/week	Observational: Did participants grab correct hold color on path **1 outcome**	- Both participants successfully learned how to rock climb††

http://dx.doi.org/10.5772/66680

Authors	Year/ country	Purpose	Participants	Method	Intervention	Outcome measure(s)/number	Main findings
MacDonald et al. [64]	2012 USA	Investigate the effectiveness of an individualized adapted bicycle intervention	ASD: N = 40 (ages 9–18, 26 male) DS: N = 30 (ages 9–18, 14 males)	Pre-post	Bicycling: 5-day intervention	Leg strength: handheld manual muscle tester Standing balance: timed trial for each leg Independent bicycle riding skills: observed **3 outcomes**	- Majority able to ride a bicycle independently upon completion†† - Leg strength greater after intervention†† - Balance not affected between riders and non-riders†
Magnusson et al. [65]	2012 New Zealand	Investigate if an individually-tailored, high-intensity exercise program would have a positive effect on physical fitness and behaviors	ASD: N = 6 (ages 9–15, 4 males; 4A, 1AS, 1 PDD-NOS)	Pre-post	Exercise program: 2x/week, 8–12 weeks	Physical testing: cardiorespiratory fitness, lower and upper body strength, abdominal strength and endurance, lower back and hamstring flexibility, and balance Behaviors: questionnaires **2 outcomes**	- Exercise program improves all physical fitness and behavioral outcomes†† - Increase in positive behaviors and reduces negative behaviors††
Morrison et al. [66]	2011 USA	Extend research on antecedent exercise by incorporating several methodological advances	A: N = 4 (ages 10–21, 2 male)	Pre-post	Preferred exercise: 10- min pre-intervention, 10-min intervention, 10-min post-intervention	Direct observation of problem behaviors **1 outcome**	- Antecedent exercise was effective in suppressing problem behavior during the intervention††
Movahedi et al. [67]	2013 Iran	Determine if teaching Karate techniques leads to improvement in social dysfunction	ASD: N = 30 (ages 5–16, 26 male)	Pre-post	Kata training: 4 sessions/week,14 weeks, 30–90 min/ session	Social interaction: GARS-2 **1 outcome**	- Exercise group demonstrated a improvement in social interaction - Social dysfunction decreased††

Authors	Year/ country	Purpose	Participants	Method	Intervention	Outcome measure(s)/number	Main findings
Neely et al. [68]	2015 USA	Evaluate effects of antecedent physical exercise on stereotypy and academic engagement	ASD: N = 2 (ages 7–8, 1 male)	Pre-post	Trampoline jumping: jumped until specified level of satiation prior to instructional session 3x/week	Stereotypy: 10-s partial interval recording procedure Academic engagement: 10s-whole interval recording procedure **2 outcomes**	- Greatest reduction in stereotypy was following exercise until satiation condition[††] - Academic engagement was highest in the exercise until satiation condition[††]
Nicholson Kehle et al. [69]	2011 USA	Examine the impact of antecedent PA on academic engagement	ASD: N = 4 (age 9, all male)	Single-subject, multiple-baseline design	Jogging: 12-min, 3x/week	Academic engagement: BOSS **1 outcome**	- Positive correlation: time spent jogging and academic engagement[††]
Oriel et al. [70]	2011 USA	Determine if aerobic exercise before classroom activities improved academic engagement and reduces stereotypic behaviors	ASD: N = 9 (ages 3–6, 7 male; 7A, 1 ID, 1 DD)	Within-subjects crossover design	Jogging: 15 min for 3 weeks	Academic engagement: direct observation of children's responses, stereotypic behaviors, and on-task behaviors **1 outcome**	- 7 of the 9 participants improved in correct responding following the treatment condition - No statistically significant improvements in on-task behavior or stereotypic behaviors[†]
Pan [71]	2011 Taiwan	Assess effects of aquatic intervention on aquatic skills and physical fitness	ASD: N = 15 Siblings: N = 15 (ages 7–12, 20 male)	Within-participant repeated-measures design	Aquatic skills program: 14 weeks, 2x/week, 60-min/session	Physical fitness: PACER Aquatic skills: HAAR checklist **2 outcomes**	- Increase in all aquatic skills[††] and physical fitness[††] subtests except body composition
Pan [72]	2010 Taiwan	Determine effectiveness of a WESP on the aquatic skills and social behaviors	ASD: N = 16 (ages 6–9, all male; 8 HFA, 8 AS)	Within-participant repeated-measures design	Swimming program: 10 weeks, 2 sessions/ week, 90-min/ session	Aquatic skills: HAAR checklist Social behaviors: SSBS-2 **2 outcomes**	- Improved aquatic skills[††] and decreased the antisocial behavior problems[††]

Authors	Year/ country	Purpose	Participants	Method	Intervention	Outcome measure(s)/number	Main findings
Pan et al. [73]	2016 Taiwan	Evaluate effects of PA intervention (table tennis exercise) on motor skill proficiency	ASD: N = 22 (ages 6–12, all male)	Pre-post	Table tennis: 12 weeks, 2x/week, 70-min/session	Motor skill proficiency: The BOT-2 Executive function: WCST **2 outcomes**	- Improvements in the experimental vs. control group in total motor composite[††] and executive functioning[††] - Effect sustained for 12 weeks
Pitetti et al. [74]	2006 USA	Determine the efficacy of a treadmill walking program in weekly academic curriculum	A: N = 10 (ages14–19, 6 male)	Pre-post	Walking: 9 months, 2–5 sessions/week, up to 20-min/session	Caloric expenditure: VO_2 and equations BMI: body measurements **2 outcomes**	- Increase in exercise capacity and monthly caloric expenditure[††] decrease in BMI[††]
Reynolds et al. [75]	2016 USA	Examine bicycle riding maintenance and differences from parent-report 1 year following bicycle camp	ASD: N = 51 (ages 9–18, 42 male)	Observation after bicycle camp, follow-up with parents 1 year after completion of camp	Bicycle camp: 5 consecutive days, 75 min/day	Parent-report: child's maintenance of riding skills one year after the camp **1 outcome**	- 86% rode 100 feet independently by the end of the week - HSC group reported higher rates of rider retention[††]
Ringenbach et al. [76]	2015 USA	Determine effects of ACT versus VC on motor and cognitive function in adolescents with ASD	ASD: N = 10 (ages: 8–16, 5 male)	Within-subjects, randomized crossover design	Cycling: Three sessions on non-consecutive days, 20 min/session	Dexterity: Purdue Pegboard test Cognitive and functional assessments: Exercise Perception Scale, Off-task Behavior Assessment, Stroop task, Trail Making Test, reaction time test, The Tower of London test **2 outcomes**	- Positive effects on motor[††] and cognitive[††] functioning in clinical populations with compromised nervous system function, low exercise motivation, and reduced cognition and motor function

Authors	Year/ country	Purpose	Participants	Method	Intervention	Outcome measure(s)/number	Main findings
Rogers et al. [77]	2010 USA	Determine if 4s CTD procedure is effective in teaching foundational swimming skills	A: N = 3 (ages 3–4, all male)	Multiple-probe design	Swimming: 2–3x/ week, 45–60-min/ session, using CTD	Target behaviors observed **1 outcome**	- CTD procedure was effective in teaching foundational swimming skills††
Sarol and Cimen [78]	2015 Turkey	Determine effect of ARPA program on the life quality	ASD: N = 59 (ages 4–18, 42 male)	Pre-post	ARPA program: 8 weeks, 2 sessions/ week, 2 h/session	Life quality: PedsQL **1 outcome**	- Increase in physical and emotional functionality, no change in social functionality or school aspects††
Strahan and Elder [79]	2015 USA	Determine feasibility and effectiveness of active video game playing	ASD: N = 1 (age 15, male)	Pre-post	Wii video game: 6 weeks, 4+ x/week, minimum of 30 min/day	Body measurements: weight, BMI, triceps skin fold, waist-to-hip ratio Stress and anxiety: Stress Survey Schedule for Persons with Autism and Other Developmental Delays, and Behavior Assessment System for Children Second Edition **2 outcomes**	- Reductions in weight after introduction of the active video gaming†† - Stress and anxiety: minimal changes from pre- to post-intervention†
Yanardag et al. [80]	2013 Turkey	Examine effectiveness of video prompting on teaching aquatic play skills, and the effect on motor performance	A: N = 3 (ages 6–8, 2 male)	Multiple-probe design across behaviors	Aquatic exercise: 12 weeks, 3 sessions/week, 1 h/session	Aquatic play skills: observation Motor skills: MABC-2 **2 outcomes**	- Increase in correct target skills, and maintenance observed†† - Aquatic training improved motor performance skills††

Note: See Appendix A for list of abbreviations used in this table.

Table 3. Articles that assessed PA interventions leading to changes in other outcome variables.

Author(s)	Year/ Country	Purpose	Participants	Method	Intervention	Outcome	Main findings
Hinckson et al. [81]	2013 New Zealand	Determine effectiveness of program on PA, dietary habits and overall health	Total: N = 17 (ages 7+, M = 14Y 4M, 10 male—A subgroup: n = 7, 5 male)	Repeated Measures (pre- /post-intervention)	10 weeks, 2x/week, 18 sessions of 1 h PA (family + students), 10 1 h healthy eating and 8 1-h motivational skills (parents/care givers)	PA (active/inactive time, PA vs. age group, time in MVPA, start a new sport, activities longer than 30 min/week), nutrition (frequency of breakfast, carbonated drinks, white bread, wholegrain, and confectionary, and cooking fresh food), 6MWT, BMI, waist circumference qualitative interview	- Trend for increased distance in 6MWT 6 24-week post-intervention
Ketcheson et al. [82]	2016 USA	Measure efficacy of motor skill intervention on motor skills and levels of PA, and changes in socialization behavior in experimental group	Experimental: n = 11 (ages 4–6, 9 male) Control: n = 9 (ages 4–6, 6 male)	Repeated Measures (pre- /post-/ follow-up)	8 weeks, 4h/day 5 days/week, weekly rotation between TGMD-2 subtests (4-week object control, 4-weeks locomotion)	All participants: TGMD-2, ActiGraph GT3X+ accelerometer (3 days, 3 h wear time) sedentary PA, LPA, MPA, VPA, MVPA Experimental group: POPE	- Experimental group: Increase in locomotor, object control, partial and gross quotient scores - Trend for decreasing min in solitary time - No difference in PA; both groups met or exceeded PA guidelines but spend majority of day (8 h) sedentary
Lalonde et al. [83]	2014 USA	Examine procedure for young adults with ASD to walk long/often enough to meet/exceed minimum guidelines for aerobic activity	ASD: N = 5 (ages 21–26, 4 male)	Multiple-baseline across participants design	Walking with specified step number goals daily; 25–42 s depending on participant	Number of steps taken: Zip Wireless Activity Tracker by FitBit Follow-up questions asked to participants about wearing the FitBit and goals Teacher asked questions from the modified TARF-F	- Differences in the number of SPD at baseline,—During treatment, all participants met the goal of 10,000 SPD
Todd and Reid [84]	2006 Canada	Investigate impact of an intervention (edible reinforcers, verbal cuing, and self-monitoring) on sustained PA	ASD: N = 3 (ages 15–20, all male)	Pre-post	Showshoeing and walking/jogging: 6-month program, 2 sessions/week, 30 min/session	Number of circuits completed at end of each session	- Instructional strategy with self-monitoring, verbal cuing, and edible reinforcers: increased sustained participation
Todd et al. [85]	2010 Canada	Investigate impact of intervention (goal setting, self-monitoring, and self-reinforcement) on sustained PA, and monitor self-efficacy	ASD: N = 3 (ages 15–17, 2 male)	Multiple-baseline changing criterion design	Cycling: 3 days/ week from March to June, 30 min/session, total 31 sessions completed	Distance and goal setting (intensity, distance, self-efficacy)	- Distance travelled increased (n = 2) - Attention to attitudes required in self-determined behavior is beneficial when designing interventions to increase PA for ASD

Note: See Appendix A for list of abbreviations used in this table.

Table 4. Articles including interventions that led to changes in PA.

24, 27, 29, 33, 37, 38, 44]. Nevertheless, studies that report no difference were also common [e.g., 17, 34]. Barriers to PA include, but are not limited to, finances, lack of resources and opportunities, poor motor skills, behavioral and learning problems, the need for supervision, family time constraints, lack of a partner, and lack of available transportation. Must et al. [39] reported a positive relationship between age and the total number of barriers. Furthermore, the number of barriers was inversely related to the number of PA hours and total number and types of activities per year. Facilitators to PA included good equipment and community programs.

There was evidence that PA interventions can improve certain outcome measures, such as communication, balance, and fitness levels [e.g., 54, 56, 71]; however, it is also important to note that others observed no effect [e.g., 62, 70]. Importantly, there was no evidence to suggest that PA interventions cause negative effects. Interventions that aimed to address levels of PA specifically found that PA interventions lead to increased PA levels, while one motor skill intervention [82] was not effective. Overall, no one intervention was suggested as optimal for decreasing negative and/or promoting positive behaviors.

Common limitations included small sample sizes with little ethnic and socioeconomic diversity that limited generalizability and underpowered analyses. Unequal sex distributions were repeatedly observed, as many participant groups were comprised of mainly males. It is important to consider that this may be a result of the intrinsic property of ASD being five times more prevalent in males than in females (CDC, 2014). Assessments of PA levels were limited, in some cases by parent-report assessments, where more objective assessments (i.e., accelerometer data) were limited by compliance, and the inability of the tool to assess all PAs (e.g., water activities). With respect to interventions, short durations were commonly reported. Furthermore, studies investigating a change in PA as the outcome variable were limited. Finally, most studies included children that were high functioning on the spectrum. Methodologically this review was limited to four search engines, and papers published within the last decade. Unpublished studies and studies published in languages other than English were not included. The quality of the studies was also not evaluated. These may have biased the results.

Future research of PA interventions should investigate the legitimacy and benefits of specific PA interventions, which may help determine the effects of distinct outcome measures. Furthermore, research on interventions leading to a change in PA should investigate non-PA interventions in the future to determine the plausibility of changing PA levels through other intervention methods (i.e., motor skill interventions). In addition, it would be beneficial to investigate the long-term changes in PA following these interventions to determine whether this effect is sustained over time. Overall, research investigating physical activity for individuals with ASD should be explored with larger sample sizes, over longer time periods and across the spectrum. This would provide more comprehensive information on the pros and cons of physical activity for this vulnerable population.

Appendix A

Abbreviations included in the tables

Word/Phrase	*Abbreviation*
Adapted Recreational Physical Activity	ARPA
Asperger's Syndrome Assisted Cycling Therapy	AS ACT
Attention Deficit/Hyperactivity Disorder	ADHD
Autism	A
Autism Spectrum Disorder	ASD
Behavioral Observation of Students in Schools	BOSS
Body Mass Index	DMI
Bone Mineral Density	BMD
Brockport Physical Fitness Test	BPFT
Bruininks-Oseretsky Test of Motor Proficiency Second Edition	BOT-2
Calcium	Ca
Child Behavior Checklist	CBCL
Child/Adolescent Activity Log	CAAL
Children's Activity Rating Scale	CARS
Children's Sleep Habits Questionnaire	CSHQ
Computer-Based Fitness Schedule Constant Time Delay	CBFS CTD
Counts Per Minute	CPM
Dance Dance Revolution	DDR
Day	d
Developmental Delay	DD
Down Syndrome	DS
Dual-Energy X-ray Absorptiometry	DXA
Energy Expenditure	EE
Gilliam Autism Rating Scale-Second Edition	GARS-2
Great Outcomes for Kids Impacted by Severe Developmental Disabilities	GO4KIDDS
Heart Rate	HR
High Functioning Autism	HFA
High Functioning Autism Spectrum Disorder Home-Support Consultation	HFASD HSC
Humpfries Assessment of Aquatic Readiness	HAAR
Intellectual Disability	ID
KorperkoordinationstestfurKinder	KTK
Light Physical Activity	LPA
Light to Moderate to Vigorous Physical Activity	LMVPA
Mean	M
Metabolic Equivalent	MET
Minute	min
Moderate Physical Activity	MPA
Moderate to Vigorous Physical Activity	MVPA

Motivation in Physical Education Scale	MPES
Movement Assessment Battery for Children Second Edition	MABC-2
National Survey of Children's Health	NSCH
Neurotypical	NT
Observational System for Recording Physical Activity of Children-Preschool	OSRAC-P
Progressive Aerobic Cardiovascular Endurance Run	PACER
Pediatric Quality of Life Inventory	PedsQL
Pervasive Developmental Disorder – Not Otherwise Specified	PDD-NOS
Physical Activity	PA
Physical Activity Heart Rate	PAHR
Physical Activity Research Questionnaire	PARQ
Physical Education	PE
Playground Observation of Peer Engagement	POPE
Salivary Alpha-Amylase	sAA
School Social Behavior Scales	SSBS-2
Six-minute Walk Test	6MWT
Social Communication Questionnaire	SCQ
Social Economic Status	SES
Social Responsiveness Scale	SRS
Special Healthcare Need	SHCN
Standard Deviation	SD
Steps Per Day	SPD
Steps Per Minute	SPM
System for Observing Children's Activity and Relationships During Play	SOCARP
Television	Td
Treatment Acceptability Rating Form Revised	TAR-F
Typically Developing	TD
United States of America	USA
Vigorous Physical Activity	VPA
Very Vigorous Physical Activity Voluntary Cycling	VVPA VC
Wake after sleep onset	WASO
Water Exercise Swimming Program	WESP
Weshsler Abbreviated Scale of Intelligence	WASI
Wisconsin Card Sorting Test	WCST
Without Disability	WD

Author details

Sara M. Scharoun[1], Kristen T. Wright[2], Jennifer E. Robertson-Wilson[2], Paula C. Fletcher[2] and Pamela J. Bryden[2,*]

*Address all correspondence to: pbryden@wlu.ca

1 Schulich School of Education, Nipissing University, North Bay, ON, Canada

2 Department of Kinesiology & Physical Education, Wilfrid Laurier University, Waterloo, Ontario, Canada

References

[1] Biddle, S. J., & Asare, M. (2011). Physical activity and mental health in children and adolescents: A review of reviews. *British Journal of Sports Medicine*, 45(11), 886–895.

[2] Janssen I, & Leblanc AG. (2010) Systematic review of the health benefits of physical activity and fitness in school-aged children and youth. *International Journal of Behavioral Nutrition and Physical Activity*. 7(40), 1–16.

[3] Tremblay, M. S., LeBlanc, A. G., Kho, M. E., Saunders, T. J., Larouche, R., Colley, R. C., Goldfield, G., & Connor Gorber, S. (2011). Systematic review of sedentary behavior and health indicators in school-aged children and youth. *International Journal of Behavioral Nutrition and Physical Activity*, 8, 98, 1–22.

[4] Moraes, A. C. F. D., Guerra, P. H., & Menezes, P. R. (2013). The worldwide prevalence of insufficient physical activity in adolescents; a systematic review. *Nutrición hospitalaria, 28*(3), 575–584.

[5] World Health Organization. (2010). Global recommendations on physical activity for health. Switzerland: WHO Press.

[6] McCoy, S. M., Jakicic, J. M., & Gibbs, B. B. (2016). Comparison of Obesity, Physical Activity, and Sedentary Behaviors Between Adolescents With Autism Spectrum Disorders and Without. *Journal of Autism and Developmental Disorders*, 1–10.

[7] World Health Organization. (2013). Autism spectrum disorders & other developmental disorders. From raising awareness to building capacity. Switzerland: WHO Press.

[8] American Psychiatric Association. (2013). Autism Spectrum Disorder. Retrieved from http://www.dsm5.org/Documents/Autism%20Spectrum%20Disorder%20Fact%20Sheet.pdf

[9] Fournier, K.A., Hass, C.J., Naik, S.K., Lodha, N., & Cauraugh, J.H. (2010). Motor coordination in autism spectrum disorders: A synthesis and meta-analysis. *Journal of Autism and Developmental Disorders*, 40, 1227–1240.

[10] Gowen, E., & Hamilton, A. (2013). Motor abilities in autism: a review using a computational context. *Journal of Autism and Developmental Disorders, 43*(2), 323–344.

[11] Goldin, R. L., Matson, J. L., Tureck, K., Cervantes, P. E., & Jang, J. (2013). A comparison of tantrum behavior profiles in children with ASD, ADHD and comorbid ASD and ADHD. *Research in Developmental Disabilities, 34*(9), 2669–2675.

[12] Richdale, A. L., & Schreck, K. A. (2009). Sleep problems in autism spectrum disorders: Prevalence, nature, & possible biopsychosocial aetiologies. *Sleep Medicine Reviews, 13*(6), 403–411.

[13] White, S. W., Oswald, D., Ollendick, T., & Scahill, L. (2009). Anxiety in children and adolescents with autism spectrum disorders. *Clinical Psychology Review, 29*(3), 216–229.

[14] Lee, L. C., Harrington, R. A., Louie, B. B., & Newschaffer, C. J. (2008). Children with autism: Quality of life and parental concerns. *Journal of Autism and Developmental Disorders, 38*(6), 1147–1160.

[15] Prupas, A., & Reid, G. (2001). Effects of exercise frequency on stereotypic behaviors of children with developmental disabilities. Education and Training in Mental Retardation and Developmental Disabilities, 26, 196–206.

[16] Pan, C.-Y., Tsai, C.-L., Chu, C.-H., & Hsieh, K.-W. (2011). Physical activity and self-determined motivation of adolescents with and without autism spectrum disorders in inclusive physical education. *Research in Autism Spectrum Disorders*, 5, 733–741.

[17] Corvey, K., Menear, K. S., Preskitt, J., Goldfarb, S., & Menachemi, N. (2016). Obesity, physical activity and sedentary behaviors in children with an autism spectrum disorder. Maternal and Child Health Journal, 20(2), 466–476.

[18] Tyler, K., Macdonald, M., & Menear, K. (2014). Physical activity and physical fitness of school-aged children and youth with autism spectrum disorders.

[19] Centers for Disease Control and Prevention (2015). Physical activity glossary of terms. Retrieved from http://www.cdc.gov/physicalactivity/basics/glossary/index.htm

[20] Ainsworth, B. E., Haskell, W. L., Whitt, M. C., Irwin, M. L., Swartz, A. M., Strath, S. J., … Leon, A. S. (2000). Compendium of physical activities: An update of activity codes and MET intensities. *Medicine & Science in Sports & Exercise, 32*(Supplement), S498–S516.

[21] Ayvazoglu, N. R., Kozub, F. M., Butera, G., & Murray, M. J. (2015). Determinants and challenges in physical activity participation in families with children with high functioning autism spectrum disorders from a family systems perspective. *Research in Developmental Disabilities, 47*, 93–105.

[22] Borremans, E., Rintala, P., & McCubbin, J. A. (2010). Physical fitness and physical activity in adolescents with asperger syndrome: a comparative study. *Adapted Physical Activity Quaterly, 27*(4), 308–320.

[23] Breslin, C. M., Rudisill, M. E., & Wadsworth, D. D. (2015). Heart rate profiles of children with and without autism spectrum disorder in response to physical play: a preliminary investigation. *Physical Educator, 72*(1), 1–19.

[24] Macdonald, M., Esposito, P., & Ulrich, D. (2011). The physical activity patterns of children with autism. *BMC Research Notes, 4*(1), 422.

[25] Pan, C. (2008b). School time physical activity of students with and without autism spectrum disorders during PE and recess, *Adapted Physical Activity Quarterly*, 25(4), 308–321.

[26] Pan, C.-Y. (2008a). Objectively measured physical activity between children with autism spectrum disorders and children without disabilities during inclusive recess settings in Taiwan. *Journal of Autism and Developmental Disorders, 38*(7), 1292–1301.

[27] Pan, C.-Y., & Frey, G. C. (2006). Physical activity patterns in youth with autism spectrum disorders. *Journal of Autism and Developmental Disorders, 36*(5), 597–606.

[28] Pan, C. Y., Hsu, P. J., Chung, I. C., Hung, C. S., Liu, Y. J., & Lo, S. Y. (2015). Physical activity during the segmented school day in adolescents with and without autism spectrum disorders. *Research in Autism Spectrum Disorders, 15–16*, 21–28.

[29] Pan, C.-Y., Tsai, C.-L., Hsieh, K.-W., Chu, C.-H., Li, Y.-L., & Huang, S.-T. (2011). Accelerometer-determined physical activity among elementary school-aged children with autism spectrum disorders in Taiwan. *Research in Autism Spectrum Disorders, 5*(3), 1042–1052.

[30] Kuo, M. H., Orsmond, G. I., Cohn, E. S., & Coster, W. J. (2011). Friendship characteristics and activity patterns of adolescents with an autism spectrum disorder. *Autism : The International Journal of Research and Practice, 17*(4), 481–500.

[31] Obrusnikova, I., & Miccinello, D. L. (2012). Parent perceptions of factors influencing after-school physical activity of children with autism spectrum disorders. *Adapted Physical Activity Quarterly, 29*(1), 63–80.

[32] Stanish, H., Curtin, C., Must, A., Phillips, S., Maslin, M., & Bandini, L. (2015). Enjoyment, barriers, and beliefs about physical activity in adolescents with and without autism spectrum disorder. *Adapted Physical Activity Quarterly : APAQ, 32*(4), 302–17.

[33] Bandini, L. G., Gleason, J., Curtin, C., Lividini, K., Anderson, S. E., Cermak, S. A., … Must, A. (2012). Comparison of physical activity between children with autism spectrum disorders and typically developing children. *Autism, 17*(1), 44–54.

[34] Boddy, L. M., Downs, S. J., Knowles, Z. R., & Fairclough, S. J. (2015). Physical activity and play behaviours in children and young people with intellectual disabilities: A cross-sectional observational study. *School Psychology International, 36*(2, SI), 154–171.

[35] Getchell, N., Miccinello, D., Blom, M., Morris, L., & Szaroleta, M. (2012). Comparing Energy Expenditure in Adolescents With and Without Autism While Playing Nintendo(®) Wii(™) Games. *Games for Health Journal, 1*(1), 58–61.

[36] Mangerud, W. L., Bjerkeset, O., Lydersen, S., & Indredavik, M. S. (2014). Physical activity in adolescents with psychiatric disorders and in the general population. *Child and Adolescent Psychiatry and Mental Health, 8*(1), 1–10.

[37] Memari, A. H., Ghaheri, B., Ziaee, V., Kordi, R., Hafizi, S., & Moshayedi, P. (2013). Physical activity in children and adolescents with autism assessed by triaxial accelerometry. *Pediatric Obesity, 8*(2), 150–158.

[38] Memari, A. H., Panahi, N., Ranjbar, E., Moshayedi, P., Shafiei, M., Kordi, R., & Ziaee, V. (2015). Children with autism spectrum disorder and patterns of participation in daily physical and play activities. *Neurology Research International*, 531906, 1–7.

[39] Must, A., Phillips, S., Curtin, C., & Bandini, L. G. (2015). Barriers to physical activity in children with autism spectrum disorders: relationship to physical activity and screen time. *Journal of Physical Activity & Health, 12*(4), 529–534.

[40] Obrusnikova, I., & Cavalier, A. R. (2011). Perceived barriers and facilitators of participation in after-school physical activity by children with autism spectrum disorders. *Journal of Developmental and Physical Disabilities, 23*(3), 195–211.

[41] Orsmond, G. I., & Kuo, H.-Y. (2011). The daily lives of adolescents with an autism spectrum disorder: Discretionary time use and activity partners. *Autism, 15*(5), 579–599.

[42] Pan, C.-Y. (2009). Age, social engagement, and physical activity in children with autism spectrum disorders. *Research in Autism Spectrum Disorders, 3*(1), 22–31.

[43] Pan, C. Y., Tsai, C. L., & Hsieh, K. W. (2011). Physical activity correlates for children with autism spectrum disorders in middle school physical education. *Research Quarterly for Exercise and Sport, 82*(3), 491–498.

[44] Pan, C. Y., Tsai, C. L., Chu, C. H., Sung, M. C., Ma, W. Y., & Huang, C. Y. (2016). Objectively measured physical activity and health-related physical fitness in secondary school-aged male students with autism spectrum disorders. *Physical Therapy, 96*(4), 511–520.

[45] Soden, S. E., Garrison, C. B., Egan, A. M., & Beckwith, A. M. (2012). Nutrition, physical activity, and bone mineral density in youth with autistic spectrum disorders. *Journal of Developmental & Behavioral Pediatrics, 33*(8), 618–624.

[46] Taheri, A., Perry, A., & Minnes, P. (2016). Examining the social participation of children and adolescents with intellectual disabilities and autism spectrum disorder in relation to peers. *Journal of Intellectual Disability Research : JIDR, 60*(5), 435–43.

[47] Dreyer Gillette, M. L. D., Borner, K. B., Nadler, C. B., Poppert, K. M., Stough, C. O., Romine, R. S., & Davis, A. M. (2015). Prevalence and health correlates of overweight and obesity in children with autism spectrum disorder. *Journal of Developmental & Behavioral Pediatrics, 36*(7), 489–496.

[48] McManus, B. M., Mandic, C. G., Carle, A. C., & Robert, S. A. (2012). The effect of parent-child function on physical activity and television viewing among adolescents with and without special healthcare needs. *International Journal of Disability, Development and Education, 59*(3), 305–319.

[49] Tatsumi, Y., Mohri, I., Shimizu, S., Tachibana, M., Ohno, Y., & Taniike, M. (2014). Daytime physical activity and sleep in pre-schoolers with developmental disorders. *Journal of Paediatrics and Child Health, 51*, 396–402.

[50] Wachob, D., & Lorenzi, D. G. (2015). Brief report: influence of physical activity on sleep quality in children with autism. *Journal of Autism and Developmental Disorders, 45*(8), 2641–2646.

[51] Anderson-Hanley, C., Tureck, K., & Schneiderman, R. L. (2011). Autism and exergaming: effects on repetitive behaviors and cognition. *Psychology Research and Behavior Management, 4*, 129–37.

[52] Arzoglou, D., Tsimaras, V., Kotsikas, G., Fotiadou, E., Sidiropoulou, M., Proios, M., & Bassa, E. (2013). The effect of a traditional dance training program on neuromuscular coordination of individuals with autism. *Journal of Physical Education and Sport, 13*(4), 563–569.

[53] Bahrami, F., Movahedi, A., Marandi, S. M., & Abedi, A. (2012). Kata techniques training consistently decreases stereotypy in children with autism spectrum disorder. *Research in Developmental Disabilities, 33*(4), 1183–1193.

[54] Bahrami, F., Movahedi, A., Marandi, S. M., & Sorensen, C. (2016). The effect of karate techniques training on communication deficit of children with autism spectrum disorders. *Journal of Autism and Developmental Disorders, 46*(3), 978–986.

[55] Brand, S., Jossen, S., Holsboer-Trachsler, E., Pühse, U., & Gerber, M. (2015). Impact of aerobic exercise on sleep and motor skills in children with autism spectrum disorders – a pilot study. *Neuropsychiatric Disease and Treatment, 11*, 1911.

[56] Casey, A. F., Quenneville-Himbeault, G., Normore, A., Davis, H., & Martell, S. G. (2015). A therapeutic skating intervention for children with autism spectrum disorder. *Pediatric Physical Therapy, 27*, 170–177.

[57] Fragala-Pinkham, M. a, Haley, S. M., & O'Neil, M. E. (2011). Group swimming and aquatic exercise programme for children with autism spectrum disorders: a pilot study. *Developmental Neurorehabilitation, 14*(4), 230–241.

[58] Fukasawa, M., & Takeda, K. (2012). Relationship between salivary -amylase activity and heart rate for evaluation of the sympathetic nervous system of children with autism. *Japanese Journal of Special Education, 49*(6), 671–684.

[59] Goodarzi, M., & Hemayattalab, R. (2012). Bone mineral density accrual in students with autism spectrum disorders: effects of calcium intake and physical training. *Research in Autism Spectrum Disorders, 6*(2), 690–695.

[60] Gruber, D. J., & Poulson, C. L. (2016). Graduated guidance delivered by parents to teach yoga to children with developmental delays. *Journal of Applied Behavior Analysis, 49*(1), 193–198.

[61] Hillier, A., Murphy, D., & Ferrara, C. (2011). A pilot study: Short-term reduction in salivary cortisol following low level physical exercise and relaxation among adolescents and young adults on the autism spectrum. *Stress and Health, 27*(5), 395–402.

[62] Judge, J. P. (2015). The effects of a computer-based fitness schedule on independent transitioning for a student with autism. *Palaestra, 29*(1), 17–21.

[63] Kaplan-Reimer, H., Sidener, T. M., Reeve, K. F., & Sidener, D. W. (2007). Using stimulus control procedures to teach indoor rock climbing to children with autism. *Behavioral Interventions, 22*(November 2006), 83–97.

[64] MacDonald, M., Esposito, P., Hauck, J., Jeong, I., Hornyak, J., Argento, A., & Ulrich, D. A. (2012). Bicycle training for youth with Down syndrome and Autism Spectrum Disorders. *Focus on Autism and Other Developmental Disabilities, 27*(August), 12–21.

[65] Magnusson, J. E., Cobham, C., & McLeod, R. (2012). Beneficial effects of clinical exercise rehabilitation for children and adolescents with autism spectrum disorder (ASD). *Journal of Exercise Physiology Online, 15*(2), 71–79.

[66] Morrison, H., Roscoe, E. M., & Atwell, A. (2011). An evaluation of antecedent exercise on behavior maintained by automatic reinforcement using a three-component multiple schedule. *Journal of Applied Behavior Analysis, 44*(3), 523–541.

[67] Movahedi, A., Bahrami, F., Marandi, S. M., & Abedi, A. (2013). Improvement in social dysfunction of children with autism spectrum disorder following long term Kata techniques training. *Research in Autism Spectrum Disorders, 7*(9), 1054–1161.

[68] Neely, L., Rispoli, M., Gerow, S., & Ninci, J. (2014). Effects of antecedent exercise on academic engagement and stereotypy during instruction. *Behavior Modification, 39*(1), 98–116.

[69] Nicholson, H., Kehle, T., Bray, M. A., & Van Heest, J. (2011). The effects of antecedent physical activity on the academic engagement of children with autism spectrum disorder. *Psychology in the Schools, 48*(2), 198–213.

[70] Oriel, K. N., George, C. L., Peckus, R., & Semon, A. (2011). The effects of aerobic exercise on academic engagement in young children with autism spectrum disorder. *Pediatric Physical Therapy : The Official Publication of the Section on Pediatrics of the American Physical Therapy Association, 23*(2), 187–193.

[71] Pan, C.-Y. (2010). Effects of water exercise swimming program on aquatic skills and social behaviors in children with autism spectrum disorders. *Autism : The International Journal of Research and Practice, 14*(1), 9–28.

[72] Pan, C. Y. (2011). The efficacy of an aquatic program on physical fitness and aquatic skills in children with and without autism spectrum disorders. *Research in Autism Spectrum Disorders, 5*(1), 657–665.

[73] Pan, C.-Y., Chu, C.-H., Tsai, C.-L., Sung, M.-C., Huang, C.-Y., & Ma, W.-Y. (2016 – online ahead of print). The impacts of physical activity intervention on physical and cognitive outcomes in children with autism spectrum disorder. *Autism*, doi:10.1177/1362361316633562

[74] Pitetti, K. H., Rendoff, A. D., Grover, T., & Beets, M. W. (2007). The efficacy of a 9-month treadmill walking program on the exercise capacity and weight reduction for adolescents with severe autism. *Journal of Autism and Developmental Disorders, 37*(6), 997–1006.

[75] Reynolds, J. L., Pitchford, E. A., Hauck, J. L., Ketcheson, L. R., & Ulrich, D. A. (2016). Outcomes of home-support consultation on the maintenance of bicycle-riding skills for youth with autism spectrum disorder. *Journal of Educational and Psychological Consultation, 26*(2), 166–185.

[76] Ringenbach, S. D. R., Lichtsinn, K. C., & Holzapfel, S. D. (2015). Assisted cycling therapy (ACT) improves inhibition in adolescents with autism spectrum disorder. *Journal of Intellectual and Developmental Disability, 0*(September), 1–12.

[77] Rogers, L., Hemmeter, M. L., & Wolery, M. (2010). Using a constant time delay procedure to teach foundational swimming skills to children with autism. *Topics in Early Childhood Special Education, 30*(2), 102–111.

[78] Sarol, H., & Çimen, Z. (2015). The effects of adapted recreational physical activity on the life quality of individuals with autism. *Anthropologist, 21*(3), 522–527.

[79] Strahan, B. E., & Elder, J. H. (2015). Video game playing effects on obesity in an adolescent with autism spectrum disorder: a case study. *Autism Research and Treatment, 2015*, 1–7.

[80] Yanardag, M., Akmanoglu, N., & Yilmaz, I. (2013). The effectiveness of video prompting on teaching aquatic play skills for children with autism. *Disability and Rehabilitation, 35*(April 2012), 1–10.

[81] Hinckson, E. A., Dickinson, A., Water, T., Sands, M., & Penman, L. (2013). Physical activity, dietary habits and overall health in overweight and obese children and youth with intellectual disability or autism. *Research in Developmental Disabilities, 34*(4), 1170–1178.

[82] Ketcheson, L., Hauck, J., & Ulrich, D. (2016 – online ahead of print). The effects of an early motor skill intervention on motor skills, levels of physical activity, and socialization in young children with autism spectrum disorder: A pilot study. *Autism*, doi: 10.1177/1362361316650611.

[83] Lalonde, K. B., MacNeill, B. R., Eversole, L. W., Ragotzy, S. P., & Poling, A. (2014). Increasing physical activity in young adults with autism spectrum disorders. *Research in Autism Spectrum Disorders, 8*(12), 1679–1684.

[84] Todd, T., & Reid, G. (2006). Increasing physical activity in individuals with autism. *Focus on Autism and Other Developmental Disabilities, 21*(3), 167–176.

[85] Todd, T., Reid, G., & Butler-kisber, L. (2010). Cycling for students with ASD self regulation promotes sustained physical activity, Adapted Physical Activity Quarterly, 27(3), 226–241.